Male Infertility for the Clinician

W0227837

Sijo J. Parekattil • Ashok Agarwal

Editors

Male Infertility
for the Clinician

A Practical Guide

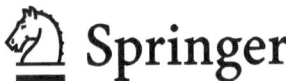 Springer

Editors
Sijo J. Parekattil, MD
Director of Urology
Winter Haven Hospital
University of Florida
Winter Haven, FL, USA

Ashok Agarwal, PhD, HCLD (ABB)
Director, Center for Reproductive Medicine
Glickman Urological and Kidney Institute
Cleveland Clinic
Cleveland, OH, USA

ISBN 978-1-4614-7851-5
Springer New York Heidelberg Dordrecht London

Library of Congress Control Number: 2013943688

Printed on acid-free paper

Springer is part of Springer Science+Business Media (www.springer.com)

Preface and Acknowledgments

The field of male infertility truly illustrates the need of a multispecialty approach to the effective diagnosis and management of such conditions. From the initial referral possibly from a reproductive endocrinology gynecologist and embryologist to the male infertility urologist, andrologist, researcher and alternative medicine specialist – this multi-disciplinary team really needs to work as a cohesive unit to provide our patients with the most effective and highest quality care.

This book was an attempt to gather experts from each of these fields and present an integrated clinical management approach with detailed descriptions of topics ranging from the initial clinical diagnosis, management, new treatment options, and scientific rational for the various approaches. The book initially focuses on the clinical aspects of male infertility diagnosis and then dives into management options. The authors come from leading institutions from around the globe in an attempt to capture a wide range of techniques and approaches. We are hoping that this text may serve as a reference guide for specialists across this team to further enhance dialogue, discussion and refinement in our multi-disciplinary approach.

We would like to thank the authors for their contributions and our families for their patience in allowing us to put together this project. We would like to acknowledge the Glickman Urological Institute at the Cleveland Clinic Foundation and the Department of Urology at University of Florida for institutional support for this endeavor as well. We would also like to thank Richard Lansing, executive editor, for his support and advice and Margaret Burns, publishing manager, for her tireless efforts in reviewing and editing each of the manuscripts.

We hope that this book will provide a concise, consolidated reference for clinical male infertility.

Winter Haven, FL, USA
Cleveland, OH, USA

Sijo J. Parekattil, MD
Ashok Agarwal, PhD, HCLD (ABB)

Contents

Contributors

Nancy L. Brackett, PhD, HCLD The Miami Project to Cure Paralysis, University of Miami Miller School of Medicine, Lois Pope Life Center, Miami, FL, USA

Jamin V. Brahmbhatt, MD Department of Urology, University of Tennessee Health Science Center, Memphis, TN, USA

Robert E. Brannigan, MD Department of Urology, Northwestern University Feinberg School of Medicine, Chicago, IL, USA

Orhan Bukulmez, MD Division of Reproductive Endocrinology and Infertility, Department of Obstetrics and Gynecology, University of Texas Southwestern Medical Center, Dallas, TX, USA

Aldo E. Calogero, MD Department of Medical and Pediatrics Sciences, University of Catania Medical School, Catania, Italy

Darby J. Cassidy, MD Department of Urology, University Hospital of Northern British Columbia, Prince George, BC, Canada

Marcello Cocuzza, MD Department of Urology, University of Sao Paulo (USP), Sao Paulo, Brazil

Marc S. Cohen, MD Department of Urology, Shands at the University of Florida, Gainesville, FL, USA

George A. de Boccard, MD Clinique Generale Beaulieu, Robot-Assisted Laparoscopic Surgery Center, Geneva, Switzerland

Peter Frank De Wil, MD Urological Department, Kliniek Sint Jan, Brussels, Belgium

Fnu Deepinder Department of Endocrinology, Diabetes and Metabolism, Cedars Sinai Medical Center, Los Angeles, CA, USA

Sandro C. Esteves, MD, PhD ANDROFERT, Andrology and Human Reproduction Clinic, Center for Male Reproduction, Campinas, SP, Brazil

Vincenzo Ficarra, MD, PhD Department of Oncological and Surgical Sciences, Urology Clinic, University of Padua, Padua, Italy

Marc Goldstein, MD Cornell Institute for Reproductive Medicine, New York Presbyterian Hospital/Weill Cornell Medical Center, Weill Cornell Medical College of Cornell University, New York, NY, USA

Ethan D. Grober, Division of Urology, Department of Surgery, University of Toronto, Mount Sinai Hospital, Toronto, ON, Canada

Sam Haywood, BA Department of Urology, Northwestern University Feinberg School of Medicine, Chicago, IL, USA

Ralf Henkel Department of Medical Biosciences, University of the Western Cape, Bellville, South Africa

Wayland Hsiao, MD Department of Urology, Emory University, Atlanta, GA, USA

Aleksey P. Ignatov, BS The Turek Clinic, San Francisco, CA, USA

Viacheslav Iremashvili, MD, PhD Department of Urology, University of Miami Miller School of Medicine, Miami, FL, USA

Keith Jarvi, MD Division of Urology, Department of Surgery, University of Toronto, Mount Sinai Hospital, Toronto, ON, Canada

Edward D. Kim, MD Division of Urology, Department of Surgery, University of Tennessee Medical Center, Knoxville, TN, USA

Tobias S. Köhler, MD, MPh Division of Urology, Southern Illinois University, Springfield, IL, USA

Rajeev Kumar, MCh Department of Urology, All India Institute of Medical Sciences, New Delhi, India

Sandro La Vignera, MD Department of Medical and Pediatrics Sciences, University of Catania Medical School, Catania, Italy

Eric L. Laborde, MD Department of Urology, Northwestern University Feinberg School of Medicine, Chicago, IL, USA

Francesco Lanzafame, MD Centro Territoriale di Andrologia, Siracusa, Italy

Kirk C. Lo, MD, CM Division of Urology, Department of Surgery, University of Toronto, Mount Sinai Hospital, Toronto, ON, Canada

Charles M. Lynne, MD Department of Urology, University of Miami Miller School of Medicine, Miami, FL, USA

Ricardo Miyaoka, MD ANDROFERT, Andrology and Human Reproduction Clinic, Center for Male Reproduction, Campinas, SP, Brazil

Ryan Mori, MD, MS Cleveland Clinic Lerner College of Medicine and Glickman Urological and Kidney Institute, Cleveland Clinic Foundation, Cleveland, OH, USA

Ray E. Moseley, PhD Department of Community Health and Family Medicine, University of Florida Health Science Center, Gainesville, FL, USA

Alexandre Mottrie Department of Urology, O.L.V. Clinic Aalst, Aalst, Belgium

Sijo J. Parekattil, MD Director of Urology, Winter Haven Hospital, University of Florida, Winter Haven, FL, USA

Henry M. Rosevear, MD Department of Urology, University of Iowa, Iowa City, IA, USA

Edmund Sabanegh Jr., MD Department of Urology, Glickman Urological and Kidney Institute, Center for Reproductive Medicine, Cleveland Clinic, Cleveland, OH, USA

Jay Sandlow, MD Department of Urology, Medical College of Wisconsin, Milwaukee, WI, USA

Peter Schlegel, MD Department of Urology, Weill Cornell Medical College, New York-Presbyterian/Weill Cornell Hospital, New York, NY, USA

Tung Shu, MD Department of Urology, Baylor College of Medicine, Center for Kidney Health at the Vanguard Urologic Institute, Houston, TX, USA

Doron Sol Stember, MD Division of Urology, Department of Surgery, Memorial Sloan-Kettering Cancer Center, New York, NY, USA

Adam F. Stewart, MD Division of Urology, Department of Surgery, University of Tennessee Medical Center, Knoxville, TN, USA

Paul J. Turek, MD, FACS, FRSM The Turek Clinic, San Francisco, CA, USA

Moshe Wald, MD Department of Urology, University of Iowa, Iowa City, IA, USA

Run Wang, MD, FACS Department of Urology, University of Texas Medical School at Houston, Houston, TX, USA

MD Anderson Cancer Center, Houston, TX, USA

Daniel H. Williams IV, MD Department of Urology, University of Wisconsin Hospital and Clinics, Madison, WI, USA

Herbert J. Wiser, MD Division of Urology, Southern Illinois University, Springfield, IL, USA

Part I
Clinical Diagnosis of Male Infertility

Chapter 1
Causes of Male Infertility

Herbert J. Wiser, Jay Sandlow, and Tobias S. Köhler

Of all sexually active couples, 12–15% are infertile [1]. When broken down by gender, a male component can be identified 50% of the time either in isolation or in combination with a female factor [2]. The majority of the causes of male infertility are treatable or preventable, so a keen understanding of these conditions is paramount. Despite advancements in assisted reproductive technologies, the goal of a male infertility specialist is not simply to retrieve sperm. Instead, the male infertility specialist attempts to optimize a male's reproductive potential and thereby allow a couple to conceive successfully through utilization of less invasive reproductive techniques. Often, this involves the use of sperm or testicular tissue cryopreservation prior to fertility insult. At the same time, the male fertility specialist is wary of underlying or causal, potentially serious medical or genetic conditions that prompted reproductive evaluation. Previous research in a US male fertility clinic analyzing 1,430 patients identified causes of infertility from most to least common: varicocele, idiopathic, obstruction, female factor, cryptorchidism, immunologic, ejaculatory dysfunction, testicular failure, drug effects/radiation, endocrinology, and all others [3]. The focus of this book on the role of reactive oxygen species (ROS) is easily applied to the majority of the listed conditions (described in detail in later chapters) which comprise this chapter's overview of pre-testicular, testicular, and post-testicular causes of male infertility.

H.J. Wiser, MD (✉) • T.S. Köhler, MD, MPh
Division of Urology, Southern Illinois University,
301 N 8th Street, Floor 4, Springfield, IL, USA
e-mail: hwiser@siumed.edu; tkohler@siumed.edu

J. Sandlow, MD
Department of Urology, Medical College of Wisconsin,
9200 West Wisconsin Avenue, Milwaukee, WI, USA
e-mail: jsandlow@mail.mcw.edu

S.J. Parekattil, A. Agarwal (eds.), *Male Infertility for the Clinician*,
© Springer Science+Business Media New York 2013

Causes of Male Infertility

Pre-testicular

Hypogonadotropic Hypogonadism

Hypogonadotropic hypogonadism affects fertility at multiple levels. Sperm production is deleteriously affected by a lack of testosterone and a lack of a stimulatory effect on the Sertoli/germ cell complex. Sexual function is also negatively impacted with effects seen at the level of erectile function, ejaculatory function, and sexual desire. There are many etiologies of hypogonadotropic hypogonadism. The most common are elevated prolactin, medications, illicit drugs, and pituitary damage. Kallmann syndrome is another, albeit rare, cause of hypogonadotropic hypogonadism.

Elevated Prolactin

Elevated prolactin may cause hypogonadism by suppressing the release of GnRH. Symptoms of hypogonadism, especially erectile dysfunction and loss of libido, are the most common presenting symptoms in males with hyperprolactinemia, though galactorrhea and gynecomastia may also be evident [4].

Elevated prolactin may be secondary to various etiologies. The most common of these is a prolactinoma, which typically arises from the pituitary. Because prolactinomas in men are more likely to manifest through mass effect, visual disturbances and headaches are more likely to be present when compared to women with prolactinomas [5].

There are other significant causes for hyperprolactinemia as well. Prolactin is elevated in renal failure, as well as in patients with hypothyroidism and cirrhosis. Prolactin levels may also be elevated in certain systemic diseases such as systemic lupus erythematosus, rheumatoid arthritis, celiac disease, and systemic sclerosis. Many drugs elevate prolactin levels, especially those which block the effects of dopamine, such as antipsychotics [6].

Pharmacologic

Various medications may cause hypogonadotropic hypogonadism. Estrogens and progestins may cause a decrease in testosterone levels via negative feedback to the hypothalamic-pituitary-gonadal axis. Marijuana is known to decrease testosterone levels by working on the endocannabinoid receptors present at multiple levels of the hypothalamic-pituitary axis [7]. Both ethanol and cannabinoids suppress GnRH secretion at the level of the hypothalamus. Endocannabinoid receptors have also been found in the pituitary and so may also affect the hypothalamic-pituitary axis at that level as well [8]. LHRH agonists and antagonists are used for the treatment of prostate cancer, precocious puberty, and gender reassignment surgeries. In the male, both induce profound hypogonadism. LHRH antagonists directly and intuitively decrease LH and FSH levels. LHRH agonists produce a tonically stimulated state which, unlike the physiologic circadian rhythmicity of normal LHRH stimulation, acts to decrease LH and FSH secretion. Narcotics may also produce profound hypogonadism. Nearly 40% of men using methadone were found to have total testosterone levels less than 230 ng/dL [9].

Kallmann Syndrome

Kallmann syndrome affects between one in 8,000–10,000 males [10, 11]. It is a spectrum of disease in which the primary manifestations are anosmia and hypogonadotropic hypogonadism which leads to an absence of puberty. Multiple genetic defects can lead to Kallmann syndrome [12]. These most commonly manifest through the same mechanism whereby GnRH secreting neurons fail to migrate to the hypothalamus. Lack of these neurons in the hypothalamus results in a lack of GnRH secretion and thus hypogonadism.

Hypergonadotropic Hypogonadism

One of the most common causes of hypergonadotropic hypogonadism is Klinefelter syndrome (Klinefelter's). Klinefelter's affects male fertility by altering spermatogenesis both directly and indirectly by altering the hormonal milieu [13–15]. Interestingly, sex hormone levels are normal until puberty. During puberty, they do rise to low-normal levels, but plateau. By adulthood, serum testosterone levels are typically below normal. Histologic studies demonstrate gradual degeneration of the testes with development, with hyperplasia of poorly functioning Leydig cells [16]. Klinefelter's also directly affects spermatogenesis, as discussed later in this chapter.

Testicular

Varicocele

A varicocele is a dilation of the pampiniform plexus likely caused by the absence or incompetence of the venous valves of the internal spermatic vein. Varicoceles have long been associated with infertility. The first written description is attributed to Celsius who noticed the association between the varicocele and testicular atrophy [17]. In the 1800s, surgical correction was seen to improve semen quality. It is currently seen to be the most common surgically correctable cause of male infertility. Roughly 12% of all men have a varicocele, but this number jumps to 25% in men with abnormal semen parameters [18].

Varicoceles affect multiple semen parameters; total sperm count, sperm motility, and sperm morphology are all negatively affected [19, 20]. There are many theories about the underlying pathophysiology of a varicocele, with heat, renal metabolites, and hormonal abnormalities all playing a role. However, most agree that disruption of the countercurrent heat exchange mechanism in the testis, causing hyperthermia, is the most likely mechanism.

Scrotal temperature in humans is variable during the day, but remains 1–2°C lower than core body temperature at 33–36°C [21]. Thermoregulation of the gonads at a temperature lower than that of body temperature is a trait that is well preserved in homeotherms and especially in mammals [22]. Nearly all mammals have a scrotum. Other mechanisms, such as the efficient heat exchange system in whales, have developed in animals in environments where the scrotum would not be efficient at keeping gonadal heat at a few degrees below body temperature. Besides this teleologic evidence that lower body temperature is necessary for testicular function, numerous studies point to impaired sperm production and a decrease in semen quality when scrotal temperatures are elevated [23–28]. One study showed that men with scrotal skin temperatures above 35°C for >75% of the day had sperm concentrations of 33 million/mL as compared with men with scrotal skin temperatures greater than 35°C for <50% of the day who had sperm concentrations of 92 million/ mL [27]. The mechanism by which heat causes decreased sperm counts is poorly understood, but one hypothesis is that increased temperature could increase the metabolic rate of testicular and epididymal sperm, secondarily increasing the amount of oxidative damage to both the structure and the DNA of the spermatocytes and spermatids [22].

Varicoceles are noted to be associated with higher scrotal temperatures [29], and cooling of the scrotum has been shown to improve semen parameters [30]. Interestingly, the temperature of the contralateral testis is also elevated in men with unilateral varicoceles. So the cause of elevated testicular temperatures, which intuitively would seem to be an impaired countercurrent flow mechanism, is less clear [31]. Hormonal abnormalities are a similarly controversial area, with no consistent hormonal changes associated with the presence of a varicocele. Testosterone, SHBG, FSH, and LH have all been examined, and different studies have produced opposing results [17].

Cryptorchidism

Cryptorchidism is well known to affect fertility. The severity of its effect on fertility is directly proportional to the severity of the cryptorchidism, with bilateral cryptorchidism having more severe effects than unilateral, and with higher testes having worse function than lower testes [32–35].

Similarly, orchidopexy has been shown to improve fertility, with the best results obtained with fixation at a young age, especially prior to 1 year of age [36]. Fixation after age 10 may not improve fertility, or may improve it only modestly, suggesting that permanent and progressive damage is done to the testis while in an abnormal position, and this is supported by histologic studies [37, 38]. Actual paternity rates in men who underwent orchidopexy for unilateral cryptorchidism are 89%, slightly less than the non-cryptorchid group, which had a 94% paternity rate. Bilaterally cryptorchid men post-orchidopexy had markedly lower paternity rates, at 62% [34, 35].

The pathophysiology of the effects of cryptorchidism is complex, with heat likely playing a partial but significant role [39, 40]. A number of other factors are also likely to come in to play, including the underlying genetics, hormonal milieu, and environmental exposures which originally led to the cryptorchidism [41–43].

Testicular Cancer

Testicular cancer is strongly associated with infertility. There are multiple ways in which testicular cancer is related to and can contribute to reduced fertility. Both testicular cancer and impaired spermatogenesis may be related in their etiology of embryologic testicular dysgenesis. The testicular dysgenesis syndrome is a spectrum of disease that may involve cryptorchidism, hypospadias, decreased spermatogenesis, and testis cancer. In this syndrome, it is thought that all of these share an origin of abnormal fetal testis development. As a result of this developmental anomaly, any number of these manifestations may be present in a boy [44]. Testicular tumors may also directly contribute to infertility by secreting hormones, which can downregulate sperm production in the contralateral testis [45–48]. This is uncommon but has been seen with Leydig and Sertoli cell tumors as well as seminomas. Tumors may also directly disrupt spermatogenesis by mass effect or by the effects of the inflammatory reaction to the tumor [49]. Cancer treatments may also decrease fertility.

At presentation, roughly 10% of men will be azoospermic, and roughly 50% will be oligospermic. While orchiectomy will result in a rebound in semen parameters in roughly 90% of these men [50], further treatment with surgery, chemotherapy, or radiation can further decrease fertility.

Ionizing Radiation

Excellent data on the effects of ionizing radiation is available from two similar studies, which are unlikely to be repeated. Researchers in these studies prospectively irradiated the testes of prisoners with single or multiple doses of radiation up to 600 cGy [51, 52]. Sperm counts were followed, and serial testicular biopsies were done. These studies showed that sperm counts declined when testes were irradiated and that decline was dose dependant. At low doses of ~7.5 cGy, a mild decline of sperm counts was seen, and this decline increased to severe oligospermia by 30–40 cGy and azoospermia by 78 cGy. The time to recovery was also seen to be dose dependant, with those receiving 20 cGy beginning to have a recovery of sperm counts by 6 months, those with 100 cGy at 7 months, 200 cGy at 11 months, and 600 cGy at 24 months. The percent of men achieving a complete recovery and time to achieve a complete recovery also declined with increasing radiation doses.

Decline to the nadir of sperm counts was seen at roughly 64 days, corresponding roughly to the time required for sperm cell production from spermatogonia. More rapid declines were seen with higher radiation doses, indicating increased damage to the more highly differentiated cells undergoing spermatogenesis. Biopsy results from these studies showed that spermatogonia numbers nadired at much lower levels with higher doses of radiation and that these nadirs took longer to achieve than those which had received lower doses of radiation.

These studies provide excellent information into the biology of the effects of radiation on spermatogenesis on the healthy young testis. Clinically, however, the effects we see are often more pronounced given the setting of the radiation, namely, cancer patients undergoing radiotherapy. Fractionated radiation has been shown to be more damaging than single dose radiation [53]. One report showed that fractionated radiation with a total dose of 200 cGy may cause permanent azoospermia [54].

As would be expected, Leydig cells are more resistant to radiation than the germinal epithelium [51]. Doses of 20 Gy are known to cause declines in testosterone [55]. Doses on the order of 2 Gy do not cause appreciable drops in testosterone [56].

Chemotherapy

Chemotherapy typically targets rapidly dividing cells and thus has profound effects on the germinal epithelium. As such, the expected outcome of acute chemotherapy is a decline in spermatogenesis, and this has been well documented since the late 1940s [57]. The mechanism by which chemotherapeutics decrease fertility and the rates of recovery is both drug and dose dependent [58–61].

Bleomycin, etoposide, and cisplatin or carboplatin (BEP) is the most commonly used chemotherapy regimen for testicular germ cell tumors. The decrease in fertility seen post-BEP chemotherapy is likely the result of a direct reduction of spermatogenesis and not as a result of any change in the hormonal milieu. Indeed, testosterone levels are not seen to be significantly reduced at 12 months post-chemotherapy, and FSH levels are appropriately elevated. FSH levels decline as spermatogenesis returns over the following 2–4 years [62]. It should be noted, however, that return of spermatogenesis is not guaranteed. In patients who were normospermic prior to chemotherapy, fewer than 4 cycles of BEP have not typically been associated with high rates of permanent infertility [63]. However, high-dose BEP is associated with approximately a 50% of permanent infertility in one study [64]. Notably, even in azoospermic men post-high dose BEP chemotherapy, nests of spermatogenesis have been found on TESE [65].

Genetic Azoospermia/Oligospermia

It is estimated that 2–8% of infertile men have an underlying genetic abnormality, with this number rising to 15% in azoospermic men [66]. Although the majority of male infertility does not have an identifiable genetic cause, two potential etiologies are Y chromosome microdeletions and karyotypic abnormalities. The two most common karyotypic abnormalities are Klinefelter's (47,XXY) and chromosomal translocations.

Y chromosome microdeletions are a common cause of these, occurring in 11–18% of azoospermic men and 4–14% of oligospermic men [67]. Currently, research is focused on the azoospermia factor (AZF) region on the long arm of the Y chromosome at Yq11. This area itself contains three separate regions, AZFa, AZFb, and AZFc, and microdeletions of these areas lead to slightly different phenotypes [68]. Deletions in the AZFa and AZFb regions both cause azoospermia, but histologically, they are different with AZFa deletions resulting in Sertoli cell-only syndrome and AZFb deletions causing an arrest of spermatogenesis at the primary spermatocyte stage [66]. AZFc deletions are the most common of the Y chromosome microdeletions and are found in 5–7% of oligospermic men [68]. Unlike the AZFa/AZFb deletions, they do not uniformly result in azoospermia; rather, a spectrum of phenotypes are seen with partial deletions being found in normospermic men, from oligospermia to azoospermia in some full deletions [66]. In men undergoing micro-TESE sperm extraction with azfC deletions, about 35% have sperm found successfully [69].

Classic and mosaic Klinefelter's are common karyotypic abnormalities found in infertile men. Klinefelter's has a prevalence of one in 660 males; thus, it is the most common genetic cause of male infertility as 75–90% of men with Klinefelter's will be azoospermic, with some with mosaic Klinefelter's being mainly oligospermic [13, 70, 71]. Studies which show higher prevalences of azoospermic men with AZF deletions than Klinefelter's are likely flawed by a selection bias as men with the obvious stigmata of Klinefelter's are not tested and included in these studies [72, 73].

As would be expected, Klinefelter's has much broader effects than Y chromosome microdeletions and affects fertility through two routes, direct effects on spermatogenesis and indirect hormonal effects on spermatogenesis [13–15]. As far as altered spermatogenesis is concerned, the majority of Klinefelter's patients actually do produce sperm, as is witnessed by the 69% TESE sperm retrieval rates [74]; however, the quantity of sperm produced is typically very low. Biopsy studies of Klinefelter's testes have demonstrated that spermatogenesis is halted pre-pachytene in the vast majority of aneuploid cells and that meiosis was seen mainly in cells with normal karyotypes [15].

Robertsonian translocations are a third significant genetic cause of infertility. They occur in 0.8% of infertile men, and this number rises to 1.6% in oligospermic men [75]. Phenotypes are highly variable given the possibilities of recombination [66].

Environmental Factors

Hyperthermia is considered to be a major contributor in the pathogenesis of infertility in men with varicocele and cryptorchidism. Many lifestyle factors also have the potential to increase scrotal temperatures, including underwear type, heated car seats, and occupational heat exposure. The role of underwear style in male infertility has been investigated. One small study of 14 normospermic men, a tight polyester scrotal support, when worn day and night, was shown to make all azoospermic at a mean time of 140 days. After removal of the scrotal support, all men regained function at a mean time of 157 days [76]. However, normal underwear, i.e., boxer or brief style, has not been shown to exert a significant influence on semen parameters [77]. Other types of heat exposure, such as occupational heat exposure in a group of welders, have been shown to decrease semen quality [78]. Sedentary posture, heated car seats, and sauna and hot tub use are all lifestyle factors that increase scrotal temperature as well and may contribute to a decline in fertility [79].

Recently, cell phones have been implicated as possibly playing a role in decreasing male fertility, and several studies show that there may be some basis for this. One observational study assessed semen parameters and cell phone usage in 361 men who presented to an infertility clinic. Sixty percent of the men in this study had greater than 2 h of cell phone use per day, with 30% using their cell phones for more than 4 h per day. They found that sperm counts, motility, viability, and morphology all worsened with increasing cell phone use [80]. The mechanism by which cell phones affect semen parameters has not yet been elucidated, but one hypothesis is that cell phone-generated electromagnetic radiation (CPEMR) alters mitochondrial function and acts to increase reactive oxygen species. This is somewhat corroborated by one study which looked at the effects of CPEMR on semen parameters and found increased levels of reactive oxygen species with decreased viability and motility in the sperm exposed to CPEMR [81].

Tobacco use has been implicated in the pathogenesis of numerous cancers and medical diseases. While the use of tobacco significantly impacts female fertility, its impact on male fertility is less clear. Semen parameters, including sperm density, motility, and morphology, have all been shown to be worsened with tobacco use [82–85]. However, a significant reduction in fertility has not yet been proven.

Testicular Injury

Injury to the testicle can be sustained either directly or indirectly. Direct trauma to the testis is typically managed by debridement of devitalized seminiferous tubules and closure of the tunica albuginea [86]. The resultant loss of volume of seminiferous tubules and possible obstruction from scarring is one possible cause of decreased fertility. Reports on testicular salvage after bilateral trauma indicated that preserved volume of testis is the key to preserving fertility [86–91].

Indirect damage to the testis may be sustained by exposure to infection or inflammation of the testis. The classic infectious agent causing infertility is mumps.

Orchitis occurs in roughly 20% of postpubertal males with mumps [92] and is bilateral in 30% of these. Of those postpubertal males with bilateral mumps orchitis, 25% will have resultant infertility. In other words, 1.5% of postpubertal males with mumps may become infertile as a result of the disease. In nations where immunization against mumps is common, this is a rare phenomenon. The mechanism by which mumps causes orchitis is via pressure atrophy. Infection of the testis with the mumps virus causes inflammation and swelling, which is limited by the tunica albuginea; this in turn leads to atrophy [93].

Other bacterial and viral pathogens may also cause infertility at the testicular level, most commonly; this is the result of spread of infection from the epididymis [94, 95]. The mechanism for infertility in these cases may be persistent inflammation which suppresses testicular function or obstruction secondary to resultant sclerosis.

Primary Ciliary Dyskinesia

Ultrastructural defects that affect sperm motility are described under the grouping of primary ciliary dyskinesia (PCD). PCD is a rare and heterogeneous genetic disease which affects one in 20,000–60,000 [96]. Many components of cilia and flagella are affected, though the defect is found in the dynein in over 80% of cases [97]. The key clinical finding is chronic respiratory infections leading to bronchiectasis. When situs inversus is present in addition to the other components, it is termed Kartagener's syndrome. Male infertility secondary to sperm dysmotility is related to the dysfunction of the flagellate tail of the sperm. It is a common finding, though not universal, and this is likely related to the heterogeneity of the genetics.

Sertoli Cell-Only Syndrome

Sertoli cell-only syndrome may be either primary or secondary, and attempts have been made to distinguish these histologically [98]. The primary form is hypothesized to result from a lack of migration of the germ cells to the seminiferous tubules during embryologic development. The secondary form is due to a gonadotoxic insult to the testis after birth. While the different etiologies of these would intuitively suggest a higher likelihood of finding sperm in biopsies of testes with secondary Sertoli cell-only syndrome, this is not borne out in the literature [99].

Antisperm Antibodies

In the normal male, sperm reside in an immunoprivileged site. The blood-testis barrier prevents proteins from the sperm from interacting with the immune system and setting up an immune reaction against them. Trauma, infection, and inflammation all may disrupt this barrier and result in immunity against the germinal epithelium and spermatozoa.

Antisperm antibodies (ASA) are very common, with 8–17% of men and 1–22% women in infertile couples testing positive for serum ASA [100, 101]. As expected, ASA are heterogeneous in their binding sites and, as such, have wide ranging effects on sperm function. Some ASA will not significantly affect fertility, and 0.9–2.5% of fertile men will test positive for serum ASA [102, 103]. ASA targeted against proteins on the head region are more likely to affect zona binding and sperm penetration, whereas ASA targeted against the tails of spermatozoa are more likely to decrease motility and cervical mucus penetration and cause sperm agglutination [104]. Antibody type also plays a significant role in the degree of reduction of fertility. In a study of ASA in men who had undergone vasectomy reversal, IgA ASA were associated with a much more significant reduction in fertility than IgG ASA [105]. While ASA clearly may affect fertility in some cases, serum ASA positivity is not a strong predictor of infertility.

DNA Damage

There are many etiologies of sperm DNA damage. Radiation, toxins, genital tract inflammation, varicocele, advanced paternal age, and testicular hyperthermia all induce significant DNA damage [106, 107] and will be discussed at length elsewhere in this book.

Post-testicular

Absence of the Vas Deferens

Congenital bilateral absence of the vas deferens (CBAVD) is a condition strongly related to cystic fibrosis (CF) and has even been considered as a diagnostic criterion for CF. However, while current dogma states that nearly all patients with CF have bilaterally absent vasa, there is little data to support this. Indeed, two recent articles suggest that CBAVD is present in half or less of CF patients. One series looking at children with CF who were undergoing inguinal hernia repair reported only a 24% (6/25) rate of CBAVD [108]. A series of 20 adults with CF and a mean age around 30 years old had a CBAVD rate of 55% [109]. In this latter series, only one man had a semen analysis consistent with possible fertility, and the more constant finding was atrophy of the seminal vesicles, which was seen in 18/20.

Nevertheless, CBAVD is strongly associated to CF, and the same genetics, mutation of the CFTR, are typically responsible for both phenomenons [110]. So, while men with CF do not necessarily have CBAVD, most men with CBAVD do have a CFTR mutation [111–113]. The pathophysiology of CBAVD thus clearly involves altered chloride transport in the majority of cases, and, like the respiratory and pancreatic sequelae seen with

CF, there is evidence that the genital abnormalities and pathology seen are a progressive disease. Namely, intentionally aborted CF fetuses demonstrate normal vas deferens, albeit with secretions filling their lumens. This suggests that the mechanism for CBAVD is atresia, and not aplasia, when a CFTR mutation is present [114]. One interesting sequela of this is that renal agenesis is not associated with CBAVD [115].

Congenital unilateral absence of the vas deferens (CUAVD) is a different entity altogether [116]. While there is still a significant rate of CFTR mutations in men with CUAVD, especially when the obstructive azoospermia is present [110], the majority of CUAVD is the result of an embryologic Wolffian duct aberrancy [117]. As such, renal agenesis is often seen with CUAVD, though CUAVD is not always seen in men with unilateral renal agenesis, as there are many other embryologic missteps that may occur to result in renal agenesis. While there is only a 20% rate of CUAVD seen in those with a unilateral renal agenesis, there is a 79% rate of unilateral renal agenesis seen in men with CUAVD. Since CUAVD not associated with a CFTR mutation is usually a unilateral and isolated phenomenon, fertility is often preserved.

Young's Syndrome

Young's syndrome is a rare disorder which presents clinically as obstructive azoospermia and chronic sinopulmonary infections [118]. Thus, it can be difficult to differentiate clinically from cystic fibrosis variants and primary ciliary dyskinesia. Indeed, definitive diagnosis of Young's syndrome requires negative CFTR genetic testing as well as investigation of ciliary ultrastructure to rule out primary ciliary dyskinesia [119]. Normal spermatogenesis is seen, and the obstructive azoospermia is due to inspissated secretions in the vas deferens.

The etiology of Young's syndrome is unclear with childhood mercury exposure having been postulated to play a role in the past [120]. Interestingly, the incidence of Young's syndrome has plummeted from estimates of one in 500 in the 1980s down to case reports and articles which question the existence of Young's syndrome today [121]. The observation that the reduced incidence over the last 50 years coincides with a decrease in mercury use and poisoning is tempered by the fact that our knowledge of genetics has rapidly advanced. Thus, the decreased incidence of Young's syndrome is more likely due to the increased correct genetic diagnosis of CF spectrum disease.

EjDO/Seminal Vesicle Dysfunction

Ejaculatory duct obstruction is a common etiology of male infertility, occurring in 1–5% of men presenting with infertility [122]. There are many causes of ejaculatory duct obstruction, including cystic fibrosis spectrum disease, Wolffian or Muellerian origin cysts, calcifications, tuberculosis and other GU infections, calculi, and urinary tract instrumentation [123, 124]. Additionally, chronic ejaculatory duct obstruction may affect the seminal vesicle in a manner analogous to the effect of bladder outlet obstruction on the bladder. Namely, with longstanding obstruction, the seminal vesicles may lose contractility, and resolution of the anatomical obstruction may not improve seminal vesicle emptying during ejaculation. Seminal vesicle dysfunction may also be seen in the absence of previous obstruction. This can be secondary to multiple sclerosis, diabetes, spinal cord injury or other neurologic insult, and medications. One interesting physical finding seen in 25–50% of men with spinal cord injuries likely related to seminal vesicle dysfunction is brown semen [125]. This brown coloration is not derived from heme and is not related to semen stasis per se.

Vasectomy and Vasectomy Reversal

Vasectomy is a procedure that is intended to produce infertility, and it is successful in over 90% of cases [126]. Some of the key determinants of success are related to aspects of surgical technique. The main reason for a correctly performed vasectomy to fail is recanalization of the vas deferens, a finding that has been histologically verified [127, 128]. Some debate remains as to which techniques provide the lowest recanalization rates. The manner of ligating the ends, non-ligation versus clipping versus suture ligation, length of vas removed, as well as whether to fold vas ends are all controversial [129, 130]. Two maneuvers which do seem to provide significant benefits are luminal cauterization and fascial interposition [131, 132].

   Vasectomy reversal may be performed in an attempt to return fertility to the sterilized man. The outcomes of vasectomy reversal are dependent on a number of factors. Surgical technique is one factor, with use of a microscope significantly improving pregnancy rates over loupe-assisted vasovasostomy [133]. Time elapsed since fertility also plays a significant role with a 97% patency rate and 76% pregnancy rate being achieved if surgery is performed at less than 3 years since vasectomy. Patency and pregnancy rates decline as time elapses, with patency and pregnancy rates of 79% and 44%, respectively, if the vasectomy was between 9 and 14 years prior and 71% and 30% if greater than 15 years elapsed [134]. Type of vasectomy reversal also plays a role with vasoepididymostomy (VE) having lower patency and pregnancy rates than vasovasostomy (VV) [135]. Presence and type of antisperm antibodies also may reduce fertility rates in men after vasectomy reversal [105]. Sperm granulomas were previously thought to decrease testicular pressure and so portend better vasectomy reversal outcomes. Though better sperm quality has been found in the vasa of men with sperm granulomas at the time of surgery, patency and pregnancy rates are not significantly different [134, 136]. Similarly, a testicular vasal remnant of 2.7 cm or longer predicts finding whole sperm in the vasal fluid [137], though research is not available as to its effect on patency and pregnancy rates. Though repeat attempts at vasectomy reversal would intuitively seem less likely to succeed, high success rates have been reported with combined VV/VE patency rates of 89% and pregnancy rates of 58% if the interval of obstruction was less than 10 years [138].

Nerve Injury

Nervous injury affecting ejaculation may occur at many levels and have a diverse etiology ranging from spinal cord injury to neural damage during retroperitoneal or pelvic surgery to neuropathy from systemic diseases. Ejaculatory dysfunction is present in 90% of spinal cord injury patients [139]. The type and severity of ejaculatory dysfunction are dependent on the level and extent of the injury. Higher cord lesions often result in an intact reflex arc which allows for penile vibratory stimulation to induce ejaculation. Men with sacral lesions or lesions of the efferent parasympathetic nerves are often not responsive to penile vibratory stimulation and may require endorectal electrical stimulation to induce ejaculation [140].

Retroperitoneal lymph node dissection (RPLND) for testicular cancer resulted in a high rate of ejaculatory dysfunction until the development of methods to spare the sympathetic nerve fibers. Both emission and bladder neck contraction are mediated by the sympathetic nervous system, and damage to the sympathetic chain and the hypogastric plexus overlying the great vessels results in a high degree of ejaculatory dysfunction. In the past, RPLND was associated with a 55–60% chance of ejaculatory dysfunction [141, 142]. Modified templates have helped to reduce the rates of retrograde ejaculation, with one study demonstrating an 82% rate of antegrade ejaculation with a modified unilateral template [143]. Another study using a modified bilateral template demonstrated an 88% rate of preservation of antegrade ejaculation [144].

Nerve sparing RPLND, developed in the late 1980s, has reduced the incidence of retrograde ejaculation even further to 0–7% [145, 146]. Nerve sparing RPLND may also be done after chemotherapy, though only 136 of 341 men qualified for this as compared to standard RPLND in one series [147]. Rates of ejaculatory dysfunction were also higher at 21%.

Medications

Medications affecting ejaculation do so by altering adrenergic signaling. This is most clearly seen with alpha-1 antagonists. Tamsulosin and silodosin, especially, are known to cause ejaculatory dysfunction [148, 149]. Previously, this was thought to be retrograde ejaculation. Recent studies have shown that the ejaculatory dysfunction induced by alpha-1 antagonists is actually a failure of emission [150, 151].

Antipsychotics have long been associated with sexual dysfunction, including ejaculatory dysfunction. Antipsychotics have effects on many different neurotransmitters including dopamine, norepinephrine, acetylcholine, and serotonin. Predictably, altered ejaculatory function with antipsychotics use correlates with anti-adrenergic actions of the antipsychotics [152]. Even atypical antipsychotics like risperidone may affect ejaculation [153, 154].

Resection of the Prostate

Surgery of the prostate is well known to cause retrograde ejaculation. Transurethral resection of the prostate as well as the laser photovaporization and enucleation all have a high likelihood of inducing retrograde ejaculation since removal of the proximal prostatic urethra severely diminishes the resistance to backflow of semen.

Coital

Abnormal coital practices may play a role in infertility when they interfere with semen deposition in the vagina or affect their timing with the female reproductive cycle. Similarly, erectile dysfunction and penile abnormalities such as hypospadias and chordee may interfere with semen deposition and thus may play a role in infertility.

Lubricants are commonly used by infertile couples, and many vaginal lubricants have been shown to negatively affect fertility. Many synthetic lubricants not only affect sperm motility but have also been shown to increase the DNA fragmentation index. In one study, FemGlide, Replens, and Astroglide all affected sperm motility, and FemGlide and K-Y jelly increased DNA fragmentation. One lubricant that has not been shown to have a significant impact on sperm motility or DNA fragmentation is Pre-Seed [155]. Another study showed similar findings with decreased motility in sperm exposed to K-Y jelly and Touch. Non-viability was seen in sperm exposed to Replens and Astroglide which was comparable to the non-viability seen when sperm were exposed to the spermicide nonoxylnol-9 [156]. In this study, canola oil was not found to affect sperm motility or viability. Yet another study showed that K-Y jelly, saliva, and olive oil all reduced sperm motility, while baby oil did not significantly affect motility [157].

Expert Commentary

This chapter has described the pre-testicular, testicular, and post-testicular spectrum of conditions known to affect male fertility. Many of the listed causes stem from or are subject to further degradation from reactive oxygen species. Pre-testicular causes often alter the normal hormonal milieu for sperm development, providing a suboptimal environment for sperm and perhaps a greater exposure or sensitivity to free radical damage. Testicular causes of infertility such as radiation, toxins, genital tract inflammation, varicocele, and testicular hyperthermia all induce significant DNA damage and thus increase reactive oxygen species. Finally, post-testicular causes of male infertility often affect sperm transit time, increasing likelihood of free radical damage of sperm. Despite our understanding of many of the conditions leading to male infertility, idiopathic infertility still comprises a large portion of the men evaluated for problems with reproduction. The proportion of idiopathic infertility will likely decrease with further understanding of the role of reactive oxygen species and clarification of the role of DNA integrity assays.

The male partners of all couples presenting with infertility must be examined and evaluated. Infertility itself is an independent risk factor for testicular cancer and genetic disease. Indeed, men of reproductive years often forego visiting physicians, and the infertility visit offers a viable platform for general health screening and recommendations. It must be remembered that the majority of the causes of male infertility are either preventable or treatable. Treatment success goes beyond simply harvesting sperm for assisted reproductive techniques. Facilitating pregnancy through intrauterine insemination with varicocele repair should be viewed with the same regard as facilitating natural pregnancy with vasectomy reversal. Finally, the importance of sperm banking cannot be understated, as cryopreservation of reproductive tissue prior to reproductive insult from chemotherapy or surgery is simple and often is the only chance of preserving future fertility.

Five-Year View

Although details and further understanding of some of the causes of male fertility conditions of male described have been elucidated in recent years, previous and future chapters in reproductive textbooks are and will be very similar to this one. However, the development and refinement of DNA integrity tests and determination of the relative importance of reactive oxygen species will likely obviate the need for male infertility evaluation. For example, if varicocele repair is definitively proven to reduce DNA damage to sperm, and decreased DNA damage to sperm is definitively proven to improve success rates with assisted reproductive techniques, referral from female fertility specialists will likely increase. Additional public and provider education on the rationale for male infertility referral and messages on the need for sperm banking will also increase the need for specialists knowledgeable in the causes and treatment of male infertility. This in itself may bring challenges because in relation to female assisted reproductive technology centers, large areas are greatly underserved by male fertility specialists [158].

Key Issues

- The majority of the causes of male infertility are either preventable or treatable.
- Male infertility is an independent risk factor for testicular cancer and genetic diseases.
- Sperm banking should be utilized liberally prior to potential gonadotoxic exposure.
- Pre-testicular causes of male infertility exert their negative effect via imbalances in the hormonal milieu of sperm production. Sexual function is also negatively

impacted with effects seen at the level of erectile function, ejaculatory function, and sexual desire.

- Medications can negatively impact pre-testicular, testicular, and post-testicular function.
- Varicocele is the most common cause of male infertility.
- For fertility potential, cryptorchidism is best treated early, especially if bilateral.
- After testicular trauma, fertility is most dependent on operative testicular volume preservation.
- Severe oligospermia or azoospermia requires genetic screening, given their high associated prevalence of Klinefelter's syndrome, karyotypic abnormalities, and microdeletion of the Y chromosome.
- CBAVD is not always seen with cystic fibrosis; evaluation for renal agenesis in CUAVD is essential.
- Many testicular causes of male infertility (radiation, toxins, environmental factors, genital tract inflammation, varicocele, testicular hyperthermia) lead directly to sperm DNA damage.
- Several post-testicular causes of male infertility stem from surgery.

References

1. Mosher WE. Reproductive impairments in the United States, 1965–1982. Demography. 1985;22:415–30.
2. Tielemans E, Burdorf A, te Velde E, Weber R, van Kooij R, Heederik D. Sources of bias in studies among infertility clients. Am J Epidemiol. 2002;156:86–92.
3. Sigman M. Male Infertility. Med Health R I. 1997;80(12):406–9.
4. Buvat J. Hyperprolactinemia and sexual function in men: a short review. Int J Impot Res. 2003;15(5):373–7.
5. Carter JN, Tyson JE, Tolis G, et al. Prolactin-screening tumors and hypogonadism in 22 men. N Engl J Med. 1978;299(16):847–52.
6. Patel SS, Bamigboye V. Hyperprolactinaemia. J Obstet Gynaecol. 2007;27(5):455–9.
7. Fasano S, Meccariello R, Cobellis G, et al. The endocannabinoid system: an ancient signaling involved in the control of male fertility. Ann N Y Acad Sci. 2009;1163:112–24.
8. Rettori V, De Laurentiis A, Fernandez-Solari J. Alcohol and endocannabinoids: neuroendocrine interactions in the reproductive axis. Exp Neurol. 2010;224(1):15–22.
9. Hallinan R, Byrne A, Agho K, et al. Hypogonadism in men receiving methadone and buprenorphine maintenance treatment. Int J Androl. 2009;32(2):131–9.
10. Dodé C, Hardelin JP. Kallmann syndrome. Eur J Hum Genet. 2009;17:139–46.
11. Fechner A, Fong S, McGovern P. A review of Kallmann syndrome: genetics, pathophysiology, and clinical management. Obstet Gynecol Surv. 2008;63(3):189–94.
12. Hardelin JP, Dode C. The complex genetics of Kallmann syndrome: KAL1, FGFR1, FGF8, PROKR2, PROK2, et al. Sex Dev. 2008;2:181–93.
13. Kamischke A, Baumgardt A, Horst J, et al. Clinical and diagnostic features of patients with suspected Klinefelter Syndrome. J Androl. 2003;24:41–8.
14. Blanco J, Egozcue J, Vidal F. Meiotic behavior of the sex chromosomes in three patients with sex chromosome abnormalities (47, XXY, mosaic 46, XY/47, XXY, and 47, XYY) assessed by flourescence in-situ hybridization. Hum Reprod. 2001;16(5):887–92.
15. Bergere M, Wainer R, Nataf V, et al. Biopsied testis cells of four 47, XXY patients: fluorescence in-situ hybridization and ICSI results. Hum Reprod. 2002;17:32–7.

16. Wikström AM, Dunkel L. Testicular function in Klinefelter syndrome. Horm Res. 2008;69(6):317–26.
17. Nagler HM, Grotas AB. Varicocele. In: Lipshultz LI, Howards SS, Niederberger CS, editors. Infertility in the male. 4th ed. New York City: Cambridge University; 2009.
18. World Health Organization. The influence of varicocele on parameters of fertility in a large group of men presenting to infertility clinics. Fertil Steril. 1992;57:1289–93.
19. MacLeod J. Seminal cytology in the presence of varicocele. Fertil Steril. 1965;16(6):735–57.
20. Paduch DA, Niedzielski J. Semen analysis in young men with varicocele: preliminary study. J Urol. 1996;156:778–90.
21. Hjollund NH, Storgaard L, Ernst E, et al. The relation between daily activities and scrotal temperature. Reprod Toxicol. 2002;16(3):209–14.
22. Ivell R. Lifestyle impact and the biology of the human scrotum. Reprod Biol Endocrinol. 2007;5:15.
23. Paul C, Murray AA, Spears N, et al. A single, mild, transient scrotal heat stress causes DNA damage, subfertility and impairs formation of blastocysts in mice. Reproduction. 2008;136(1):73–84.
24. Dada R, Gupta NP, Kucheria K. Spermatogenic arrest in men with testicular hyperthermia. Teratog Carcinog Mutagen. 2003;S1:235–43.
25. Esfandiari N, Saleh RA, Blaut AP, et al. Effects of temperature on sperm motion characteristics and reactive oxygen species. Int J Fertil Womens Med. 2002;47(5):227–33.
26. Bedford JM. Effects of elevated temperature on the epididymis and testis: experimental studies. Adv Exp Med Biol. 1991;286:19–32.
27. Hjollund NH, Bonde JP, Jensen TK, et al. Diurnal scrotal skin temperature and semen quality. The Danish first pregnancy planner study team. Int J Androl. 2000;23(5):309–18.
28. Wang C, McDonald V, Leung A, et al. Effect of increased scrotal temperature on sperm production in normal men. Fertil Steril. 1997;68(2):334–9.
29. Zorgniotti AW, MacLeod J. Studies in temperature, human semen quality, and varicocele. Fertil Steril. 1973;24(11):854–63.
30. Jung A, Eberl M, Schill WB. Improvement of semen quality by nocturnal scrotal cooling and moderate behavioral change to reduce genital heat stress in men with oligoasthenoteratozoospermia. Reproduction. 2001;121(4):595–603.
31. Goldstein M, Eid JF. Elevation of intratesticular and scrotal skin surface temperature in men with varicocele. J Urol. 1989;142(3):743–5.
32. Trsinar B, Muravec UR. Fertility potential after unilateral and bilateral orchidopexy for cryptorchidism. World J Urol. 2009;27(4):513–9.
33. Gracia J, Sánchez Zalabardo J, Sánchez García J, et al. Clinical, physical, sperm and hormonal data in 251 adults operated on for cryptorchidism in childhood. BJU Int. 2000;85(9):1100–3.
34. Lee PA, O'Leary LA, Songer NJ, et al. Paternity after unilateral cryptorchidism: a controlled study. Pediatrics. 1996;98:676–9.
35. Lee PA, O'Leary LA, Songer NJ, et al. Paternity after bilateral cryptorchidism. A controlled study. Arch Pediatr Adolesc Med. 1997;151(3):260–3.
36. Canavese F, Mussa A, Manenti M, et al. Sperm count of young men surgically treated for cryptorchidism in the first and second year of life: fertility is better in children treated at a younger age. Eur J Pediatr Surg. 2009;19(6):388–91.
37. Wiser A, Raviv G, Weissenberg R, et al. Does age at orchidopexy impact on the results of testicular sperm extraction? Reprod Biomed Online. 2009;19(6):778–83.
38. Cooper ER. The histology of the retained testis in the human subject at different ages and its comparison to the testis. J Anat. 1929;64:5–10.
39. Murphy F, Paran TS, Puri P. Orchidopexy and its impact on fertility. Pediatr Surg Int. 2007;23(7):625032. Epub 13 Mar 2007.
40. Setchell BP. The Parkes Lecture: heat and the testis. J Reprod Fertil. 1998;114(2):179–94.
41. Leissner J, Filipas D, Wolf HK, et al. The undescended testis: considerations and impact on fertility. BJU Int. 1999;83(8):885–91.
42. Hadziselimovic F, Zivkovic D, Bica DTG, et al. The importance of mini-puberty for fertility in cryptorchidism. J Urol. 2005;174:1536–9.
43. Kurpisz M, Havryluk A, Nakonechnyj A, et al. Cryptorchidism and long-term consequences. Reprod Biol. 2010;10(1):19–35.

44. Jørgensen N, Meyts ER, Main KM, Skakkebaek NE. Testicular dysgenesis syndrome comprises some but not all cases of hypospadias and impaired spermatogenesis. Int J Androl. 2010;33(2):298–303. Epub 4 Feb 2010.
45. Abe T, Takaha N, Tsujimura A, et al. Leydig cell tumor of the testis presenting male infertility: a case report. Hinyokika Kiyo. 2003;49(1):39–42.
46. Shiraishi Y, Nishiyama H, Okubo K, et al. Testicular Leydig cell tumor presenting as male infertility: a case report. Hinyokika Kiyo. 2009;55(12):777–81.
47. Chovelidze S, Kochiashvili D, Gogeschvili G, et al. Cases of Leydig cell tumor in male infertility. Georgian Med News. 2007;143:76–9.
48. Hayashi T, Arai G, Hyochi N, et al. Suppression of spermatogenesis in ipsilateral and contralateral testicular tissues in patients with seminoma by human chorionic gonadotropin beta subunit. Urology. 2001;58(2):251–7.
49. Ho GT, Gardner H, DeWolf WC, et al. Influence of testicular carcinoma on ipsilateral spermatogenesis. J Urol. 1992;148(3):821–5.
50. Carmignani L, Gadda F, Paffoni A, et al. Azoospermia and severe oligospermia in testicular cancer. Arch Ital Urol Androl. 2009;81(1):21–3.
51. Rowley MJ, Leach DR, Warner GA, et al. Effect of graded doses of ionizing radiation on the human testis. Radiat Res. 1974;59(3):665–78.
52. Paulsen CA. The study of radiation effects on the human testis: including histologic, chromosomal and hormonal aspects. Final progress report of AEC contract AT(45-1)-2225, Task Agreement 6. RLO-2225-2. 1973.
53. Speiser B, Rubin P, Casarett G. Aspermia following lower truncal irradiation in Hodgkin's disease. Cancer. 1973;32(3):692–8.
54. Ash P. The influence of radiation on fertility in man. Br J Radiol. 1980;53:271–8.
55. Giwercman A, von der Maase H, Berthelsen JG, et al. Localized irradiation of testes with carcinoma in situ: effects of Leydig cell function and eradication of malignant germ cells in 20 patients. J Clin Endocrinol Metab. 1991;73(3):596–603.
56. Shapiro E, Kinsella TJ, Makuch RW, et al. Effects of fractionated irradiation on endocrine aspects of testicular function. J Clin Oncol. 1985;3(9):1232–9.
57. Spitz S. The histological effects of nitrogen mustard on human tumours and tissues. Cancer. 1948;1(3):383–98.
58. Watson AR, Rance CP, Bain J. Long term effects of cyclophosphamide on testicular function. BMJ. 1985;291:1457–60.
59. Pryzant RM, Meistrich ML, Wilson G, et al. Long-term reduction in sperm count after chemotherapy with and without radiation therapy for non-Hodgkin's lymphomas. J Clin Oncol. 1993;11(2):239–47.
60. da Cunha MF, Meistrich ML, Fuller LM, et al. Recovery of spermatogenesis after treatment for Hodgkin's disease: limiting dose of MOPP chemotherapy. J Clin Oncol. 1984;2(6):571–7.
61. Meistrich ML, Chawla SP, Da Cunha MF, et al. Recovery of sperm production after chemotherapy for osteosarcoma. Cancer. 1989;63(11):2115–23.
62. Pectasides D, Pectasides M, Farmakis D. Testicular function in patients with testicular cancer treated with Bleomycin-Etoposide-Carboplatin (BEC90) combination chemotherapy. Eur Urol. 2004;45(2):187–93.
63. Pont J, Albrect W. Fertility after chemotherapy for testicular germ cell cancer. Fertil Steril. 1997;68:1–5.
64. Ishikawa T, Kamidono S, Fujisawa M. Fertility after high-dose chemotherapy for testicular cancer. Urology. 2004;63:137–40.
65. Sakamoto H, Oohta M, Inoue K, et al. Testicular sperm extraction in patients with persistent azoospermia after chemotherapy for testicular germ cell tumor. Int J Urol. 2007;14(2):167–70.
66. Ferlin A, Raicu F, Gatta V, Zuccarello D, Palka G, Foresta C. Male infertility: role of genetic background. Reprod Biomed Online. 2007;14(6):734–45.
67. Foresta C, Moro E, Ferlin A. Y chromosome microdeletions and alterations of spermatogenesis. Endocr Rev. 2001;22(2):226–39.
68. Vogt PH. Azoospermia factor (AZF) in Yq11: towards a molecular understanding of its function for human male fertility and spermatogenesis. Reprod Biomed Online. 2005;10(1):81–93.

69. Stahl PJ, Masson P, Mielnik A, et al. A decade of experience emphasizes that testing for Y microdeletions is essential in American men with azoospermia and severe oligozoospermia. Fertil Steril. 2010;94(5):1753–6.
70. Bojesen A, Gravholt CH. Klinefelter syndrome in clinical practice. Nat Clin Pract Urol. 2007;4(4):192–204.
71. Ferlin A, Garolla A, Foresta C. Chromosome abnormalities in sperm of individuals with constitutional sex chromosomal abnormalities. Cytogenet Genome Res. 2005;111:310–6.
72. Zhou-Cun A, Yang Y, Zhang SZ, et al. Chromosomal abnormality and Y chromosome microdeletion in Chinese patients with azoospermia or severe oligozoospermia. Yi Chuan Xue Bao. 2006;33(2):111–6.
73. Foresta C, Garolla A, Bartoloni L, Bettella A, Ferlin A. Genetic abnormalities among severely oligospermic men who are candidates for intracytoplasmic sperm injection. J Clin Endocrinol Metab. 2005;90(1):152–6.
74. Schiff JD, Palermo GD, Veeck LL, et al. Intracytoplasmic sperm injection in men with Klinefelter syndrome. J Clin Endocrinol Metab. 2005;90(11):6263–7.
75. O'FlynnO'Brien KL, Varghese AC, Agarwal A. The genetic causes of male factor infertility: a review. Fertil Steril. 2010;93(1):1–12.
76. Shafik A. Contraceptive efficacy of polyester-induced azoospermia in normal men. Contraception. 1992;45(5):439–51.
77. Munkelwitz R, Gilbert BR. Are boxer shorts really better? A critical analysis of the role of underwear type in male subfertility. J Urol. 1998;160(4):1329–33.
78. Bonde JP. Semen quality in welders exposed to radiant heat. Br J Ind Med. 1992;49(1):5–10.
79. Jung A, Schuppe HC. Influence of genital heat stress on semen quality in humans. Andrologia. 2007;39:203–15.
80. Agarwal A, Deepinder F, Sharma RK, et al. Effect of cell phone usage on semen analysis in men attending infertility clinic: an observational study. Fertil Steril. 2008;89:124–8.
81. Agarwal A, Desai NR, Makker K, et al. Effects of radiofrequency electromagnetic waves (RF-EMW) from cellular phones on human ejaculated semen: an in vitro pilot study. Fertil Steril. 2009;92:1318–25.
82. Collodel G, Capitani S, Pammolli A, et al. Semen quality of male idiopathic infertile smokers and nonsmokers: an ultrastructural study. J Androl. 2010;31:108–13.
83. Calogero A, Polosa R, Perdichizzi A, et al. Cigarette smoke extract immobilizes human spermatozoa and induces sperm apoptosis. Reprod Biomed Online. 2009;19:564–71.
84. Gaur DS, Talekar MS, Pathak VP. Alcohol intake and cigarette smoking: impact of two major lifestyle factors on male fertility. Indian J Pathol Microbiol. 2010;53:35–40.
85. Künzle R, Mueller MD, Hänggi W, et al. Semen quality of male smokers and nonsmokers in infertile couples. Fertil Steril. 2003;79:287–91.
86. Brandes SB, Buckman RF, Chelsky MJ, et al. External genitalia gunshot wounds: a ten-year experience with fifty-six cases. J Trauma. 1995;39:266–71.
87. Cass AS, Ferrara L, Wolpert J, et al. Bilateral testicular injury from external trauma. J Urol. 1988;140:1435–6.
88. Kuhlmann J, Bohme H, Tauber R. Bilateral testicular gunshot injuries. Urologe A. 2005; 44:918–20.
89. Tomomasa H, Oshio S, Amemiya H, et al. Testicular injury: late results of semen analyses after uniorchiectomy. Arch Androl. 1992;29:59–63.
90. Lin WW, Kim ED, Quesada ET, et al. Unilateral testicular injury from external trauma: evaluation of semen quality and endocrine parameters. J Urol. 1998;159:841–3.
91. Kukadia AN, Ercole CJ, Gleich P, et al. Testicular trauma: potential impact on reproductive function. J Urol. 1996;156:1643–6.
92. Philip J, Selvan D, Desmond A. Mumps orchitis in the non-immune postpubertal male: a resurgent threat to male fertility? BJU Int. 2006;97:138–41.
93. Masarani M, Wazait H, Dinneen M. Mumps orchitis. J R Soc Med. 2006;99:573–5.
94. Osegbe DN. Testicular function after unilateral bacterial epididymo-orchitis. Eur Urol. 1991;19:204–8.
95. Schuppe HC, Meinhardt A, Allam JP, et al. Chronic orchitis: a neglected cause of male infertility? Andrologia. 2008;40:84–91.

96. Zariwala MA, Knowles MR, Omran H. Genetic defects in ciliary structure and function. Annu Rev Physiol. 2007;69:423–50.
97. Leigh MW, Pittman JE, Carson JL, et al. Clinical and genetic aspects of primary ciliary dyskinesia/Kartagener syndrome. Genet Med. 2009;11:473–87.
98. Terada T, Hatakeyama S. Morphological evidence for two types of idiopathic "Sertoli-cell-only" syndrome. Int J Androl. 1991;14(2):117–26.
99. Weller O, Yogev L, Yavetz H, et al. Differentiating between primary and secondary Sertoli-cell-only syndrome by histologic and hormonal parameters. Fertil Steril. 2005;83(6):1856–8.
100. Collins JA, Burrows EA, Yeo J, et al. Frequency and predictive value of antisperm antibodies among infertile couples. Hum Reprod. 1993;8(4):592–8.
101. Menge AC, Medley NE, Mangione CM, et al. The incidence and influence of antisperm antibodies in infertile human couples on sperm-cervical mucus interactions and subsequent fertility. Fertil Steril. 1982;38:439–46.
102. Sinisi AA, Di Finizio B, Pasquali D, et al. Prevalence of antisperm antibodies by SpermMARtest in subjects undergoing a routine sperm analysis for infertility. Int J Androl. 1993;16:311–4.
103. Heidenreich A, Bonfig R, Wilbert DM, et al. Risk factors for antisperm antibodies in infertile men. Am J Reprod Immunol. 1994;31:69–76.
104. Walsh T, Turek P. Immunologic infertility. In: Lipshultz LI, Howards SS, Niederberger CS, editors. Infertility in the male. 4th ed. New York City: Cambridge University; 2009.
105. Meinertz H, Linnet L, Fogh-Andersen P, et al. Antisperm antibodies and fertility after vasovasostomy: a follow-up study of 216 men. Fertil Steril. 1990;54:315–21.
106. Hammiche F, Laven J, Boxmeer J, et al. Semen quality decline among men below 60 years of age undergoing IVF or ICSI treatment. J Androl. 2010;32:70–6. Epub ahead of print.
107. Belloc S, Benkhalifa M, Junca AM, et al. Paternal age and sperm DNA decay: discrepancy between chromomycin and aniline blue staining. Reprod Biomed Online. 2009;19:264–9.
108. Escobar MA, Grosfeld JL, Burdick JJ, et al. Surgical considerations in cystic fibrosis: a 32-year evaluation of outcomes. Surgery. 2005;138:560–71.
109. Wilschanski M, Corey M, Durie P, et al. Diversity of reproductive tract abnormalities in men with cystic fibrosis. JAMA. 1996;276:607–8.
110. Lissens W, Mercier B, Tournaye H, et al. Cystic fibrosis and infertility caused by congenital bilateral absence of the vas deferens and related clinical entities. Hum Reprod. 1996;S4:55–78.
111. Donat R, McNeill AS, Fitzpatrick DR, et al. The incidence of cystic fibrosis gene mutations in patients with congenital bilateral absence of the vas deferens in Scotland. Br J Urol. 1997;79:74–7.
112. Sokol RZ. Infertility in men with cystic fibrosis. Curr Opin Pulm Med. 2001;7:421–6.
113. Dörk T, Dworniczak B, Aulehla-Scholz C, et al. Distinct spectrum of CFTR gene mutations in congenital absence of vas deferens. Hum Genet. 1997;100:365–77.
114. Gaillard DA, Carré-Pigeon F, Lallemand A. Normal vas deferens in fetuses with cystic fibrosis. J Urol. 1997;158:1549–52.
115. Radpour R, Gourabi H, Gilani M, et al. Correlation between CFTR gene mutations in Iranian men with congenital absence of the vas deferens and anatomical genital phenotype. J Androl. 2008;29:35–40.
116. Donohue RE, Fauver HE. Unilateral absence of the vas deferens. A useful clinical sign. JAMA. 1989;261:1180–2.
117. Shapiro E, Goldfarb DA, Ritchey ML. The congenital and acquired solitary kidney. Rev Urol. 2003;5:2–8.
118. Handelsman DJ, Conway AJ, Boylan LM, et al. Young's syndrome. Obstructive azoospermia and chronic sinopulmonary infections. N Engl J Med. 1984;310:3–9.
119. Domingo C, Mirapeix RM, Encabo B, et al. Clinical features and ultrastructure of primary ciliary dyskinesia and Young syndrome. Rev Clin Esp. 1997;197:100–3.
120. Goeminne PC, Dupont LJ. The sinusitis-infertility syndrome: Young's saint, old devil. Eur Respir J. 2010;35:698.

121. Arya AK, Beer HL, Benton J, et al. Does Young's syndrome exist? J Laryngol Otol. 2009;123:477–81.
122. Smith JF, Walsh TJ, Turek PJ. Ejaculatory duct obstruction. Urol Clin North Am. 2008;35: 221–7.
123. Paick JS, Kim SH, Kim SW. Ejaculatory duct obstruction in infertile men. BJU Int. 2000;85:720–4.
124. Carson CC. Transurethral resection for ejaculatory duct stenosis and oligospermia. Fertil Steril. 1984;41:482–4.
125. Wieder JA, Lynne CM, Ferrell SM, et al. Brown-colored semen in men with spinal cord injury. J Androl. 1999;20:594–600.
126. Labrecque M, Nazerali H, Mondor M, et al. Effectiveness and complications associated with 2 vasectomy occlusion techniques. J Urol. 2002;168:2495–8.
127. Freund MJ, Weidmann JE, Goldstein M, et al. Microrecanalization after vasectomy in man. J Androl. 1989;10:120–32.
128. Cruickshank B, Eidus L, Barkin M. Regeneration of vas deferens after vasectomy. Urology. 1987;30:137–42.
129. Hallan RI, May AR. Vasectomy: how much is enough? Br J Urol. 1988;62:377–9.
130. Adams CE, Wald M. Risks and complications of vasectomy. Urol Clin North Am. 2009;36:331–6.
131. Sokal DC, Labrecque M. Effectiveness of vasectomy techniques. Urol Clin North Am. 2009;36:317–29.
132. Cook LA, Van Vliet H, Lopez LM, et al. Vasectomy occlusion techniques for male steriliza- tion. Cochrane Database Syst Rev. 2007;2:CD003991.
133. Jee SH, Hong YK. One-layer vasovasostomy: microsurgical versus loupe-assisted. Fertil Steril. 2010;94(6):2308–11.
134. Belker AM, Thomas Jr AJ, Fuchs EF, et al. Results of 1,469 microsurgical vasectomy rever- sals by the Vasovasostomy Study Group. J Urol. 1991;145:505–11.
135. Nagler HM, Jung H. Factors predicting successful microsurgical vasectomy reversal. Urol Clin North Am. 2009;36:383–90.
136. Magheli A, Rais-Bahrami S, Kempkensteffen C, et al. Impact of obstructive interval and sperm granuloma on patency and pregnancy after vasectomy reversal. Int J Androl. 2010;41(1):52–7.
137. Witt MA, Heron S, Lipshultz LI. The post-vasectomy length of the testicular vasal remnant: a predictor of surgical outcome in microscopic vasectomy reversal. J Urol. 1994;151: 892–4.
138. Hollingsworth MR, Sandlow JI, Schrepferman CG, et al. Repeat vasectomy reversal yields high success rates. Fertil Steril. 2007;88:217–9.
139. Talbot HS. The sexual function in paraplegia. J Urol. 1955;73:91–100.
140. Utida C, Truzzi JC, Bruschini H, et al. Male infertility in spinal cord trauma. Int Braz J Urol. 2005;31:375–83.
141. Narayan P, Lange PH, Fraley EE. Ejaculation and fertility after extended retroperitoneal lymph node dissection for testicular cancer. J Urol. 1982;127:685–8.
142. Lange PH, Narayan P, Vogelzang NJ, et al. Return of fertility after treatment for nonsemino- matous testicular cancer: changing concepts. J Urol. 1983;129:1131–5.
143. Pizzocaro G, Salvioni R, Zanoni F. Unilateral lymphadenectomy in intraoperative stage I nonseminomatous germinal testis cancer. J Urol. 1985;134:485–9.
144. Richie JP. Clinical stage 1 testicular cancer: the role of modified retroperitoneal lymphade- nectomy. J Urol. 1990;144:1160–3.
145. Donohue JP, Foster RS, Rowland RG, et al. Nerve-sparing retroperitoneal lymphadenectomy with preservation of ejaculation. J Urol. 1990;144:287–91.
146. Heidenreich A, Albers P, Hartmann M, et al. Complications of primary nerve sparing retro- peritoneal lymph node dissection for clinical stage I nonseminomatous germ cell tumors of the testis: experience of the German Testicular Cancer Study Group. J Urol. 2003;169: 1710–4.

24   H.J. Wiser et al.

147. Pettus JA, Carver BS, Masterson T, et al. Preservation of ejaculation in patients undergoing nerve-sparing postchemotherapy retroperitoneal lymph node dissection for metastatic testicular cancer. Urology. 2009;73:328–31.
148. Hellstrom WJ, Sikka SC. Effects of acute treatment with tamsulosin versus alfuzosin on ejaculatory function in normal volunteers. J Urol. 2006;176:1529–33.
149. Marks LS, Gittelman MC, Hill LA, et al. Rapid efficacy of the highly selective alpha1A-adrenoceptor antagonist silodosin in men with signs and symptoms of benign prostatic hyperplasia: pooled results of 2 phase 3 studies. J Urol. 2009;181:2634–40.
150. Hisasue S, Furuya R, Itoh N, et al. Ejaculatory disorder caused by α-1 adrenoceptor antagonists is not retrograde ejaculation but a loss of seminal emission. Int J Urol. 2006;13:1311–6.
151. Kobayashi K, Masumori N, Hisasue S, et al. Inhibition of seminal emission is the main cause of an ejaculation induced by a new highly selective α1A-blocker in normal volunteers. J Sex Med. 2008;5:2185–90.
152. Smith SM, O'Keane V, Murray R. Sexual dysfunction in patients taking conventional antipsychotic medication. Br J Psychiatry. 2002;181:49–55.
153. Loh C, Leckband SG, Meyer JM, et al. Risperidone-induced retrograde ejaculation: case report and review of the literature. Int Clin Psychopharmacol. 2004;19:111–2.
154. Haefliger T, Bonsack C. Atypical antipsychotics and sexual dysfunction: five case-reports associated with risperidone. Encéphale. 2006;32:97–105.
155. Agarwal A, Deepinder F, Cocuzza M, et al. Effect of vaginal lubricants on sperm motility and chromatin integrity: a prospective comparative study. Fertil Steril. 2008;89:375–9.
156. Kutteh WH, Chao CH, Ritter JO, et al. Vaginal lubricants for the infertile couple: effect on sperm activity. Int J Fertil Menopausal Stud. 1996;41:400–4.
157. Anderson L, Lewis SE, McClure N. The effects of coital lubricants on sperm motility in vitro. Hum Reprod. 1998;13:3351–6.
158. Nangia AK, Likosky DS, Wang D. Distribution of male infertility specialists in relation to the male population and assisted reproductive technology centers in the United States. Fertil Steril. 2010;94(2):599–609.

Further Reading

Blau H, Freud E, Mussaffi H, et al. Urogenital abnormalities in male children with cystic fibrosis. Arch Dis Child. 2002;87:135–8.
Chen-Mok M, Bangdiwala SI, Dominik R, et al. Termination of a randomized controlled trial of two vasectomy techniques. Control Clin Trials. 2003;24:78–84.
Fejes I, Závaczki Z, Koloszár S, et al. Hypothesis: safety of using mobile phones on male fertility. Arch Androl. 2007;53:105–6.

Chapter 2
Laboratory Evaluation for Male Infertility

Ryan Mori and Edmund Sabanegh Jr.

The diagnosis and treatment options for male infertility have recently undergone a sea of change as advancements in technology and understanding in the fields of molecular biology, genetics, and laboratory medicine have grown. Further, advancements in assisted reproductive technologies (ART) have rendered previously subfertile and infertile couples with various options for pregnancy. Such changes in the understanding and treatment of fertility and infertility have necessitated a much more detailed assessment of the couple presenting with infertility. At the basis of this assessment is a sophisticated and methodological evaluation of male factor infertility including laboratory assessment of urine, serum, and semen, as well as radiological and genetic studies.

Conception requires a balanced coordination between the endocrinologic and reproductive systems of both the male and the female partners. Studies in normal individuals demonstrate that within 1 year of unprotected intercourse, 60–75% of couples will achieve conception, whereas 90% will achieve conception after 1 year [1]. Based on such studies, the currently accepted definition of infertility by the American Society for Reproductive Medicine (ASRM) is the absence of conception after 12 months of regular, unprotected intercourse [2].

The workup and diagnosis of infertility is unique in medicine in that it involves multiple organ systems of two individuals. Pathology is often difficult to isolate given this complexity. Isolated male factor has been shown to be causative in 20% of infertility cases and is a contributing factor in conjunction with female factor pathology in an additional 30% of cases [3]. These estimates have changed little over time despite great diagnostic advancements [4, 5].

R. Mori, MD, MS (✉)
Cleveland Clinic Lerner College of Medicine and Glickman Urological and Kidney Institute, Cleveland Clinic Foundation, Cleveland, OH, USA

E. Sabanegh Jr., MD
Department of Urology, Glickman Urological and Kidney Institute, Center for Reproductive Medicine, Cleveland Clinic, 9500 Euclid Avenue/Q10-1, Cleveland, OH 44195, USA
e-mail: sabanee@ccf.org

S.J. Parekattil, A. Agarwal (eds.), *Male Infertility for the Clinician,*
© Springer Science+Business Media New York 2013

A workup of couples presenting for evaluation of failure to conceive after 12 months of unprotected intercourse should consist of concurrent male and female partner evaluation. Further, as recommended by the practice committees of both the American Urological Association (AUA) and the ASRM, workup for infertility should be started earlier than 12 months in the setting of (1) male risk factors for infertility, (2) advanced maternal age (>35y), or (3) there is concern about male factor infertility [2]. The initial workup of the male partner should be basic, methodological, and cost-effective. Isolated pathology should be isolated and treated when possible given the high cost of ART. The initial evaluation of the male may suggest the need to proceed with more costly advanced testing. Many treatments of male factor infertility and subfertility allow pregnancy using the patient's own sperm with or without ART. Options for uncorrectable causes of male factor infertility include donor sperm insemination in a healthy female partner as well as adoption.

Clinical and Laboratory Evaluation of Male Factor Infertility

Initial Evaluation of Male Factor Infertility

The initial evaluation of a male presenting with infertility mandates a thorough general history, physical exam, and review of systems as well as a focused and targeted reproductive history and physical exam. A plethora of general medical conditions may contribute to infertility or altered sexual function and may be undiagnosed prior to urological evaluation (Table 2.1). Up to 1.3% of men undergoing evaluation for infertility are diagnosed with a significant and potentially life-threatening general medical condition [6]. Basic laboratory testing is a critical component of the initial evaluation of male factor and includes urinalysis, basic semen analysis, and a routine serum hormone analysis. Data from the initial evaluation will guide more advanced testing in infertility and should proceed in a methodological and cost-effective fashion.

History and Review of Systems

A complete medical history is important to obtain as a variety of medical conditions can contribute to abnormal fertility and sexual function in the male, as detailed in Table 2.1. Recent acute systemic illness such as viremia or fever should be noted. The human spermatogenesis cycle has a length of 64 days with an additional 5–10 days needed for epididymal sperm transit [7–9]. Thus, any insult to spermatogenesis such as a febrile illness may not be manifested for 2–3 months in semen analysis. In addition, medical conditions such as diabetes mellitus, hypertension, diseases of the thyroid, certain neoplasms, and diseases of the central and peripheral nervous systems may have substantial impact on fertility, erectile or ejaculatory function.

Table 2.1 Pertinent components of the history for male infertility evaluation

Past medical history
- Infertility
  Previous conceptions
  Duration
  Previous evaluations/treatments
  Female partner fertility status: previous conceptions/outcomes, evaluation, previous
    treatments
- Sexual
  Erectile/ejaculatory function
  Lubrications
  Intercourse timing/knowledge
- Childhood
  Infectious: mumps orchitis, sexually transmitted infections/urethritis
  Trauma: groin/testicular trauma, torsion, prior inguinal surgery
  Onset of puberty
- Adult
  General/systemic: obesity, hypertension
  Metabolic/endocrinologic: DM, metabolic syndrome, thyroid function
  Infectious: sexually transmitted infections/urethritis, urinary tract infections, epididymo-
    orchitis/prostatitis
  Neoplasms: treatments (radiation, chemotherapy)
  Neurological: spinal cord, MS
  Trauma: testicular, CNS/PNS

Past surgical history
- Inguinal: orchidopexy, herniorrhaphy
- Pelvic/retroperitoneal: prostate, bladder/bladder neck, RPLND
- Scrotal: vasectomy, hydrocele

Social history
- Environmental/occupational exposures
- Tobacco use
- Alcohol use
- Recreational drugs: marijuana, cocaine, anabolic steroids

Family history
- Chromosomal abnormalities: Klinefelter's syndrome
- Infertility
- Cystic fibrosis

Medications
- Ejaculatory dysfunction: antihypertensives, alpha-blockers
- Erectile dysfunction: antidepressants, psychotropics
- Hypogonadism: anabolic steroids
- Spermatogenesis: antibiotics

A reproductive history should focus on identification of primary versus secondary infertility, details of prior conceptions of both partners, previous fertility treatments, and evaluation of libido, erectile function, and ejaculatory function. Primary infertility is by definition the absence of previous conception, whereas secondary infertility represents conception in the past with the current or previous partner. A sexual history should be addressed and include timing and frequency of coitus. As sperm survive within cervical mucus for 2–5 days [10], optimal timing of inter-course is at least every 48 h during the periovulatory period [11]. Commercially available ovulation prediction kits aid the couple in determining accurate time of ovulation. Attention should also be paid to types of lubricants used as many com-mercially available sexual lubricants have been shown to adversely affect sperm quality [12, 13].

Attention should be paid to the past medical history of the patient as well as a number of childhood diseases and conditions which may adversely affect future fertility including but not limited to mumps orchitis, cryptorchidism, testicular tor-sion or trauma, and previous inguinal surgery. Studies suggest that paternity rates for unilateral cryptorchidism are only slightly decreased, but significantly reduced in cases of bilateral cryptorchidism [14]. Controversy exists regarding future sperm quality and paternity after orchidopexy. The timing of the onset of puberty should be assessed as either delayed or precocious puberty may be indicative of underlying endocrinologic abnormalities.

A thorough review of systems and family medical history can identify genetic diseases which may affect fertility including Klinefelter's syndrome, Kallmann syn-drome, and cystic fibrosis. The existence of male siblings with infertility may sug-gest Y chromosome microdeletions or other chromosomal abnormalities, although most genetic diseases present as de novo rather than inherited mutations. Cystic fibrosis (CF) is associated with congenital absence of the vas deferens bilaterally (CBAVD). Genetic causes of infertility can be transmissible, especially with the advent of ART. With the growing use of ART, we can expect the incidence of genet-ically derived infertility to increase in the future.

Past surgical history should focus on surgery involving the male genitourinary tract, the retroperitoneum, or the inguinal region as such surgeries can be associated with ejaculatory dysfunction or obstruction or erectile dysfunction. Previous expo-sure to ionizing radiation should be noted as this has been shown to affect sperm quality. Social history should identify any hazardous occupational exposures as well as ingestion of potentially gonadotoxic substances including ETOH, tobacco, mari-juana, and other recreational drugs. Use of anabolic steroids or other performance-enhancing drugs should be assessed in appropriate patient populations. A review of medications is valuable and should include both prescribed substances as well as over-the-counter and herbal substances. Specific attention should be given to medi-cations that can lead to impaired ejaculation (alpha-blockers, antihypertensives) or sexual dysfunction (antidepressants, antipsychotic agents).

Physical Examination

The physical examination consists of a general examination as well as a detailed genital examination. The general overall appearance and degree of virilization can offer clues about possibly androgen deficiency. Assessment of body habitus, hair growth patterns, and gynecomastia should be noted and may suggest underlying endocrinological or hormonal abnormalities. A man with a history of primary infertility presenting with disproportionately long extremities and low volume testes is highly suggestive of Klinefelter's syndrome.

The genital exam includes a thorough evaluation of the phallus and testes as well as the paratesticular structures. The phallus should be evaluated for potential causes of altered deposition of ejaculate including penile curvature, hypospadias, or meatal stenosis. The testes should be examined in both the supine and standing positions. The exam is often facilitated by warming of the scrotum via either room temperature or a scrotal warming pack to prevent retraction of the testes from the cremasteric reflex. The testes should be palpated for masses, and attention should be paid to the volume of the testis and any discrepancies in symmetry. Normal adult testis volume should be at least 20 cm^3, or 4 × 3 cm [15], and an orchidometer or calipers can assist in measurement. Enlargement or tenderness of the epididymides may suggest obstruction or inflammation. The spermatic cord should be evaluated with the patient in the upright position to aid in identification of abnormally dilated spermatic veins, which by definition is a varicocele. Classically, a prominent varicocele is described as having a "bag of worms" feel on physical exam. Examination during a Valsalva maneuver is required to correctly grade the varicocele if present. A grade I varicocele is only detectable during the Valsalva maneuver. Grade II varicoceles are palpable without Valsalva maneuver, and grade III varicoceles are visible through the scrotal skin. Varicoceles are common findings, present in up to 15% of normal males. In men presenting for evaluation of infertility, 19–41% have been shown to have varicoceles. Ninety percent of unilateral varicoceles are left sided, thought to be secondary to the more acute insertion of the left gonadal vein into the renal vein. An isolated moderate to severe unilateral right varicocele raises suspicion of a retroperitoneal process obstructing the insertion of the gonadal vein more proximally such as a retroperitoneal mass or large renal mass with a vein thrombus.

During examination of the spermatic cord, the vas deferens should be palpated. Absence of the vas deferens raises suspicion of genetic causes of infertility, such as mutation in cystic fibrosis transmembrane regulator gene (CFTR). The prostate should be palpated for midline cysts, or Mullerian duct cysts, which can be associated with ejaculatory duct obstruction. The seminal vesicles are not normally palpable, but may be in the setting of obstruction.

Laboratory Evaluation of Male Factor Infertility

Basic Testing

The initial assessment of a man presenting for an evaluation of male factor infertility should include a basic laboratory assessment of the semen. Further testing such as serum endocrine assays or genetic tests is suggested and guided by the results of the physical and laboratory evaluations.

Semen Analysis. A semen analysis is a critical component of the initial workup of male infertility. It can offer great insight into the etiology of infertility or

Table 2.2 Comparison of 1999 and 2010 WHO normal reference values for semen parameters

Semen parameter	Normal values: 1999 WHO	2010 WHO lower reference limit (5th centile + 95% CI)
Semen volume (mL)	2–6	1.5 (1.4–1.7)
Total motility PR + NP (%)	50+	40 (38–42)
Progressive motility PR (%)	25+	32 (31–34)
Vitality (% live spermatozoa)	50+	58 (55–63)
Sperm number (10^6 sperm/ejaculate)	>40	39 (33–46)
Sperm concentration (10^6 sperm/mL)	20	15 (12–16)
Morphology (% normal)	>30	4 (3.0–4.0)

Data from World Health Organization [21]. WHO Laboratory Manual for the Examination of Human Semen and Sperm-Cervical Mucus Interaction, 1999; World Health Organization, Department of Reproductive Health and Research [59]. WHO Laboratory Manual for the Examination and Processing of Human Semen, 5th edn. 2010; Cooper et al. [19]

Table 2.3 WHO nomenclature related to semen quality

Aspermia	No semen
Asthenospermia	<32% Progressively motile spermatozoa
Asthenoteratospermia	Percentages of both progressively motile and morphologically normal spermatozoa below the reference limits
Azoospermia	No spermatozoa present in the ejaculate
Cryptozoospermia	Spermatozoa not found in fresh preparations but found in centrifuged pellet
Hematospermia	Erythrocytes in ejaculate
Leukospermia	Presence of leukocytes in ejaculate > threshold (1 mil/cm^3)
Necrospermia	Low percentage of live and high percentage of immotile spermatozoa in ejaculate
Normozoospermia	Within normal limits for spermatozoa number and motility
Oligoasthenospermia	Total number of spermatozoa and percentage of progressively motile spermatozoa below lower reference limits
Oligoasthenoteratospermia	Total number of, percentage of progressively motile, and percentage of morphologically normal spermatozoa below the lower reference limits
Oligoteratospermia	Total number of and percentage of progressively motile spermatozoa below the lower reference limits
Oligospermia	Total number of spermatozoa below the lower reference limit
Teratospermia	Percentage of morphologically normal spermatozoa below the reference limit

Adapted from Appendix 1 Reference values and semen nomenclature. World Health Organization, Department of Reproductive Health and Research [59] with permission

subfertility; however, it serves as a surrogate rather than a true measure of fertility. An abnormal semen analysis can yield a viable pregnancy, and normal semen parameters can be associated with failure to conceive. As few as 15% of men presenting with infertility have currently recognizable abnormalities on semen analysis [16]. Table 2.2 reports a distribution of abnormalities in semen analyses in men presenting for infertility evaluation, and Table 2.3 lists the currently accepted

Table 2.4 Components of the macroscopic semen assessment

Macroscopic variable	Normal quality
Liquefaction	Homogenous, <60 min
Appearance	Homogenous, gray opalescent
Viscosity	Thread < 2 cm
Volume	>1.5 mL
pH	>7.2

nomenclature of diagnoses set forth by the World Health Organization (WHO). Beyond just the appearance of semen and spermatozoa microscopically, it is often necessary to obtain functional studies of sperm to assess the true fertilizing potential. In addition, guided by the basic semen analysis, more advanced testing may be needed and will be explored in greater depth below.

Evaluation of Basic Semen Analyses

Collection. Prior to analysis, semen must be properly collected into a sterile container. Sperm count and semen volume are variable from day to day; thus, it is essential to evaluate at least 2 samples to characterize baseline data for a patient [17]. Semen parameters and ejaculate volume can also vary widely based on the frequency of ejaculation, and it is currently recommended that a period of 2–5 days of ejaculatory abstinence precede sample collection. This period of abstinence should remain a constant with further semen samples to maintain comparability.

Optimally, the sample should be collected via self-stimulation in a private room near the laboratory to reduce the time between collection and analysis and to ensure constant temperature of the specimen. Lubricants should be avoided if possible as they may lead to altered sperm motility. The semen sample should be complete, and the man should be cautioned to collect all fractions of the ejaculate, as the first fraction contains sperm-rich prostatic fluids [18]. Coitus interruptus should be avoided as this first fraction is often loss. Semen collection devices that are free of spermicidal lubricants are less than ideal, but may be necessary if the patient has barriers to conventional collection methods. Semen should be analyzed within 1 h of collection to prevent alteration in semen parameters secondary to delayed analysis. Patients unable to provide a sample on location should be instructed to bring the sample to the lab at a constant temperature near body temperature for analysis within 1 h.

Some patients will be unable to provide a semen sample due to erectile or ejaculatory dysfunction and may require oral or intracavernosal injection therapy to produce a specimen. Discussion of such techniques is beyond the scope of this chapter.

Macroscopic Assessment. Semen analysis begins with a macroscopic assessment after liquefaction occurs. The time to liquefaction should be noted and considered abnormal if greater than 60 min. The five macroscopic variables are semen volume, viscosity, color, coagulation, and pH (Table 2.4).

The semen volume is best measured by weight, but can also be measured directly. The volume of the ejaculate is supplied mainly by the seminal vesicles and prostate gland, with some contribution from the bulbourethral glands and the epididymides.

Table 2.5 Distribution of semen analysis parameters in men presenting for initial evaluation of infertility

Semen parameter	Incidence (%)
Any abnormality	37
Motility	26
Asthenospermia	24
Oligospermia	8
Agglutination	2
Volume	2
Morphology	1
Azoospermia	8
Normal semen analysis	55

From Lipshultz [58] with permission of Elsevier

The viscosity can be measured by drawing the sample into a wide-bore 1.5-mm pipette and letting the semen drop. A thread length of greater than 2 cm is abnormally viscous. While viscosity is a consistently measured parameter, the significance of an abnormal assessment is controversial with many experts discounting the importance of this finding. A normal liquefied semen sample is described as homogenous and gray opalescent in color. Seminal pH results from the balance of acidic prostatic secretion and alkaline seminal vesicular secretions. This principle can be clinically valuable in the setting of low semen volume and abnormal pH, as the location of obstruction can be logically deduced to be at the level of the ejaculatory duct.

Microscopic Assessment. A wet prep of the semen next examined under light microscopic magnification. A basic microscopic semen analysis assesses agglutination/aggregation, sperm count, motility, morphology, and presence of non-sperm cells. The World Health Organization has set forth "normal" reference ranges for each of the above semen parameters. There has been some lack of consensus as to the utility and applicability of previously accepted lower limits of normal. The lower reference values have been recently updated based on analysis of semen samples of men with proven fertility and time to pregnancy less than 12 months [19]. Distributions of semen parameters across these men were obtained using standardized WHO laboratory criteria, and the lower reference limit, taken as the 5th centile, is presented in comparison with previous lower limits from the 1999 WHO criteria [20] in Table 2.5.

- Sperm aggregation and agglutination: Semen is first analyzed as a wet prep specimen. Agglutination or clumping of spermatozoa with either sperm or non-sperm semen elements is noted as well as site of binding (head to head, tail to tail, or mixed fashion). Though some degree of sperm agglutination is considered normal, more considerable amounts could represent the presence of antisperm antibodies (ASA) [21]. Aggregation refers to the clumping together of nonmotile spermatozoa. The presence of agglutination may also be suggestive of ASA. Sperm agglutination with non-sperm semen elements may occur in the presence of infection. Thus, the presence of agglutination on microscopic assessment should trigger further testing with seminal white blood cell assessment and antisperm antibody measurement.

- Motility: The degree of progressive sperm motility is related to pregnancy rates [22]. Sperm are classified as either being motile or immotile. Further, motile sperm are assessed for their degree of progressive motility. Movement is considered progressively motile (PR) if the spermatozoa is moving actively either linearly or in a large circle. Nonprogressive motility (NP) refers to motion with absence of progression such as movement in small circles. Total motility (PR + NP) and progressive motility (PR) are reported in the basic semen analysis as percentages of total sperm. Complete absence of motility may be suggestive of ultrastructural cilia abnormalities such as Kallmann syndrome as well as necrospermia. Necrospermia is assessed via sperm vitality testing as detailed below.
- Sperm vitality: Sperm vitality is measured as a function of the membrane integrity of sperm cells and is expressed as a percentage of total sperm. This measurement is especially important when a large number of immotile sperm are present in order to rule out necrospermia [16]. The 2 methods commonly employed to assess the integrity of the cell membrane are the dye exclusion test and hypotonic swelling. The dye exclusion test is based on the principle that an intact membrane will not take in dye. In the latter test, a hypotonic solution is utilized, and spermatozoa with intact membrane swell within 5 min. This test is particularly useful if viable sperm are being identified for use in ICSI. Recently published lower reference limit for sperm vitality is 58% which is in agreement with previous assessments [19].
- Sperm count and concentration: Of paramount importance in the evaluation of male factor infertility is the presence of sperm in the ejaculate. Azoospermia, or the absence of sperm in the ejaculate, may occur from ejaculatory dysfunction, obstruction of the reproductive tract, or as a result of abnormal sperm production. Both the number of sperm per ejaculate and the sperm concentration have been correlated with both time to pregnancy and pregnancy rates [23]. Sperm concentration is directly measured and expressed in terms of millions per milliliter, whereas total sperm number is a calculated value based on semen volume and concentration. The total number of spermatozoa in the ejaculate has been correlated with testis volume; however, the concentration is heavily influenced by the volume of the glandular secretions. The normal sperm concentration is commonly accepted as > 20 million sperm per mL semen based on the 1999 WHO cutoff [20]. However, according to this threshold, 20% of 18-year-old males would be classified as oligospermic [24]. As demonstrated in Table 2.5, more recent data by the WHO sets the lower reference limit of sperm concentration to 15 million/mL in a population of fertile men [19]. Oligospermia is still commonly accepted by definition as a sperm concentration of less than 20 million sperm per mL. For an exhaustive list of current WHO infertility nomenclature and definition, refer to Table 2.3.
- Non-sperm cells: The number of non-sperm cells present in a semen sample should be estimated and may have implications regarding underlying pathology. The most commonly encountered non-sperm cells in semen are epithelial cells, immature germ cells, and leukocytes [25]. The latter two cell types are referred to collectively as round cells due to their appearance microscopically and are not easily

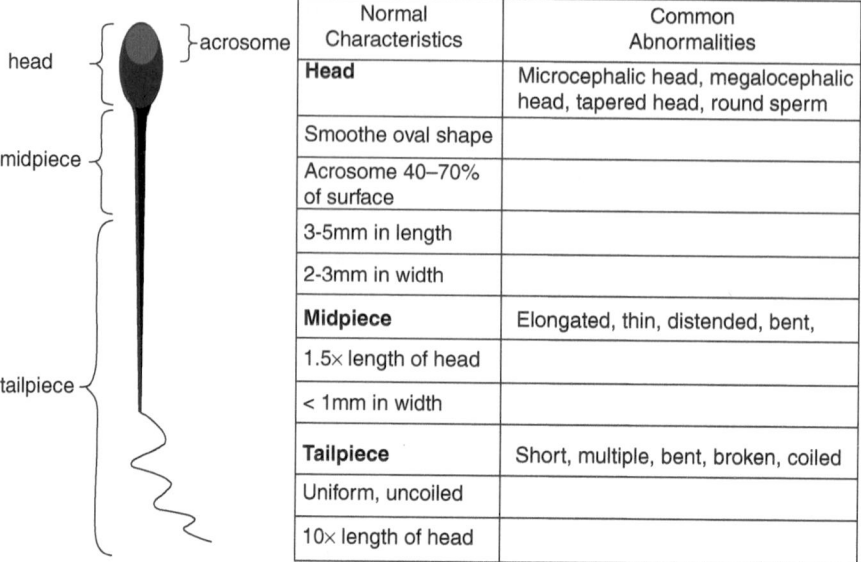

	Normal Characteristics	Common Abnormalities
	Head	Microcephalic head, megalocephalic head, tapered head, round sperm
	Smoothe oval shape	
	Acrosome 40–70% of surface	
	3-5mm in length	
	2-3mm in width	
	Midpiece	Elongated, thin, distended, bent,
	1.5× length of head	
	< 1mm in width	
	Tailpiece	Short, multiple, bent, broken, coiled
	Uniform, uncoiled	
	10× length of head	

Fig. 2.1 Sperm morphology (Kruger Strict Criteria)

differentiated by microscopy alone. If the estimated round cell concentration exceeds 1×10^6/mL, then further testing should be done to assess the nature of the cell types. This is most reliably done by using immunohistochemistry to stain for specific leukocyte markers. However, the Endtz test allows a cost-effective method of identifying leukocytes by measuring peroxidase enzyme activity visualized with orthotoluidine dye [26]. The presence of leukocytes in semen may have detrimental effects on semen quality including reductions in sperm motility and DNA integrity [27, 28] as well as elevations in seminal reactive oxygen species [29].

• Sperm morphology: Sperm cells by nature have varying morphologies during maturation. Assessment is operator dependent and thus more subjective than other components of the basic semen analysis. Studies of sperm taken from postcoital cervical mucus or zona pellucida offer insight about the morphology of sperm with fertilizing potential [30–32]. Multiple classification schemata exist, but the currently most widely used are the WHO criteria and Kruger's strict criteria. Kruger and colleagues demonstrated that in men with sperm concentrations greater than 20 million sperm per mL and greater than 30% motility, fertilization rates were significantly higher for those men with greater than 14% normal sperm by the rigid criteria [13]. By WHO criteria, teratospermia represents less than 15% of sperm with normal morphology [20]. There remains substantial controversy regarding the predictive implications of abnormal morphology on assisted reproductive outcomes with both intrauterine insemination and intracytoplasmic sperm injection.

Normal spermatozoa consist of a head, midpiece, and a tailpiece (Fig. 2.1). A spermatozoa must have both a normal head and tail to be considered morphologically normal. The head should be a smooth ovoid shape with a well-defined acrosomal region (more lightly stained region) comprising about 40–70% of the head volume and containing no large vacuoles. The head should taper into a midpiece aligned along the same axis of the head. The tail should be of uniform caliber and approximately 10 times the length of the head. Looping of the tail is acceptable, but any sharp abnormalities are abnormal. Excess residual cytoplasm is also a morphologic abnormality. Common abnormalities of spermatozoa head, midpiece, and tail are demonstrated in Fig. 2.1.

Abnormal sperm morphology is commonly seen with defective spermatogenesis or with certain epididymal pathologies. They generally have less fertilizing potential and have been linked with increased DNA fragmentation [33] and chromosomal abnormalities [34].

All intact spermatozoa per area surveyed should be assessed, and the percentage of normal sperm should be recorded. Recently updated lower reference limits for normal forms in fertile men is 4% by strict criteria [19, 21], which is considerably lower than the previously accepted reference range. Some spermatozoa may have multiple defects; thus, percentages of specific defects should be based on total sperm count.

Computer-Assisted Semen Analysis (CASA). With advances in technology, it is now feasible to measure sperm motility, kinematics, and concentration using computer-aided sperm analysis (CASA). The potential advantages over more traditional methods are its precision and ability to quantify the kinematic properties of the spermatozoa. At present, this technology requires costly equipment and training and is more commonly a tool used in research settings rather than basic pathology laboratories.

Functional Sperm Testing

The fertilizing potential of a sperm cell cannot always be inferred from a basic semen analysis. Functional sperm tests assess various processes in the normal fertilization cycle to include sperm transit, penetration of the zona pellucida of the oocyte, and, ultimately, fertilization. Sperm-mucous interaction can be assessed by a cervical mucus migration assay where the rate of sperm transit through mucous is measured. The sperm penetration assay (SPA) measures the ability of a human sperm to penetrate a specially prepared hamster egg that has been stripped of the outer zona pellucida, allowing cross-species fertilization. This yields useful information about a sperm's ability to successfully undergo capacitation, acrosome reaction, membrane fusion with oocytes, and chromatin decondensation. A good result on SPA suggests proceeding with a trial of spontaneous conception or intrauterine insemination (IUI), whereas a poor SPA result might suggest the need for IVF with ICSI.

The acrosome reaction test measures the ability of the sperm cell to mount an effective acrosome reaction and may be useful in the setting of profound teratospermia with head predominant abnormalities where IVF is not successful. Currently, this test may be recommended in the setting of abnormal sperm head morphology or failure to fertilize oocytes in conventional IVF cycles. However, this test has been difficult to standardize, limiting its role at the present time.

Additional/Advanced Semen Testing

Antisperm Antibody Testing. Under normal anatomical circumstances, the seminiferous tubules are immunologically protected from the humoral environment as the tight junctions between the Sertoli cells form the blood-testis barrier. However, following a breech of this barrier such as after orchitis, scrotal trauma, or surgery, the immune system may be exposed to these "foreign" sperm antigens, and antisperm antibodies (ASA) may develop. The presence of sperm agglutination, especially head to head, should suggest the possibility of ASA. In addition, low sperm motility in the setting of previous injury or surgery (i.e., vasectomy), leukocytospermia, or otherwise unexplained infertility should also lower the clinician's threshold for evaluating for ASA.

Antisperm antibodies may be found in the serum and in the seminal plasma and bound to the sperm themselves. They can cause agglutination and immotility or can be spermatotoxic depending on the type of antibody. In previous reports, up to 10% of infertile men present with ASA versus only 2% of fertile men [35]. However, men can have normal semen parameters with presence of ASA as well [36]. The direct ASA test detects sperm-bound immunoglobulins, while indirect testing detects the biological activity of circulating ASA. Direct assays of sperm-bound immunoglobulins are preferred since most agree that sperm-bound antibodies are the most clinically relevant. Serum ASA testing, once widely used, has been largely discarded due to the much greater sensitivity of semen testing.

Sperm DNA Damage. Sperm DNA damage has been shown to have a positive correlation with abnormal semen parameters. [37]. Various factors and agents have been associated with sperm DNA damage including testicular cancers, tobacco use, and certain chemotherapeutic agents [27]. The etiology of sperm DNA damage at this time is thought to involve abnormal chromatin packing, elevated reactive oxygen species [27], and apoptosis [38]. There are several tests currently available to assess sperm DNA integrity by assessing strand breaks in situ [39]. The single cell gel electrophoresis assay, or comet assay, uses gel electrophoresis to assess DNA fragmentation. With the terminal deoxynucleotidyl transferase-mediated deoxyuridine triphosphate nick-end labeling (TUNEL) assay, a fluorescent-labeled nucleotide is transferred to the hydroxyl end of a broken DNA strand, and flow cytometry is used to assess DNA nicks. The sperm chromatin structure assay (SCSA) uses low pH to denature sperm DNA at the site of DNA breaks and is followed by acridine orange staining and flow cytometry to measure percentage of denatured DNA. Meta-analyses have shown that couples with sperm DNA fragmentation indices (DNI) less than 30% [40, 41] are twice as likely to achieve pregnancy using IVF. Although tests of DNA integrity are not part of the basic semen analysis, they can be useful especially in the setting of unexplained infertility but normal bulk semen parameters.

ROS Testing

Reactive oxygen species (ROS), also known as free radicals, are by-products of normal intercellular and intracellular metabolism and have been implicated in the etiology of multiple diseases across multiple organ systems. They are a necessary result of oxygen metabolism, which takes place in all healthy tissues, and are formed by the addition of unpaired electrons to the oxygen molecule through the process of reduction. The addition of an electron to molecular O_2 produces a superoxide anion radical (O_2-) that is reactive. Secondary ROS include hydroxyl radical (OH), peroxyl radical (ROO), and hydrogen peroxide (H_2O_2). ROS are critical to normal cell physiology, but excessive levels are detrimental to cell survival and function. In excess, they induce cellular damage by the oxidation of cellular and cell membrane components and cause DNA damage by modification of bases, deletions, frameshifts, and chromosomal relocations.

Oxidative stress by definition refers to the imbalance between reactive oxygen species and their scavengers, known generally as antioxidants. Antioxidants are the crux of the host defense against ROS and are formed via both enzymatic and non-enzymatic pathways. The primary enzymatic antioxidants include superoxide dismutases, catalase, and glutathione peroxidase. The superoxide dismutases convert superoxide into O_2 and H_2O_2. Catalase and glutathione peroxidase further degrade H_2O_2 into water and O_2. Glutathione is the main nonenzymatic antioxidant, and its cysteine subunit contains a sulfhydryl group which directly scavenges free radicals. Vitamins E and C are also important nonenzymatic scavengers of free radicals.

Reactive oxygen species have been shown to be critical throughout normal spermatogenesis and conception, specifically during sperm capacitation [42] and sperm-oocyte fusion [43]. Seminal fluid contains superoxide dismutase, catalase, glutathione peroxidase, and glutathione reductase. High levels of ROS are correlated with poor sperm quality and function. Spermatozoa which have been incubated with ROS overnight have increased lipid peroxidation. Further, addition of free radical scavengers like alpha tocopherol has been shown to revive sperm motility both in vitro [11] and in vivo.

Sperm are exposed to free radicals both by intrinsic production, extrinsic production in the semen, and via external and environmental sources including cigarette smoking, exposure to certain industrial compounds, and increased intrascrotal temperatures.

In normal semen, there is a low level of oxidative stress, as the free radicals necessary for certain cell signaling processes are kept in check by the antioxidants in order to avoid cellular damage. However, this balance is lost in conditions where there is either increased production of free radicals or decreased buffering capacity by available antioxidants. Leukocytes and spermatozoa are both significant sources of free radicals in the semen. Normal semen contains some white blood cells, predominantly neutrophils. Neutrophils exert their normal cytotoxic function partly by releasing high concentrations of ROS. Although the relationship is incompletely defined, leukospermia, defined as peroxidase positive leukocytes at a concentration greater than $1\times10\times6$ per mL by the WHO [21], has been associated with altered semen parameters including decreased sperm concentration, motility, and morphology [4]. Although there is a correlation between seminal leukocytes and infertility [10], some studies have failed to show an alteration of sperm parameters in the presence of leukospermia [5]. However, several studies have linked proinflammatory cytokines including IL-6, IL-8, and TNF-alpha to altered sperm function [38, 44, 45].

In addition to seminal leukocytes, spermatozoa themselves are source of ROS. As sperm mature, they extrude cytoplasm rich in reducing molecules. Abnormalities in sperm maturation lead to retention of cytoplasm and increased levels of ROS in semen. The effects of the ROS on over all sperm function may correlate with the site of ROS production, intrinsic or extrinsic to the sperm. Some authors suggest that higher levels of extrinsic ROS, such as that produced by leukospermia, have greater effects on sperm count, motility, and morphology, whereas increased intrinsic ROS production is associated with higher levels of DNA fragmentation [37].

Testing for reactive oxygen species is not a part of the standard initial evaluation of male factor infertility. However, there is increasing research being conducted in this area, and despite the lack of randomized control trials, it is becoming evident that men presenting with infertility with increased oxidative stress in the semen may benefit from antioxidant therapy [46, 47]. Additionally, infertile men with varicoceles have been shown to have elevated seminal ROS [48] with levels that correlate with varicocele grade [49], and several studies have shown that surgical varicocelectomy is correlated with decreased seminal oxidative stress, increased seminal antioxidants, and improved sperm quality [20, 50, 51].

Various direct and indirect testing modalities exist to determine the level of oxidative stress in the semen. The most commonly employed method of ROS testing is a chemiluminescence probe assay, which is used to quantify redox activities of spermatozoa [52]. Using this technique, a luminol probe (5-amino-2,3-dihydro-1,4-phthalazinedione), used to measure both intracellular and extracellular ROS, or a lucigen probe measuring superoxide radicals released extracellularly is employed. Direct assays of oxidative stress are available, but cost and practicality issues have rendered these assays tools of research with limited clinical application at this time.

Hormonal Assessment

In addition to a basic semen analysis, many patients may warrant a serum hormonal analysis at time of presentation. The goal of such an analysis is to evaluate the hypothalamic-pituitary-gonadal axis and to rule out an underlying endocrinopathy or primary testicular failure. Controversy exists as to the necessity of a hormonal evaluation in all patients presenting with infertility. However, there is a consensus that basic hormonal testing including serum follicle-stimulating hormone (FSH) and early morning serum total testosterone should be done in the setting of (1) abnormally low sperm count (<10 million/cm^3), (2) impaired sexual function, and

(3) clinical findings suggestive of an endocrine abnormality such as reduced testicular volume or gynecomastia [1, 53].

The pituitary and gonadal hormones are released in a pulsatile fashion, and this rhythm is orchestrated by the hypothalamus, which receives diffuse input from multiple cortical and subcortical brain regions. The hypothalamus communicates to the anterior pituitary both via neuronal input as well as via the portal vascular system which allows direct delivery of hypothalamic hormones in high concentration to the anterior pituitary. The most important of these hypothalamic hormones is luteinizing hormone-releasing hormone (LHRH) or gonadotropin-releasing hormone (GNRH) which stimulates the secretion of luteinizing hormone (LH) and FSH. GNRH secretion is modulated by many factors and is under direct negative feedback control by circulating gonadal hormones including testosterone and inhibin.

LH, FSH, and prolactin are the primary hormones released from the anterior pituitary into the systemic circulation. LH stimulates the Leydig cells in the testes to produce testosterone, while FSH acts on the Sertoli cells of the testes and promotes development and growth of the seminiferous.

The testes are composed primarily of Leydig cells, Sertoli cells, and seminiferous tubules. The bulk of the testicular volume is comprised of seminiferous tubules and germinal elements; thus, reduced testicular size suggests impaired spermatogenesis [54]. Within the testes, Leydig cells are responsible for androgen synthesis. Testosterone, the primary circulating male androgen, is secreted in a pulsatile fashion with a regular circadian cycle peaking in the early morning. Only 2% of the serum testosterone is free in the systemic circulation with the remainder bound in roughly equal proportions to sex hormone-binding globulin (SHBG) and albumin. Alterations in serum SHBG will increase free testosterone in the serum. SHBG levels are influenced by a number of conditions including liver and thyroid disease, medications, advanced age, and obesity. Peripherally, testosterone is reduced to dihydrotestosterone (DHT) by 5 alpha-reductase and is also converted to estradiol by aromatases.

Sertoli cells line the seminiferous tubules and are linked by tight junctions, forming the blood–testis barrier which provides an immunologically naïve environment for spermatogenesis. The Sertoli cells are under the control of FSH and produce multiple paracrine factors important in stimulating and supporting spermatogenesis. Inhibin B is released from Sertoli cells in response to FSH stimulation and is important as regulator of the HGP axis via negative feedback at the pituitary and hypothalamus. The Sertoli cells also express androgen-binding protein in response to FSH stimulation and allow for very high intraluminal testosterone levels to support spermatogenesis via paracrine mechanisms

The most common abnormality encountered on hormonal analysis in the infertile man is an elevated serum FSH. This finding is suggestive of impaired spermatogenesis; however, the finding of elevated FSH is not always present in cases of testicular failure [55]. Abnormal preliminary screening tests should prompt a more involved endocrinologic workup consisting of total and free testosterone, prolactin, TSH, LH, and FSH. Clinical findings of headaches or visual field changes or findings of an elevated prolactin level necessitate an MRI of the sella turcica to evaluate for a potential macroadenoma of the pituitary.

Genetic Evaluation

In patients who present with azoospermia or severe oligospermia, where obstructive etiologies have been ruled out, evaluation of chromosome number and structure becomes important. A karyotype will rule out genetic conditions most commonly associated with infertility, including Klinefelter's syndrome (47, XXY), 46XX, 47XXY, and Noonan's syndrome. The chromosome structure of the Y chromosome should be assessed as well. This is done with the Y chromosome-linked microdeletion assay. Disruptions or deletions in various loci of the Y chromosome have been associated with severe defects in spermatogenesis. Early studies identified an area on the short arm of the Y chromosome critical for spermatogenesis referred to as the azoospermic factor (AZF) [56]. Subsequently, this has been divided into 3 regions: AZFa, AZFb, and AZFc [57]. Deletions in the regions of AZFa and AZFb are less common and usually associated with poor sperm retrieval rates for ART. AZFc microdeletions are the most commonly found microdeletion in azoospermic men and are associated with the most promising sperm retrieval rates [36]. Although Y chromosome microdeletions have no apparent impact on the health of the patient, the possibility of an inheritable form of infertility in male offspring via ART should prompt appropriate genetic counseling.

Expert Commentary

The purpose of this chapter was to delineate the evaluation of a man presenting with infertility with a focus on the laboratory evaluation. In the new era of the human genome project and with a better understanding of molecular biology and genetics, advances in both the diagnostic capabilities and the management options for male factor infertility are quickly advancing the field. In addition, enhancements in assisted reproductive technology are allowing many couples the opportunity to conceive when it would have been otherwise impossible. As conception is more reliant on laboratory technology, the laboratory evaluation of a man or couple presenting with infertility will remain of paramount importance.

Five-Year View

Conventional semen parameters continue to provide poor prognostic information regarding both frequency and quality of conception. Over the near term, marked research efforts will be dedicated to further elucidating sperm function. Emphasis will continue on the role of oxidative stress and sperm DNA fragmentation on subfertility. Novel research efforts in the field of metabolomics, metabolic profiling of semen, hold promise in elucidating the cause of heretofore idiopathic infertility.

Key Issues

- Infertility is the absence of conception after 12 months or regular unprotected intercourse, and male factor plays a role in up to 50% of cases.
- The initial clinical evaluation of male factor infertility should include a detailed and complete history and physical examination as well as a focused sexual history and genitourinary examination.
- Initial assessment should include a basic microscopic and macroscopic assessment of 2 separate semen analyses collected properly. Further testing should be based on the findings of the initial evaluation.
- New data on lower reference limits of semen parameters in fertile males suggests that there is a broader range of normal parameters than previously thought.
- Advanced semen testing should not be routine, but may be warranted based on the evaluation and includes antisperm antibody detection, assays of sperm DNA damage, and analysis of seminal oxidative stress and seminal antioxidant levels.
- Further testing with basic and extensive hormonal analysis as well as genetic testing may be warranted based on the initial evaluation.
- Reactive oxygen species derived from both intrinsic and extrinsic sources are being increasingly implicated in many cases of subfertility and infertility and have been shown to affect semen quality through several mechanisms including DNA fragmentation and lipid peroxidation. Antioxidant therapy as well as modification of exposures to extrinsic sources of ROS may have a role in the management of infertility.

Acknowledgments The authors would like to thank Eric Klein, MD, Chairman, Glickman Urological and Kidney Institute, Cleveland Clinic Foundation, for his support.

References

1. The optimal evaluation of the infertile male: American Urological Society Best Practice Statement. American Urological Society, Education and Research Inc. 2010.
2. Said TM, Agarwal A, Sharma RK, Thomas AJ, Sikka SC. Impact of sperm morphology on DNA damage caused by oxidative stress induced by beta-nicotinamide adenine dinucleotide phosphate. Fertil Steril. 2005;83:95–103.
3. Slama R, et al. Time to pregnancy and semen parameters: a cross-sectional study among fertile couples from four European cities. Hum Reprod. 2002;17(2):503–15.
4. Moskovtsev SI, Willis J, White J, Mullen JB. Leukocytospermia: relationship to sperm deoxyribonucleic acid integrity in patients evaluated for male factor infertility. Fertil Steril. 2007;88(3):737–40. Epub 6 Mar 2007.
5. Tomlinson MJ, Barratt CL, Cooke ID. Prospective study of leukocytes and leukocyte subpopulations in semen suggests they are not a cause of male infertility. Fertil Steril. 1993;60:1069–75.
6. Kolettis PN, Sabanegh ES. Significant medical pathology discovered during a male infertility evaluation. J Urol. 2001;166(1):178–80.
7. Franca LR, Avelar GF, Almeida FFL. Spermatogenesis and sperm transit through the epididymis with emphasis on pigs. Theriogenology. 2005;63:300–18.

8. Mortimer D, Leslie EE, Kelly RW, Templeton AA. Morphological selection of human spermatozoa in vivo and in vitro. J Reprod Fertil. 1982;64:391–9.
9. Clermont Y, Heller C. Spermatogenesis in man: an estimate of its duration. Science. 1963;140:184–5.
10. Wolff H. The biologic significance of white blood cells in semen. Fertil Steril. 1995 Jun;63(6):1143–57. Review.
11. Verma A, Kanwar KC. Effect of vitamin E on human sperm motility and lipid peroxidation in vitro. Asian J Androl. 1999;1(3):151–4.
12. Agarwal A, Deepinder F, Cocuzza M, Short RA, Evenson DP. Effect of vaginal lubricants on sperm motility and chromatin integrity: a prospective comparative study. Fertil Steril. 2008;89(2):375–9.
13. Kruger TF, Acosta AA, Simmons KF, et al. Predictive value of abnormal sperm morphology in in vitro fertilization. Fertil Steril. 1988;49:112–7.
14. Cendron M, Keating MA, Huff DS, et al. Cryptorchidism, orchiopexy and infertility: a critical long-term retrospective analysis. J Urol. 1989;142:559–62.
15. Charny CW. The spermatogenic potential of the undescended testis before and after treatment. J Urol. 1960;83:697.
16. Misell LM, Holochwost D, Boban D, et al. A stable isotope/mass spectrometric method for measuring the kinetics of human spermatogenesis in vivo. J Urol. 2006;175:242–6.
17. Carlsen E, et al. Effects of ejaculatory frequency and season on variations in semen quality. Fertil Steril. 2004;82(2):358–66.
18. Bjorndahl L, Kvist U. Sequence of ejaculation affects the spermatozoon as a carrier and its message. Reprod Biomed Online. 2003;7(4):440–8.
19. Cooper TG, Noonan E, von Eckardstein S, Auger J, et al. World Health Organization reference values for human semen characteristics. Hum Reprod Update. 2010;16(3):231–45.
20. Zini A, Blumenfield A, Libman J, Willis J. Beneficial effect of microsurgical varicocelectomy on human sperm DNA integrity. Hum Reprod. 2005;20:1018–21.
21. World Health Organization. World Health Organization: WHO Laboratory Manual for the Examination of Human Semen and Sperm-Cervical Mucus Interaction. 1999.
22. Jouannet P, Ducot B, Feneux D, Spira A. Male factors and the likelihood of pregnancy in infertile couples. I. Study of sperm characteristics. Int J Androl. 1988 Oct;11(5):379–94.
23. Spira A. Epidemiology of human reproduction. Hum Reprod. 1986;1:111–5.
24. Andersen AG, Jensen TK, Carlsen E, Jørgensen N, Andersson AM, Krarup T, Keiding N, Skakkebaek NE. High frequency of sub-optimal semen quality in an unselected population of young men. Hum Reprod. 2000 Feb;15(2):366–72.
25. Fedder J. Nonsperm cells in human semen: with special reference to seminal leukocytes and their possible influence on fertility. Arch Androl. 1996;36(1):41–65.
26. Sigma M, Jarow J. Male infertility. In: Wein AJ, Kavoussi LR, Novick AC, Partin AW, Peters CA, editors. Campbell-Walsh urology. 9th ed. Philadelphia: Saunders Elsevier; 2007.
27. Agarwal A, Saleh RA, Bedaiwy MA. Role of reactive oxygen species in the pathophysiology of human reproduction. Fertil Steril. 2003;79:829–43.
28. Zini A, Libman J. Sperm DNA damage: importance in the era of assisted reproduction. Curr Opin Urol. 2006;16(6):428–34.
29. Athayde KS, et al. Development of normal reference values for seminal reactive oxygen species and their correlation with leukocytes and semen parameters in a fertile population. J Androl. 2007;28(4):613–20.
30. Fredricsson B, Bjork G. Morphology of postcoital spermatozoa in the cervical secretion and its clinical significance. Fertil Steril. 1977;28:841–5.
31. Mosher WD, Pratt WF. Fecundity and infertility in the United States: incidence and trends. Fertil Steril. 1991;56:192.
32. Marks JL, McMahon R, Lipshultz LI. Predictive parameters of successful varicocele repair. J Urol. 1986;136:609–12.
33. Gandini L, Lombardo F, Paoli D, Caponecchia L, Familiari G, Verlengia C, Dondero F, Lenzi A. Study of apoptotic DNA fragmentation in human spermatozoa. Hum Reprod. 2000;15(4): 830–9.

34. Lee JD, Kamiguchi Y, Yanagimachi R. Analysis of chromosome constitution of human spermatozoa with normal and aberrant head morphologies after injection into mouse oocytes. Hum Reprod. 1996 Sep;11(9):1942–6.
35. Guzick DS, Overstreet JW, Factor-Litvak P, Brazil CK, Nakajima ST, Coutifaris C, Carson SA, Cisneros P, Steinkampf MP, Hill JA, Xu D, Vogel DL, National Cooperative Reproductive Medicine Network. Sperm morphology, motility, and concentration in fertile and infertile men. N Engl J Med. 2001;345(19):1388–93.
36. Oates RD, Silber S, Brown LG, Page DC. Clinical characterization of 42 oligospermic or azoospermic men with microdeletion of the AZFc region of the Y chromosome, and of 18 children conceived via ICSI. Hum Reprod. 2002;17(11):2813–24.
37. Agarwal A, Said TM. Role of sperm chromatin abnormalities and DNA damage in male infertility. Hum Reprod Update. 2003;9(4):331–45.
38. Sanocka D, et al. Male genital tract inflammation: The role of selected interleukins in regulation of pro-oxidant and antioxidant enzymatic substances in seminal plasma. J Androl. 2003;24:448–55.
39. Evenson DP, Wixon R. Clinical aspects of sperm DNA fragmentation detection and male infertility. Theriogenology. 2006;65:979–91.
40. Evenson DP, Larson KL, Jost LK. Sperm chromatin structure assay: Its clinical use for detecting sperm DNA fragmentation in male infertility and comparisons with other techniques. J Androl. 2002;23:25–43.
41. Li Z, Wang L, Cai J, Huang H. Correlation of sperm DNA damage with IVF and ICSI outcomes: a systematic review and meta-analysis. J Assist Reprod Genet. 2006;23(9–10):367–76. Epub 4 Oct 2006.
42. Griveau JF, Grizard G, Boucher D, Le Lannou D. Influence of oxygen tension on function of isolated spermatozoa from ejaculates of oligozoospermic patients and normozoospermic fertile donors. Hum Reprod. 1998;13(11):3108–13.
43. O'Flaherty C, de Lamirande E, Gagnon C. Positive role of reactive oxygen species in mammalian sperm capacitation: triggering and modulation of phosphorylation events. Free Radic Biol Med. 2006;41(4):528–40.
44. Camejo MI, Segnini A, Proverbio F. Intgerleukin-6 in seminal plasma of infertile men, and lipid peroxidation in their sperm. Arch Androl. 2001;47:97–101.
45. Martinez P, Proverbio F, Camejo MI. Sperm lipid peroxidation and pro-inflammatory cytokines. Asian J Androl. 2007;9:102–7.
46. Silver EW, et al. Effect of antioxidant intake on sperm chromatin stability in healthy non-smoking men. J Androl. 2005;26:550–6.
47. Keskes-Ammar L, Feki-Chakroun N, Rebai T, et al. Sperm oxidative stress and the effect of an oral vitamin E and selenium supplement on semen quality in infertile men. Arch Androl. 2003;49: 83–94.
48. Köksal IT, Tefekli A, Usta M, Erol H, Abbasoglu S, Kadioglu A. The role of reactive oxygen species in testicular dysfunction associated with varicocele. BJU Int. 2000 Sep;86(4):549–52.
49. Allamaneni SS, Naughton CK, Sharma RK, Thomas Jr AJ, Agarwal A. Increased seminal reactive oxygen species levels in patients with varicoceles correlate with varicocele grade but not with testis size. Fertil Steril. 2004;82(6):1684–6.
50. Mostafa T, et al. Varicocelectomy reduces reactive oxygen species levels and increases antioxidant activity of seminal plasma from infertile men with varicocele. Int J Androl. 2001;24:261–5.
51. Evers JLH, Collins JA. Assessment of efficacy of varicocele repair for male subfertility: A systematic review. Lancet. 2003;361: 1849–52.
52. Baker MA, Aitken RJ. Reactive oxygen species in spermatozoa: methods for monitoring and significance for the origins of genetic disease and infertility. Reprod Biol Endocrinol. 2005;3:67.
53. Report on optimal evaluation of the infertile male. AUA Best Practice Policy and ASRM Practice Committee Report, Volume 1, 2001. http://www.auanet.org. Accessed 20 Dec 2009.
54. Lipshultz LI, Corriere Jr JN. Progressive testicular atrophy in the varicocele patient. J Urol. 1977 Feb;117(2):175–6.

55. Turek PJ, Kim M, Gilbaugh 3rd JH, Lipshultz LI. The clinical characteristics of 82 patients with Sertoli cell-only testis histology. Fertil Steril. 1995;64(6):1197–200.
56. Tiepolo L, Zuffardi O. Localization of factors controlling spermatogenesis in the nonfluorescent portion of the human Y chromosome long arm. Hum Genet. 1976;34:119–24.
57. Vogt PH. Human chromosome deletions in Yq11, AZF candidate genes and male infertility: history and update. Mol Hum Reprod. 1998;4(8):739–44.
58. Lipshultz L. Subfertility. In: Kaufman JJ, editor. Current urologic therapy. Philadelphia: WB Saunders; 1980.
59. World Health Organization, Department of Reproductive Health and Research. WHO laboratory manual for the examination and processing of human semen. 5th ed. Geneva: World Health Organization; 2010.

Further Reading

Griveau JF, Renard P, Le Lannou D. Superoxide anion production by human spermatozoa as a part of the ionophore-induced acrosome reaction process. Int J Androl. 199;18(2):67–74.

Kefer JC, Agarwal A, Sabanegh EC. Role of antioxidants in the treatment of male infertility. Int J Urol. 2009;16:449–57.

Kutteh WH, Chao CH, Ritter JO, et al. Vaginal lubricants of the infertile couple: effect on sperm activity. Int J Fertil Menopausal Stud. 1996;41:400–4.

Lampiao F, du Plessis SS. TNF-alpha and IL-6 affect human sperm function by elevating nitric oxide production. Reprod Biomed Online. 2008;17(5):628–31.

Liu DY, Baker HW. Morphology of spermatozoa bound to the zona pellucida of human oocytes that failed to fertilize in vitro. J Reprod Fertil. 1992;94:71–84.

McLachlan RI, et al. Semen analysis: its place in modern reproductive medical practice. Pathology. 2003;35(1):25–33.

Munuce MJ, Berta CL, Pauluzzi F, Caille AM. Relationship between antisperm antibodies, sperm movement, and semen quality. Urol Int. 2000;65(4):200–3.

Sakkas D, Mariethoz E, Manicardi G, Bizzaro D, Bianchi PG, Bianchi U. Origin of DNA damage in ejaculated human spermatozoa. Rev Reprod. 1999;4(1):31–7.

Shekarriz M, Sharma RK, Thomas Jr AJ, Agarwal A. Positive myeloperoxidase staining (Endtz test) as an indicator of excessive reactive oxygen species formation in semen. J Assist Reprod Genet. 1995;12(2):70–4.

Simmons FA. Human infertility. New Engl J Med. 1956;255:1140.

Thonneau P, Marchand S, Tallec A, et al. Incidence and main causes of infertility in a resident population (1,850,000) of three French regions (1988–1989). Hum Reprod. 1991;6:811–6.

Tur-Kaspa I, Maor Y, Levran D, et al. How often should infertile men have intercourse to achieve conception? Fert Steril. 1994;62(2):370–5.

Wilcox AJ, Weinberg CR, Baird DD. Timing of sexual intercourse in relation to ovulation. Effects on the probability of conception, survival of the pregnancy, and sex of the baby. New Engl J Med. 1995;333(23):1517–21.

World Health Organization, Department of Reproductive Health and Research. WHO Laboratory Manual for the Examination and Processing of Human Semen. 5th ed. Geneva: World Health Organization; 2010.

Chapter 3
Imaging Modalities in the Diagnosis of Male Infertility

Marcello Cocuzza and Sijo J. Parekattil

Infertility affects approximately 15% of couples desiring conception, and male infertility underlies almost half of the cases. Assisted reproductive techniques (ART) are increasingly being used to overcome multiple sperm deficiencies and because of their effectiveness have been suggested by some to represent the treatment for all cases of male factor infertility regardless of etiology. Although the use of these technologies may allow infertile couples to achieve pregnancy rapidly, associated higher cost, potential safety issues, and the fear of transferring the unnecessary burden of invasive treatment on healthy female partners weigh down this treatment option heavily.

Diagnostic imaging techniques may be indicated as part of the complete male fertility evaluation. Productive therapy can be instituted only after completion of a thorough evaluation that begins with a detailed, direct history and physical examination. Due to the introduction and enhancement of newer imaging modalities, reliable adjuncts to clinical examination can be obtained to diagnose a variety of causes of male infertility including varicocele, epididymal blockage, testicular microlithiasis, seminal vesicle agenesis, and ejaculatory obstruction. Imaging plays a key role in the evaluation of the hypospermia or azoospermic man. It can detect correctable abnormalities, which can lead to a successful conception. It can also reveal potentially life-threatening disorders in the course of an infertility evaluation such as testicular tumors. The goal of this article is to provide the reader with a foundation for a comprehensive evaluation of the male partner as well as emerging technologies that can improve the treatment of correctable causes of male infertility.

M. Cocuzza, MD (✉)
Department of Urology, University of Sao Paulo (USP),
Ave. Dr. Eneas de Carvalho Aguiar, 255, 7 andar, Sala 710F, Sao Paulo, Brazil
e-mail: mcocuzza@uol.com.br

S.J. Parekattil, MD
Director of Urology, Winter Haven Hospital, University of Florida,
200 Avenue F. N.E., Winter Haven, FL 33881, USA
e-mail: sijo.parekattil@winterhavenhospital.org

S.J. Parekattil, A. Agarwal (eds.), *Male Infertility for the Clinician*,
© Springer Science+Business Media New York 2013

Testicular Tissue Imaging for Guided Sperm Retrieval

Doppler Duplex Flow Imaging

Testis biopsy with cryopreservation of sperm is a procedure performed in men with possible nonobstructive azoospermia (NOA), and at times, in men with a previous vasectomy (who do not want a reversal) and men with spinal cord injuries (who fail electro-ejaculation or vibratory ejaculation). Recent studies have illustrated that it is likely to find active spermatogenesis in areas with good blood supply within the testicle. These studies utilized detailed color Doppler ultraso-nography and needle guidance techniques to localize possible areas of spermatogenesis within the testicle. We have been exploring the efficacy of using a percutaneous handheld Doppler phase shift measurements of the testicle at the time of biopsy to localize areas of spermatogenesis.

A prospective blinded controlled trial of six patients who underwent testis biopsy from September 2008 to August 2009 for NOA (two men), previous vasectomy (two men), and spinal cord injury (two men) was performed. Percutaneous handheld Doppler (Vascular Technology™, Nashua, NH) blood flow shift measurements were taken from 12 different marked regions of one testicle (one testicle scanned on each patient—the larger testicle was chosen). The surgeon then obtained 12 biopsies from the same testicle in these marked regions (blinded to the Doppler analysis). The findings from the biopsies were then compared to the pre-biopsy Doppler phase shift mapping to assess if the Doppler readings had any predictive value in detecting spermatogenesis.

The Doppler phase shift readings were analyzed and an algorithm developed to identify areas of the testicle with specific flow patterns. These flow patterns were then analyzed to assess for any correlation with spermatogenesis. A predictive model optimized to identify areas of sperm production was then created. The model was 85% accurate (ROC 0.8, 95% CI 0.6–0.9) in identifying areas within the testicle that had sperm based on Doppler phase shift readings.

Our preliminary evaluation of handheld Doppler phase shift flow mapping of the testicle at the time of biopsy appears to have promise in detecting areas of spermatogenesis. However, further data analysis on more patients has now shown that the predictive value was not as high as we initially had expected, and so there is still more work that has to be done in this area before conclusions can be made about the use of this technology for this application.

MRI Spectral Imaging

Patients with idiopathic oligospermia or azoospermia, especially those with normal serum gonadotrophins and physical examination, always present a diagnostic dilemma. Both situations can represent a ductal obstruction or a testicular failure, but they have completely different prognoses. Testicular functions are currently evaluated in rather indirect ways, by seminal parameters and hormonal assays. Histo-logical analysis, which involves obtaining specimens by biopsies or surgical explorations, can directly evaluate testicular tissue. However, it cannot be widely used in clinical situations due to possible damage to testicular functions and its invasive character. Therefore, noninvasive techniques for evaluating testicular functions in vivo are needed [1].

Ultrasound is the initial radiological method that is used to evaluate the testis. However, the increased availability of magnetic resonance imaging (MRI) has allowed this noninvasive diagnostic tool to further evaluate testicular function. This technique was already used in a number of experimental studies on testis [1, 2]. On humans, there are few magnetic resonance spectroscopy (MRS) reports; one describes its application on a patient with testicular non-Hodgkin's lymphoma to monitor response to irradiation [3], and the other reveals the in vivo tissue characterization of the testis in patients with carcinoma in situ [4]. Also, differentiation between normal healthy testes and those with markedly decreased spermatogenesis presenting with oligospermia or azoospermia in whom spermatogenesis is completely absent was achieved [5, 6].

MRI spectroscopy is a noninvasive technique for obtaining metabolic information from living tissue based upon differences in the ratio of peaks of lipid and choline levels [7]. These metabolites may be used to evaluate the state of fertility and to investigate ischemia–reperfusion disorders.

More recently, in vivo hydrogen MR spectroscopy using stimulated echo acquisition mode measurements was performed with a short echo time, improving the detection of signals from low-molecular-weight metabolites including glutamate, choline, creatinine, and glycine not only in the normal state but also in diseased conditions such as ischemia [8]. In addition to these metabolites, a lactate signal could be observed in the ischemic testis. The presence of a lactate signal in the H spectra could be utilized to distinguish between normal and ischemic testes [8].

MR spectroscopy is a sensitive tool for assessment of testicular metabolic integrity and differentiation of normal testicles from those with markedly decreased spermatogenesis. MRS may improve sperm retrieval rates by better identifying isolated foci of spermatogenesis during testicular sperm retrieval in men presenting with nonobstructive azoospermia. MR spectroscopy of the testis might be a promising new modality that warrants further clinical studies to assess its diagnostic and therapeutic capability.

Testicular Artery Mapping During Varicocelectomy

Current data supports the statement that varicocele repair does indeed have a beneficial effect in reversing the harmful effects of varicocele upon testicular function in selected patients by improving seminal parameters in the majority of controlled studies [9]. A diversity of open surgical techniques has been used to repair this condition, including retroperitoneal, inguinal, and subinguinal. Recently, open

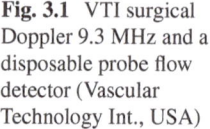 **Fig. 3.1** VTI surgical Doppler 9.3 MHz and a disposable probe flow detector (Vascular Technology Int., USA)

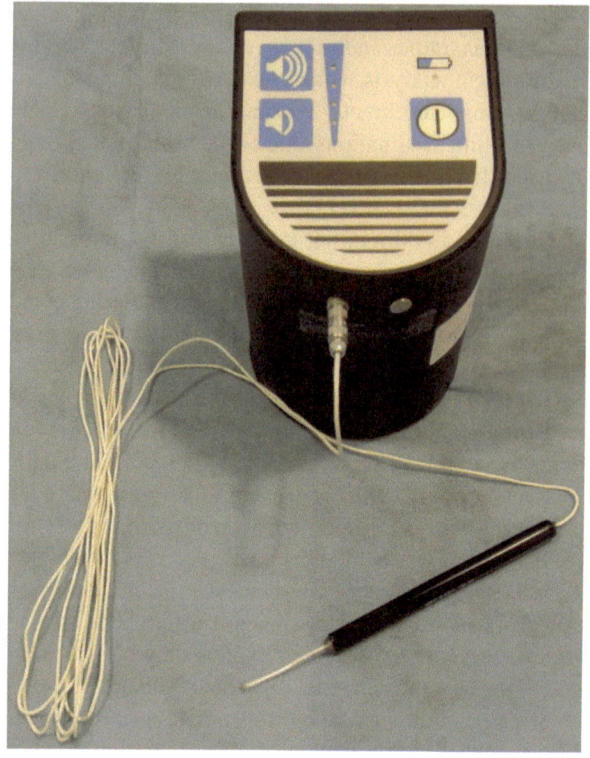

microsurgical inguinal or subinguinal varicocelectomy techniques have been shown to result in higher spontaneous pregnancy rates and fewer recurrences and postoperative complications than conventional varicocelectomy techniques in infertile men [10]. The subinguinal approach has the same principles as the inguinal approach but is performed through an incision below the external inguinal obviating to the need to open the aponeurosis of the external oblique causing less postoperative pain.

The microsurgical subinguinal varicocelectomy is the preferred approach for most experts. The use of an operating microscope allows the preservation of the testicular artery and lymphatics vessels, resulting in lower recurrence rates as well as hydrocele after the procedure [11]. On the other hand, the spermatic cord at the subinguinal level has a greater number of internal spermatic veins and an increased likelihood of encountering multiple spermatic arteries [12]. Previous studies reported that multiple spermatic arteries are identified in approximately 40% of the spermatic cords during microsurgical varicocelectomy at the subinguinal level [12, 13]. The recognition of the main spermatic artery can be confirmed by visualization of clear pulsatile movement and/or evidence of antegrade, pulsatile blood flow with gentle lifting and partial occlusion of the vessel. However, the identification of tiny secondary arteries is not at all times apparent, and a sterile intraoperative probe attached to a 9.3-MHz VTI surgical Doppler and a disposable probe flow detector (Vascular Technology Inc., USA) (Fig. 3.1) have been used at this point [14, 15].

Fig. 3.2 Using a vascular
Doppler probe to preserve all
testicular arterial branches
during varicocele repair

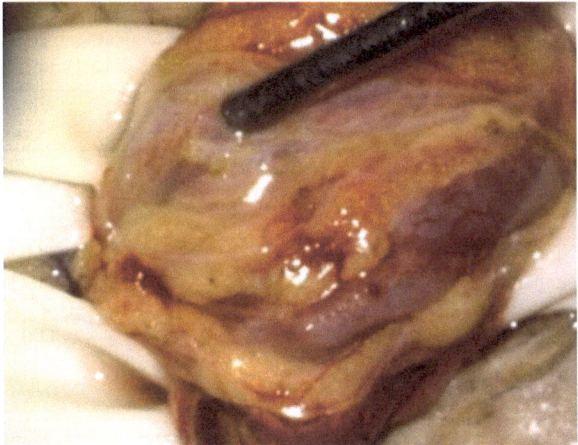

Consequently, it is possible that an inadvertent unrecognized ligation of a small
internal spermatic artery occurs more frequently than reported [16]. Following are
some of the reasons that could explain how the injury occurs: First, the size of the
arteries may be so small that the pulsation is difficult to identify. Second, aggressive
manipulation of the vessels during dissection can lead to spasm, making it difficult
to identify arterial pulsation. Third, the arteries tend to be in close proximity to or
buried under complex branches of veins [16]. In all these situations, the use of vascular Doppler may help to preserve the arterial branches (Fig. 3.2). Even though
there is no agreement about the necessity to preserve all testicular arterial branches
during varicocele surgery [17, 18], not doing so might be responsible for suboptimal
improvement in seminal parameters in some cases [19].

A recent study showed that concomitant use of intraoperative vascular Doppler
during subinguinal varicocelectomy allows a higher number of arterial branches to
be identified and therefore preserved [20]. Data concerning surgery using the
Doppler vascular device and without it show that a solitary artery is identified in
45.5% and 69.5% of cords, respectively, 2 arteries are identified in 43.5% and
28.5%, respectively, and 3 or more arteries are identified in 11% and 2%, respectively. Also, the authors reported that a higher number of internal spermatic veins
were ligated when Doppler was used (Table 3.1). The use of intraoperative Doppler
gives the surgeon more confidence during dissection of a dense complex of adherent veins surrounding the artery present in 95% of cases when the subinguinal
approach is used [12]. Accidental artery ligation documented by a pulsatile twitch-
ing of the ligated vessel stump under magnification is less common when Doppler
is applied [20].

The clinical implication of these findings can be supported by recent studies
showing that the total number of veins ligated was significantly positive correlated
with improvements in total sperm motility and sperm concentration [21, 22]. These
results suggest that ligating a larger number of veins should decrease reflux, which
in turn would lead to diminished insult to spermatogenesis.

Table 3.1 Intraoperative evaluation of internal spermatic veins ligated, number of lymphatic spared, and arteries preserved and injured in 377 spermatic cord dissections during microsurgical subinguinal varicocele repair with and without vascular Doppler

Variable	With Doppler (no. spermatic cords = 225)	Without Doppler (no. spermatic cords = 152)	P value
Number of veins ligated[a]	8.0 (3.1)	7.3 (2.8)	0.02
Number of arteries preserved[a]	1.6 (0.6)	1.3 (0.5)	<0.01
Number of arteries injured[b]	0	2 (1.1%)	0.06
Number of lymphatics spared[a]	2.2 (1.2)	2.0 (1.5)	0.21
Operative time unilateral repair (min)[a]	52.8 ± 17.8	53.0 ± 36.7	0.98
Operative time bilateral repair (min)[a]	101.0 ± 16.2	101.9 ± 16.3	0.37

[a]Values are mean and SD. Compared using student's unpaired t test
[b]Data presented as number (percentage) of patients. Compared using chi-square test. $P < 0.05$ was considered statistically significant
From Cocuzza et al. [20], with permission of Elsevier, Inc.

Management of Testicular Lesions in Infertile Patients

Organ-Sparing Microsurgical Resection of Testicular Tumors in Infertile Patients

Epidemiologic studies have given attention to a worldwide possible increase in testicular cancer incidence in the last two decades, particularly in industrialized developed countries [23]. One of the possible explanations for this augmented detection of testicular lesions is the widespread use of ultrasound as a screening method in all fields of medical practice, including scrotal ultrasonography in urology [24, 25].

In patients presenting with bilateral tumors (Fig. 3.3) or tumors in a solitary testis, the gold-standard procedure is to perform a radical orchiectomy which leads to permanent sterility, lifelong dependence on androgen replacement therapy, and psychological problems of castration at a young age [26]. As a result, organ-sparing surgery has been reported as a safe procedure in selected patients, especially for infertile men desiring to preserve their fertility [27–29]. The German Testicular Cancer Study Group established a guideline for organ-sparing surgery for testis tumors that includes cold ischemia during spermatic cord clamping, restriction of the procedure for organ-confined tumors of less than 20 mm that do not infiltrate the rete testis, performance of multiple biopsies of the tumor bed, and application of adjuvant local radiotherapy to eradicate carcinoma in situ and avoid local recurrence [29].

Testicular germ cell tumors are the most common type of malignancy during the reproductive age [30, 31]. However, as the majority of incidental testicular nonpalpable lesions with negative markers diagnosed in scrotal ultrasonography

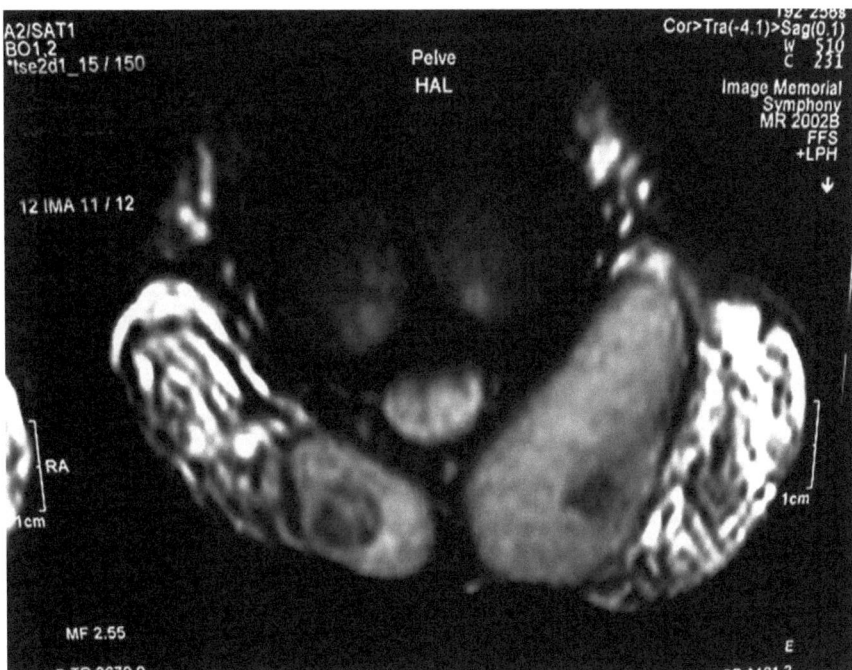

Fig. 3.3 Magnetic resonance showing a solid bilateral testicular lesion

performed during andrology investigation show a benign histology, surgical approach must be as conservative as possible for the testicular parenchyma [32]. In such cases, the most important step is the confirmation that frozen section analysis is an oncologically useful method for assessing small incidental testicular tumors when performed by an experienced pathologist [33]. The high degree of oncological efficiency achieved by the frozen section analysis during resection of testicular masses supports organ-sparing approaches that reduce the chances of facing difficult decisions intraoperatively [34].

Due to the advances of microsurgical techniques, partial orchiectomy was appointed as first-line therapy in infertile men even for nonpalpable small testicular lesions [27, 35, 36]. Also, infertile patient presenting with azoospermia and incidental testicular lesions now can experience the chance to father their own genetic offspring [37]. The combination of organ-sparing surgery, microdissection for TESE, cryopreservation, and assisted reproductive technologies represents a powerful tool to preserve fertility even for azoospermic men [38]. The complete procedure was meticulously described by Hallak et al. as follows [35]: During the procedure, the testis can be delivered through the inguinal incision, respecting principles for oncological procedures to avoid any potential spillage of tumor cells. Vas deferens must be carefully isolated from the spermatic cord and blood circulation interrupted by a delicate vascular clamp placed across the spermatic cord (Fig. 3.4). Slugged ice may be used to prevent warm ischemia and a temperature probe inserted far from the

Fig. 3.4 Blood circulation
was interrupted by a delicate
vascular clamp placed across
the spermatic cord after the
vas deferens was carefully
isolated

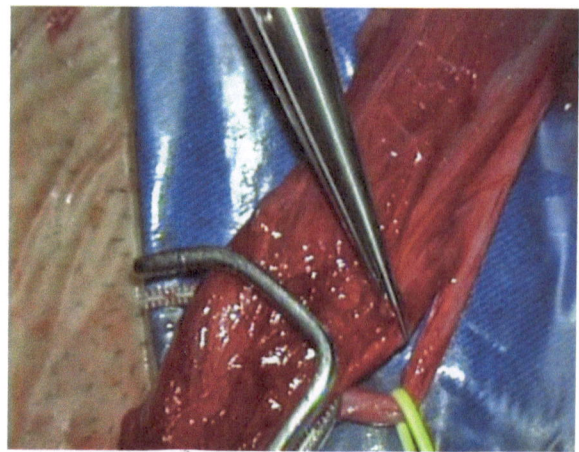

Fig. 3.5 Slugged ice
wrapped the testicle, thus
preventing from warm
ischemia

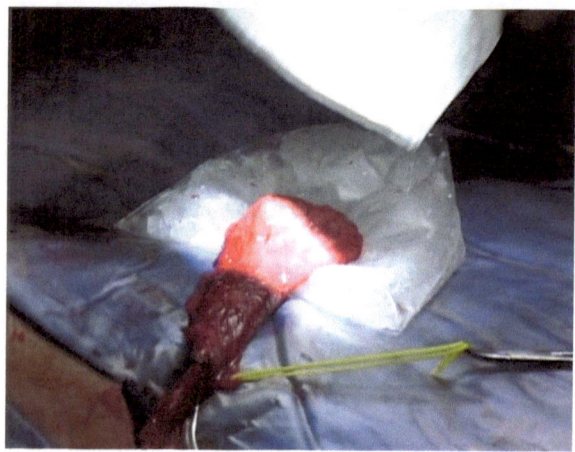

tumor location controls temperature at 12–15°C (Figs. 3.5 and 3.6). A linear ultrasound transducer at 15 MHz guides real-time intraoperative placement of a 30-gauge
10-cm-long stereotaxic hook-shaped needle (Guiding-Marker System; Hakko,
Tokyo, Japan) adjacent to the tumor to guide microsurgical resection (Figs. 3.7 and
3.8). Using a surgical operating microscope, the tumor can be gently dissected and
removed along with the adjoining parenchymal tissue (Fig. 3.9). Frozen section
studies must be performed, and if malignancy is confirmed, biopsies of the tumor
cavity margins and remaining parenchyma must be obtained to ensure absence of
residual tumors. After biopsies are sent for frozen section, the testicular parenchyma
must be meticulously microdissected for identification of functioning seminiferous
tubules, as reported by Schlegel [38]. After excision of selected enlarged and opaque
tubules, viable spermatozoa can be retrieved for cryopreservation in 80% of cases
[35]. This procedure integrates modern skills accumulated in the field of male

Fig. 3.6 A temperature probe was inserted far from the tumor location in the upper pole of the testicle

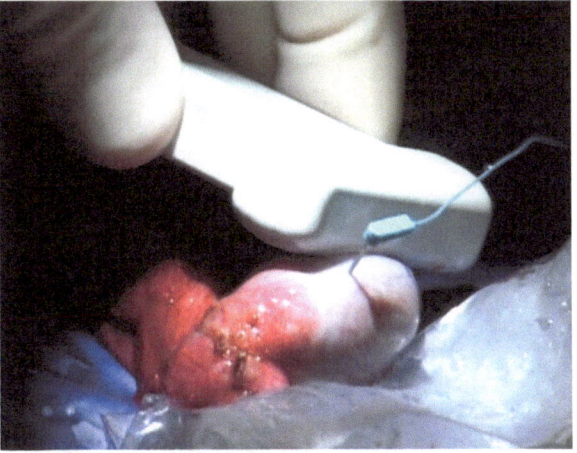

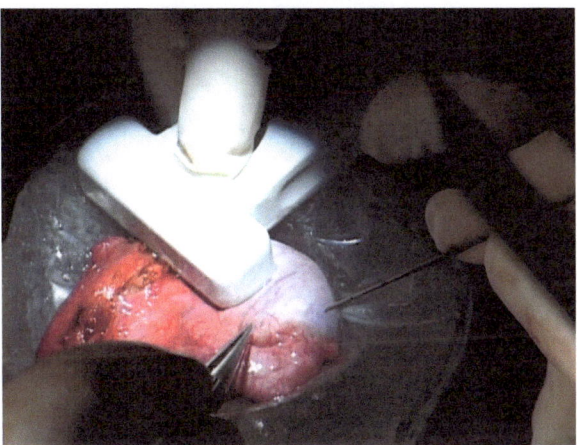

Fig. 3.7 A linear ultrasound transducer at 15-MHz guides real-time intraoperative placement of the stereotaxic hook-shaped needle adjacent to the nodule. The 30-gauge stereotaxic hook-shaped needle that permits the hook to be completely contained in and pass through the needle lumen. The introducing needle can thus be optimally positioned prior to engaging the hook. The hook is ejected and released from the needle tip reforming to hook and anchoring into the tissue adjacent to the tumor

infertility, combining knowledge in testicular vascular anatomy, oncology, micro-surgery, organ preservation, tissue preparation, and sperm cryopreservation.

The possibility of intracytoplasmic sperm injection with cryopreserved testicular sperm has given infertile azoospermic men the chance to have their own genetic offspring [37]. It is very important to keep in mind that this approach is only appropriate in centers experienced in managing testicular cancer for patients who want to preserve fertility.

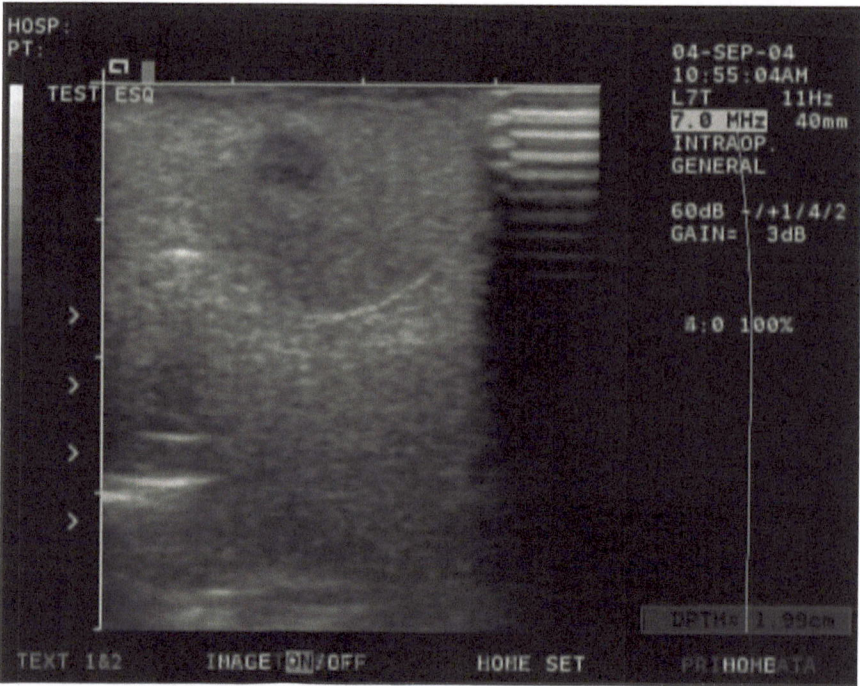

Fig. 3.8 Intraoperative ultrasound image showing a nonpalpable hypoechoic intratesticular lesion to guide real-time needle placement

Fig. 3.9 After the tunica albuginea is incised in an avascular region using an operating microscope, dissection respecting testicular lobules and arteries is conducted. Seminiferous tubules were separated carefully by blunt dissection following the needle until the lesion that is excised using micro-instruments is found, leaving 2–3-mm borders as safe margins around the nodule

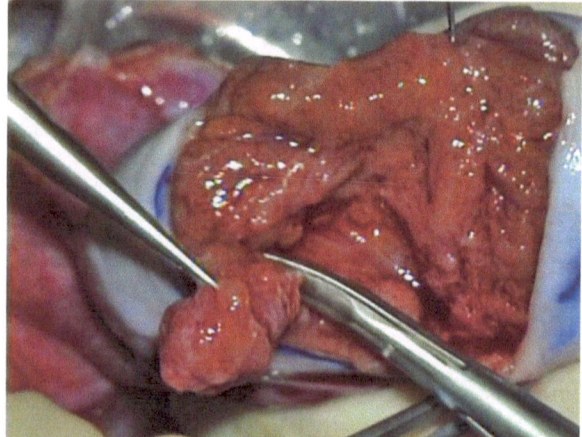

Testicular Microlithiasis

Testicular microlithiasis (TM) is an entity of unknown etiology that results in the formation of intratubular calcifications. TM is detected in 0.6% of adult males with clinical indications for scrotal ultrasonography [39]. Although TM is uncommon, it has been associated with several conditions such as Klinefelter's syndrome, cryptorchidism, varicocele, testicular atrophy, torsion, tumors, and infertility [40–43]. The mechanism by which microlithiasis affects spermatogenesis is unknown [43]. Scrotal ultrasound is diagnostic, and typically, there are small echogenic foci (1–3 mm).

The clinical significance of TM is debatable since inconsistencies exist in the literature. Therefore, there are conflicting recommendations regarding the appropriate interval and duration of subsequent surveillance of patients with testicular microlithiasis, as well as initial management strategies. It is of concern to the urologist due to its possible association with testis cancer [44]. Although commonly present in patients with germ cell tumors, there appears to be no definitive association with TM and cancer [45]. Therefore, follow-up at this time should be dictated based on risk factors for developing testis cancer more than on the presence of TM [46]. Casteren et al. suggested taking a testicular biopsy in a selected patient population with at least one additional risk factor for testicular germ cell tumors [47]. Similarly, there is no definitive proof that TM by itself can cause infertility. Probably, decrease seminal function is not directly due to the TM but rather to an underlying testicular abnormality or associated condition such as cryptorchidism [48].

Seminal Vesicle and Ejaculatory Duct Imaging

Turek et al. [49] recently presented a technique of transrectal vasodynamics (pressure-flow study of the seminal vesicle) to assess for partial ejaculatory duct obstruction (EDO). We have been exploring the use of a 3D transrectal ultrasound imaging and needle targeting system to perform vasodynamics for the treatment of necrospermia with partial EDO (Target Scan Touch, Envisioneering, St. Louis, MO).

A patient with necrospermia (viability staining of sperm) and low ejaculatory volume (<0.5 cc) was evaluated for EDO by vasodynamics performed utilizing a 3D transrectal ultrasound needle guidance system (Target Scan™, Envisioneering) in January 2008. This system was utilized to access and maintain a flexible needle within the seminal vesicle (SV) during vasodynamics. The decision to perform transurethral unroofing of the ejaculatory duct would be based on the pressure readings obtained during vasodynamics.

The patient had no visible left SV and a dilated right SV (>1.5 cm). The system provided an easy stable guided platform to place and maintain a flexible needle within the right SV. A pressure reading of 41 cm H_2O was achieved with delayed emptying of the right SV (on simultaneous cystoscopic examination of the ejaculatory ducts within the urethra). Transurethral (TUR) unroofing of the right ejaculatory duct was performed, and the post-TUR SV pressure reading dropped to 31 cm H_2O. The right SV drained promptly post-TUR on cystoscopic examination. Postoperatively, the patient initially had retrograde ejaculation. At 1 year post-op, the patient now has an ejaculate volume of 1 cc with 70 million sperm/hpf with 64% motility.

The use of a 3D transrectal ultrasound needle guidance system to perform vasodynamics is feasible for the treatment of patients with necrospermia and partial EDO, and it enhances a surgeon's ease in performing vasodynamics. Further testing and evaluation is needed.

Expert Commentary

In approximately half of infertility cases, a male factor is involved. Thus, identifying the pathology and treating the male may allow couples to regain fertility and conceive through natural intercourse. The goal of infertility management is to diagnose reversible causes of infertility and treat them to achieve seminal improvement and pregnancy. Despite advancements in the diagnostic workup of infertile men, up to 25% of patients exhibit abnormal semen analyses for which no etiology can be identified [50]. This condition is referred to as idiopathic male infertility, and non-specific treatments are usually applied that are based on theoretical concepts. A variety of empiric medical therapies have been recommended to treat these patients. However, the majority of these therapies have been shown to be effective in repeated controlled randomized studies. Even though the available assisted reproduction techniques can help overcome severe male factor infertility, the application of these methods in infertile couples classified as *idiopathic* infertility would definitely represent overtreatment.

We look toward the future with excitement and hope that the advanced technologies discussed will not only provide new treatment options but will reduce the number of couples without a definitive diagnosis of the cause of failure to conceive. There is no hesitation that all technical advances such as those explained in this chapter will drive the development of pioneering approaches to the management of the infertile male by andrologists. The use of imaging in the field of infertility is no longer just for diagnosis but also as part of the arsenal that provides more precise surgery procedures as described above.

Five-Year View

Numerous advances have been made in reproductive medicine in the last few years. Infertile couples who previously were considered untreatable now have a chance at genetic paternity. ART provide a great opportunity to families with infertility, and their use has become routine in the treatment of infertile couples. The increasing use of ICSI as an efficient therapy for cases of male infertility has become an applicable means to overcome multiple sperm deficiencies. Even men with potentially treatable causes of infertility can be treated with ART instead of a specific therapy.

The objective of this chapter was to discuss the potential role of imaging modalities in the management of male infertility. Collaborations with radiologists have provided a rich opportunity to explore and expand imaging techniques for intraoperative use during urologic surgery. Due to the continual improvement of a variety of imaging and tissue characterization modalities, the surgeons of tomorrow will have a number of tools at their disposal to improve intraoperative surgical decision-making. Only through the application of evidence-based assessment and evaluation, however, will there be a firm understanding of the true impact of these new technologies on the field of urology. However, further studies will be needed to confirm whether or not these techniques can evolve into widespread clinical practice.

As a result, the application of technological advances during varicocelectomy including optical magnification, microsurgery skills and vascular Doppler may offer patients maximal preservation of the arterial blood supply to the testes. However, additional research is needed to better clarify whether the use of Doppler during varicocelectomy is likely to improve testicular function and seminal parameters.

New methods for testicular screening, such as MRS, appear to be promising for testicular sperm extraction procedures. By identifying testicular locations that are likely to contain viable spermatozoa in the testes of nonobstructive azoospermic men, the potential for testicular damage may be reduced.

Key Issues

MR spectroscopy is a sensitive tool for assessment of testicular metabolic integrity and differentiation of normal testicles from those with markedly decreased spermatogenesis. MRS may improve sperm retrieval rates by better identifying isolated foci of spermatogenesis during testicular sperm extraction in men presenting with nonobstructive azoospermia. MR spectroscopy of the testis might be a promising new contribution that warrants further clinical studies to assess its full diagnostic and therapeutic capability.

Microsurgical technique remains the gold-standard procedure for the varicocele repair, but the concomitant use of intraoperative Doppler should be seriously considered as a tool to improve surgical outcome and safety.

Use of intraoperative vascular Doppler during microsurgical varicocelectomy allows a higher number of arterial branches to be preserved, and more internal spermatic veins are likely to be ligated.

Microsurgical organ-sparing testicular tumor resection associated with microdissection for TESE and tissue cryopreservation techniques may be considered an attractive option for infertile patients presenting with azoospermia and incidental testicular lesions, especially for those with solitary testicles and bilateral tumors. The technique described in the chapter in a precise manner can be easily reproduced by others.

Despite greater awareness of TM, a clear definition is currently missing, and the etiology is still obscure. This causes confusion in management and follow-up. There is no convincing evidence that TM alone is premalignant. However, when it accompanies other potentially premalignant features, we recommend annual ultrasound follow-up. With longer follow-up of patients with TM, its true likelihood of leading to cancer will be elucidated, and more evidence-based guidelines can be established.

Acknowledgments The authors are grateful to Ashok Agarwal, Cleveland Clinic, for his support and encouragement.

References

1. Sasagawa I, Nakada T, Kubota Y, Ishigooka M, Uchida K, Doi K. In vivo 31P magnetic resonance spectroscopy for evaluation of testicular function in cryptorchid rats. J Urol. 1995; 154(4):1557–9.
2. Srinivas M, Degaonkar M, Chandrasekharam VV, et al. Potential of MRI and 31P MRS in the evaluation of experimental testicular trauma. Urology. 2002;59(6):969–72.
3. Kiricuta IC, Bluemm RG, Ruhl J, Beyer HK. 31-P MR spectroscopy and MRI of a testicular non-Hodgkin lymphoma recurrence to monitor response to irradiation. A case report. Strahlenther Onkol. 1994;170(6):359–64.
4. Thomsen C, Jensen KE, Giwercman A, Kjaer L, Henriksen O, Skakkebaek NE. Magnetic resonance: in vivo tissue characterization of the testes in patients with carcinoma-in-situ of the testis and healthy subjects. Int J Androl. 1987;10(1):191–8.
5. Chew WM, Hricak H, McClure RD, Wendland MF. In vivo human testicular function assessed with P-31 MR spectroscopy. Radiology. 1990;177(3):743–7.
6. van der Grond J, Laven JS, te Velde ER, Mali WP. Abnormal testicular function: potential of P-31 MR spectroscopy in diagnosis. Radiology. 1991;179(2):433–6.
7. Navon G, Gogol E, Weissenberg R. Phosphorus-31 and proton NMR analysis of reproductive organs of male rats. Arch Androl. 1985;15(2–3):153–7.
8. Yamaguchi M, Mitsumori F, Watanabe H, Takaya N, Minami M. In vivo localized 1 H MR spectroscopy of rat testes: stimulated echo acquisition mode (STEAM) combined with short TI inversion recovery (STIR) improves the detection of metabolite signals. Magn Reson Med. 2006;55(4):749–54.
9. Agarwal A, Deepinder F, Cocuzza M, et al. Efficacy of varicocelectomy in improving semen parameters: new meta-analytical approach. Urology. 2007;70(3):532–8.
10. Cayan S, Shavakhabov S, Kadioglu A. Treatment of palpable varicocele in infertile men: a meta-analysis to define the best technique. J Androl. 2009;30(1):33–40.
11. Goldstein M, Gilbert BR, Dicker AP, Dwosh J, Gnecco C. Microsurgical inguinal varicocelectomy with delivery of the testis: an artery and lymphatic sparing technique. J Urol. 1992; 148(6):1808–11.
12. Hopps CV, Lemer ML, Schlegel PN, Goldstein M. Intraoperative varicocele anatomy: a microscopic study of the inguinal versus subinguinal approach. J Urol. 2003;170(6 Pt 1):2366–70.
13. Grober ED, O'Brien J, Jarvi KA, Zini A. Preservation of testicular arteries during subinguinal microsurgical varicocelectomy: clinical considerations. J Androl. 2004;25(5):740–3.
14. Minevich E, Wacksman J, Lewis AG, Sheldon CA. Inguinal microsurgical varicocelectomy in the adolescent: technique and preliminary results. J Urol. 1998;159(3):1022–4.
15. Wosnitzer M, Roth JA. Optical magnification and Doppler ultrasound probe for varicocelectomy. Urology. 1983;22(1):24–6.
16. Chan PT, Wright EJ, Goldstein M. Incidence and postoperative outcomes of accidental ligation of the testicular artery during microsurgical varicocelectomy. J Urol. 2005;173(2):482–4.
17. Matsuda T, Horii Y, Yoshida O. Should the testicular artery be preserved at varicocelectomy? J Urol. 1993;149(5 Pt 2):1357–60.

18. Student V, Zatura F, Scheinar J, Vrtal R, Vrana J. Testicle hemodynamics in patients after laparoscopic varicocelectomy evaluated using color Doppler sonography. Eur Urol. 1998;33(1):91–3.
19. Penn I, Mackie G, Halgrimson CG, Starzl TE. Testicular complications following renal transplantation. Ann Surg. 1972;176(6):697–9.
20. Cocuzza M, Pagani R, Coelho R, Srougi M, Hallak J. The systematic use of intraoperative vascular Doppler ultrasound during microsurgical subinguinal varicocelectomy improves precise identification and preservation of testicular blood supply. Fertil Steril. 2010;93(7):2396–9.
21. Belani JS, Yan Y, Naughton CK. Does varicocele grade predict vein number and size at microsurgical subinguinal repair? Urology. 2004;64(1):137–9.
22. Pasqualotto FF, Lucon AM, de Goes PM, et al. Relationship between the number of veins ligated in a varicocelectomy with testicular volume, hormonal levels and semen parameters outcome. J Assist Reprod Genet. 2005;22(6):245–9.
23. Huyghe E, Matsuda T, Thonneau P. Increasing incidence of testicular cancer worldwide: a review. J Urol. 2003;170(1):5–11.
24. Horstman WG, Haluszka MM, Burkhard TK. Management of testicular masses incidentally discovered by ultrasound. J Urol. 1994;151(5):1263–5.
25. Carmignani L, Gadda F, Mancini M, et al. Detection of testicular ultrasonographic lesions in severe male infertility. J Urol. 2004;172(3):1045–7.
26. Fossa SD, Opjordsmoen S, Haug E. Androgen replacement and quality of life in patients treated for bilateral testicular cancer. Eur J Cancer. 1999;35(8):1220–5.
27. Colpi GM, Carmignani L, Nerva F, Guido P, Gadda F, Castiglioni F. Testicular-sparing microsurgery for suspected testicular masses. BJU Int. 2005;96(1):67–9.
28. Yossepowitch O, Baniel J. Role of organ-sparing surgery in germ cell tumors of the testis. Urology. 2004;63(3):421–7.
29. Heidenreich A, Weissbach L, Holtl W, et al. Organ sparing surgery for malignant germ cell tumor of the testis. J Urol. 2001;166(6):2161–5.
30. Bokemeyer C, Schmoll HJ, Schoffski P, Harstrick A, Bading M, Poliwoda H. Bilateral testicular tumours: prevalence and clinical implications. Eur J Cancer. 1993;29A(6):874–6.
31. Coleman MP, Esteve J, Damiecki P, Arslan A, Renard H. Trends in cancer incidence and mortality. IARC Sci Publ. 1993;121:1–806.
32. Carmignani L, Gadda F, Gazzano G, et al. High incidence of benign testicular neoplasms diagnosed by ultrasound. J Urol. 2003;170(5):1783–6.
33. Leroy X, Rigot JM, Aubert S, Ballereau C, Gosselin B. Value of frozen section examination for the management of nonpalpable incidental testicular tumors. Eur Urol. 2003;44(4):458–60.
34. Steiner H, Holtl L, Maneschg C, et al. Frozen section analysis-guided organ-sparing approach in testicular tumors: technique, feasibility, and long-term results. Urology. 2003;62(3):508–13.
35. Hallak J, Cocuzza M, Sarkis AS, Athayde KS, Cerri GG, Srougi M. Organ-sparing microsurgical resection of incidental testicular tumors plus microdissection for sperm extraction and cryopreservation in azoospermic patients: surgical aspects and technical refinements. Urology. 2009;73(4):887–91. discussion 891–82.
36. Binsaleh S, Sircar K, Chan PT. Feasibility of simultaneous testicular microdissection for sperm retrieval and ipsilateral testicular tumor resection in azoospermic men. J Androl. 2004;25(6):867–71.
37. Oates RD, Mulhall J, Burgess C, Cunningham D, Carson R. Fertilization and pregnancy using intentionally cryopreserved testicular tissue as the sperm source for intracytoplasmic sperm injection in 10 men with non-obstructive azoospermia. Hum Reprod. 1997;12(4):734–9.
38. Schlegel PN. Testicular sperm extraction: microdissection improves sperm yield with minimal tissue excision. Hum Reprod. 1999;14(1):131–5.

60   M. Cocuzza and S.J. Parekattil

39. Hobarth K, Susani M, Szabo N, Kratzik C. Incidence of testicular microlithiasis. Urology. 1992;40(5):464–7.
40. Ganem JP, Workman KR, Shaban SF. Testicular microlithiasis is associated with testicular pathology. Urology. 1999;53(1):209–13.
41. Aizenstein RI, DiDomenico D, Wilbur AC, O'Neil HK. Testicular microlithiasis: association with male infertility. J Clin Ultrasound. 1998;26(4):195–8.
42. Vrachliotis TG, Neal DE. Unilateral testicular microlithiasis associated with a seminoma. J Clin Ultrasound. 1997;25(9):505–7.
43. Qublan HS, Al-Okoor K, Al-Ghoweri AS, Abu-Qamar A. Sonographic spectrum of scrotal abnormalities in infertile men. J Clin Ultrasound. 2007;35(8):437–41.
44. Ringdahl E, Claybrook K, Teague JL, Northrup M. Testicular microlithiasis and its relation to testicular cancer on ultrasound findings of symptomatic men. J Urol. 2004;172(5 Pt 1): 1904–6.
45. Rashid HH, Cos LR, Weinberg E, Messing EM. Testicular microlithiasis: a review and its association with testicular cancer. Urol Oncol. 2004;22(4):285–9.
46. Dagash H, Mackinnon EA. Testicular microlithiasis: what does it mean clinically? BJU Int. 2007;99(1):157–60.
47. van Casteren NJ, Looijenga LH, Dohle GR. Testicular microlithiasis and carcinoma in situ overview and proposed clinical guideline. Int J Androl. 2009;32(4):279–87.
48. Miller RL, Wissman R, White S, Ragosin R. Testicular microlithiasis: a benign condition with a malignant association. J Clin Ultrasound. 1996;24(4):197–202.
49. Eisenberg ML, Walsh TJ, Garcia MM, Shinohara K, Turek PJ. Ejaculatory duct manometry in normal men and in patients with ejaculatory duct obstruction. J Urol. 2008;180(1):255–60. discussion 260.
50. Greenberg SH, Lipshultz LI, Wein AJ. Experience with 425 subfertile male patients. J Urol. 1978;119(4):507–10.

Chapter 4
Genetic Aspects of Male Infertility

Orhan Bukulmez

Genetic abnormalities may account for 15–30% of male factor infertility [1]. Genes and genomic regulation involved in male genital tract development, gonadal development, and function including those related to spermatogenesis may be involved with male infertility. Although many of the genetic factors are still to be elucidated and many of the predicted genetic perturbations are yet to find their place for clinical applications, it is essential to appraise the current information on genetic basis of male reproductive system disorders.

Genomic Regulation of Male Sexual Development

The gender-specific development simply relies on whether testes or ovaries form in the embryo from paired omnipotent structures known as genital ridges. Male developmental pathway depends on the presence and correct function of a male-determining gene from Y chromosome called *Sry* (sex-determining region Y) which functions in a specific set of genital ridge cells to stimulate them to differentiate as Sertoli cells, which are the cells that interact with and nurture the germ cells. Sertoli cells play a role in orchestrating the differentiation of other cell types required for testis formation such as germ cells and steroid hormone-producing cells [2]. In the absence of *Sry* function, the developmental pathway proceeds to female differentiation, although in reality the sexual development is more complex involving multiple networks of molecular signals and fragility of these pathways are reflected to the

O. Bukulmez, MD
Division of Reproductive Endocrinology and Infertility, Department of Obstetrics and Gynecology, University of Texas Southwestern Medical Center, 5323 Harry Hines Boulevard, Dallas, TX 75390-9032, USA
e-mail: orhan.bukulmez@utsouthwestern.edu, obukulmez@obgyn.ufl.edu

S.J. Parekattil, A. Agarwal (eds.), *Male Infertility for the Clinician,*
© Springer Science+Business Media New York 2013

fact that disorders of sexual development are among the most common birth defects. These disorders range from hypospadias to complete sexual ambiguity and sex reversal which are often associated with infertility.

Testicular Development

Early formation of indifferent genital ridges is a requirement before testicular development. Studies in mice have shown that several transcription factor genes are required for this process. These genes include empty spiracles homologue 2 (Emx2), GATA-binding protein-4 (GATA4), Lim homeobox protein 9 (Lhx9), steroidogenic factor 1 (SF-1/NR5A1), dosage-sensitive sex reversal, adrenal hypoplasia critical region, X chromosome, gene 1 (DAX-1/Nr0b1), and Wilms' tumor 1 (WT-1) [3–8]. WT-1 and SF-1 are crucial for formation of genital ridges in humans. Furthermore, they are both important in sex-specific gonadal development [9, 10]. DAX-1 levels and expression thresholds on the other hand are important for male versus female functional development [8].

Timely expression of *Sry* is important for testicular development [11]. Spatially dynamic *Sry* expression begins in waves within the genital ridge, peaks for a short time, and then declines as demonstrated in mice [12, 13]. The mechanism of this specific and tight regulation of *Sry* regulation remains elusive. Decreased expression of *Sry* was noted in the presence of splice variant mutants of WT-1, GATA4, friend of GATA (FOG2), and insulin receptor family [14, 15]. Delayed expression of *Sry* has been implicated in XY sex reversals, unilateral or bilateral ovotestes, to delayed testis formation [16, 17]. It is thought that *Sry* expression must reach a certain threshold within a specific temporal window of competence in the precursors of supporting cells for proper testicular development. *Sry* encodes for a nuclear high-mobility group (HMG) domain protein that binds and bends DNA.

Downstream of *Sry*, other factors such as SRY-box containing gene 9 (SOX9), SOX8, DAX-1, and fibroblast growth factor 9 (FGF9) have important roles in Sertoli cell differentiation and function [2]. SOX9 is considered as an early acting and essential component of male development pathway.

Peritubular myoid cells of testis are necessary for testicular cord development and integrity. Differentiation of these cells correlates with Sertoli cell-specific secretion of desert hedgehog (DHH). DHH receptor patched (PTC) is expressed on peritubular myoid cells and Leydig cells. It has been demonstrated that null mutation of DHH in mice leads to impaired differentiation of peritubular myoid cells and Leydig cells leading to feminized males [18, 19]. DHH mutations in humans lead to partial or pure XY gonadal dysgenesis accompanied by impaired cord formation and decreased testosterone levels [20, 21].

Fetal Leydig cell development is essential for male sexual differentiation. The candidate genes important in Leydig cell differentiation include aristaless-related homeobox gene (ARX), α-thalassemia/mental retardation syndrome, X-linked (ATRX) and platelet-derived growth factors (PDGFs), and their receptor PDGFRA [22–24].

Primordial germ cells migrate from their origin at the posterior part of the embryo through hindgut to populate genital ridges where they interact with somatic cells to form primitive sex cords. Germ-cell migration is facilitated by interferon-induced transmembrane proteins 1 and 3 (IFITM1 and IFITM3) [25]. Stromal cell-derived factor 1 (SDF1) and its receptor CXCR4 function in the colonization of genital ridges [26].

Testicular Descent

Testicular descent occurs in two phases. Transabdominal phase of testicular descent happens at 8–15 weeks of gestation in humans and controlled by insulin-like 3 (INSL3) hormone produced by Leydig cells, acting via its receptor LGR8 (also known as GREAT) [27]. Inguinoscrotal phase is usually completed by 35th week of gestation and is facilitated by the neurotransmitter calcitonin gene-related peptide (CGRP or CALCA) released by genitofemoral nerve under the influence of androgens. Mutations in genes involved with androgen signaling and those encode transcription factors homeobox A10 (HOXA10), HOXA11, and developmentally and sexually retarded with transient immune abnormalities (DESRT) lead to second-stage arrest in testicular descent [28].

Spermatogenesis

There are many genes and molecules involved in spermatogenesis. For instance, the number of sperm-specific membrane proteins alone has been estimated to be greater than 200 [29]. Through the use of cDNA microarrays in humans, over 100 genes seem to be involved in the regulation of spermatogenesis [30]. One study showed that of 1,652 genes whose expression increased with onset of meiosis, 351 of them were expressed only in the male germ line [31]. There are many genes involved in DNA condensation, sperm maturation, adhesion, and motility as well. The genes and proteins involved with male germ cells and spermatogenesis have been reviewed extensively [32]. This review presents 178 genes associated with spermatogonia, spermatocytes, and Sertoli cells [32]. These genes are located on both autosomal and sex chromosomes.

In patients with azoospermia, deleted regions on Yq has attracted clinical attention. Deleted in azoospermia (DAZ) gene on Y chromosome belongs to a family of three members: DAZ, BOULE, and DAZ-like. Their proteins contain a highly conserved RNA-binding motif [33]. DAZ proteins bind to RNAs and may be involved in posttranscriptional regulation of mRNA expression [34]. The DAZ gene family is expressed exclusively in germ cells.

Many forms of partial deletions occur on Y chromosome in some male infertility cases [35]. These infertility-related deletions are not considered to be inherited [36], and most infertile males do not show any mutations or deletions on the Yq. Majority of genes involved with spermatogenesis are actually located on autosomal chromosomes [32, 37]. For instance, mutations in protamine (PRM) and transition protein (TPN) genes involved with histone to protamine replacement located on autosomes have been found in 1/200–1/300 of male infertility cases in Japan [37].

As shown in mice, X chromosome is also enriched for spermatogenic genes functioning both in premeiotic and in postmeiotic germ cells [38]. In human, the examples of genes in X chromosome important in spermatogenesis include structural maintenance of chromosomes 1A (component of meiotic cohesion complex, SMC1A) on Xp11.22–p11.21 and testis-expressed 11 (binding protein expressed only in male germ cells, TEX11) on Xq13.1. The X chromosome seems to play more important role in the premeiotic stages of mammalian spermatogenesis.

Male Genital Tract Development

The Wolffian (mesonephric) ducts (WDs) lead to mature male genital tract. Urogenital sinus contributes to the genital tract by developing prostate. In XY embryo, Mullerian ducts degenerate in an active process facilitated by anti-Mullerian hormone (AMH) which is secreted by Sertoli cells. AMH binds to its receptor AMHR2 on the surface of Mullerian duct mesenchymal cells inducing secretion of matrix metalloproteinase 2 (MMP2) leading to apoptosis of Mullerian duct epithelial cells [39]. Failure of this process in humans results in persistent Mullerian duct syndrome (PMDS), an autosomal recessive condition which can lead to male infertility [40, 41].

Wolffian ducts differentiate under the influence of testosterone into epididymis, vas deferens, and seminal vesicle [42]. Mice lacking androgen receptor (AR) show agenesis of epididymis, vas deferens, and seminal vesicles. Bone morphogenic protein 4 (BMP4), BMP7, BMP8, HOXA10, and HOXA11 genes play important roles in epididymis development. Fibroblast growth factor 10 (FGF10) and growth and differentiation factor 7 (GDF7) are essential in proper development of seminal vesicles [2].

Male External Genitalia Development

Male external genitalia largely depends on the expression of 5α-reductase in the genital tubercle mesenchyme-converting testosterone to 5α-dihydrotestosterone (DHT) which is the most potent ligand for AR. Mutations of 5α-reductase result in abnormalities in male external genitalia and prostate development.

Complete androgen insensitivity syndrome due to X-linked AR gene mutation leads to XY sex reversal, but partial forms may present with various phenotypes ranging from ambiguous genitalia to male infertility. Other mediators important in male external genitalia include cell surface molecules like ephrins and their receptors (Ephs), Wnts, FGFs, BMPs, noggin, and Hox genes [2, 43]. Urethral fusion defects lead to hypospadias. HOXA13 and HOXD13 gene mutations reported in hand-foot-genital syndrome suggest that these genes are important in pathogenesis of hypospadias [44].

Genetic Defects Associated with Male Infertility

Numerical and Structural Chromosomal Abnormalities

Infertile men have an eight- to tenfold higher prevalence of chromosomal abnormalities than fertile men [45]. Chromosomal abnormalities can be detected in about 5% of infertile men, and the same frequency in azoospermic men was estimated to at 15% [1]. In a review of studies involving 9,766 azoospermic and severely oligospermic men, sex and autosomal chromosomal anomalies were found in 4.2% and 1.5% of infertile men, as compared with 0.14% and 0.25%, respectively, in control population [46]. It should also be noted that 0.37% of sperm donors with normal sperm parameters have been reported to have chromosomal translocations [47].

Aneuploidy is the most common error resulting from chromosomal anomalies in infertile men [48]. Although many autosomal and sex chromosomes can be involved, most common of those are Klinefelter syndrome, XYY syndrome, XX male syndrome, mixed gonadal dysgenesis, autosomal translocations, and Y-chromosome microdeletions. Especially, men with nonobstructive azoospermia present with high incidence of aneuploidy of up to 13.7% being predominantly numerical or structural defects [49]. In men with oligospermia, a 4.6% prevalence of autosomal translocations and inversions was reported [50]. Sex chromosomal aneuploidy may account for approximately two-thirds of chromosomal abnormalities observed in infertile men [51].

Klinefelter Syndrome

Klinefelter syndrome is seen in about 1 in 500 male live deliveries and is the most common known genetic cause of azoospermia accounting for up to 14% of all cases [52]. It results from X-chromosomal aneuploidy in which 90% of cases carry an extra X chromosome (47, XXY) and 10% are mosaics as 47XXY/46XY. In about half of the Klinefelter syndrome cases, extra X chromosome is paternally derived. The classic triad associated with the syndrome includes small and firm testes, azoospermia, and gynecomastia. It is also associated with eunuchoid body habitus with increased height, low intelligence quotation scores, varicosities, obesity, diabetes, increased incidence of extragonadal germ-cell tumors, leukemia, and breast cancer. There is high phenotypic variation, and many patients may not demonstrate these classic findings. The only invariant finding of non-mosaic form is that of small testes volume of 2–4 ml. The laboratory findings include severe oligospermia or azoospermia and low testosterone levels with increased LH and FSH. Testicular histopathology is consistent with seminiferous tubular sclerosis and hyalinization and sometimes Sertoli cell only. In some cases, remarkable small islands of spermatogenesis can be observed creating opportunity to obtain testicular sperm [53, 54].

Mosaic forms of the syndrome are associated with spontaneous fertility. Testicular sperm extraction (TESE) with intracytoplasmic sperm injection (ICSI) has been successful in achieving successful pregnancies in non-mosaic forms. The success with TESE in those cases ranges from 27% to 69% [54, 55]. Interestingly, 80–100% of mature sperm obtained from 47XXY patients show normal haploid sex chromosome with either X or Y [56, 57]. This may be either due to somatic germ line mosaicism or abnormal germ cells that simply do not develop due to meiotic arrest. Nevertheless, the rates of aneuploid sperm, although low in absolute terms, are increased in men with Klinefelter syndrome as is the prevalence of aneuploid embryos (both sex and autosomal) making genetic and preimplantation genetic diagnosis (PGD) counseling an important component of management [58–60].

XYY Syndrome

This syndrome is seen in 1/1,000 live male births. Phenotypic characteristics include increased height, decreased intelligence, higher risk of some malignancies like leukemia, and aggressive or antisocial behavior [52]. XYY syndrome is associated with severe oligospermia or azoospermia with elevated FSH but normal testosterone and LH levels. Testis biopsies were found consistent with maturation arrest or Sertoli cell only. Although, as similar to Klinefelter syndrome, majority of the sperm obtained from these patients show normal haploid sex chromosomes, higher rates of both sex and autosomal chromosomal imbalances have been reported in 47XYY men [61, 62].

XX Male Syndrome

Its main characteristics are gynecomastia at puberty and azoospermia. It is less frequent than Klinefelter or XYY syndromes with a frequency of 1 in 20,000 live male births. Patients usually show elevated FSH and LH levels with low testosterone. Testicular histology shows absent spermatogenesis with hyalinization of seminiferous tubules, fibrosis, and Leydig cell clumping [52]. It is thought that the translocation of *Sry* to X chromosome results in testes development; however, there is no spermatogenesis since Yq is totally lacking [63]. Since there is no spermatogenesis, any surgical or medical treatment will not be successful for fertility purposes. These patients may require testosterone treatment for hypogonadism.

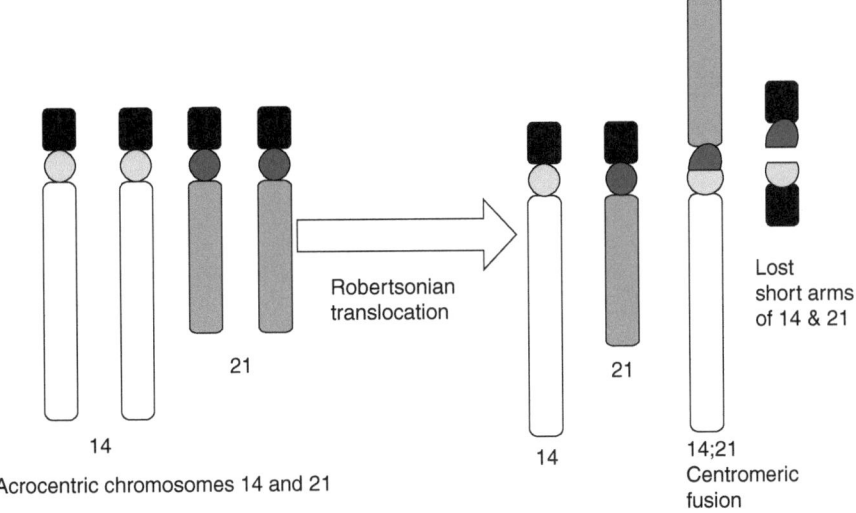

Fig. 4.1 A Robertsonian translocation involves centromeric fusion of the long arms of the acrocentric chromosomes, while the short arms are lost

Mixed Gonadal Dysgenesis

This is a rare condition with male or female phenotype usually with a unilateral testis and a contralateral streak gonad. Patients may have ambiguous genitalia and abdominal testes showing Sertoli cell only. The gonads are predisposed to malignant germ-cell tumors and need to be removed prior to puberty. The karyotype may be 45X/46XY or 46XY. The mutations of Sry have not been detected in majority of the cases with some suspect genes downstream to *Sry* [52].

Translocations and Inversions

Translocations or inversions of autosomal chromosomes can be detected in 1 in 600 to 1 in 1,000 live deliveries. Exchanges between chromosomes may interrupt important genes at the break point or may interfere with normal chromosomal pairing during meiosis. Robertsonian translocations involving chromosomes 13, 14, 15, 21, and 22 and reciprocal translocations are at least eightfold more common in infertile men [52].

Robertsonian translocations occur when two acrocentric chromosomes fuse with loss of the short arm material, hence the chromosome number will be 45. They are the most common chromosomal abnormalities in humans seen in 0.1% of newborns. Most commonly, they involve chromosomes 13;14 and 14;21 (Fig. 4.1). Robertsonian translocations may be seen in 1.5% of oligospermic and 0.2% of azoospermic men [1, 64, 65]. Furthermore, carriers of Robertsonian translocations are at risk of pregnancies with miscarriages or birth defects. Interestingly, within some families, fertility is unaffected despite the same apparent translocation of t(13;14)

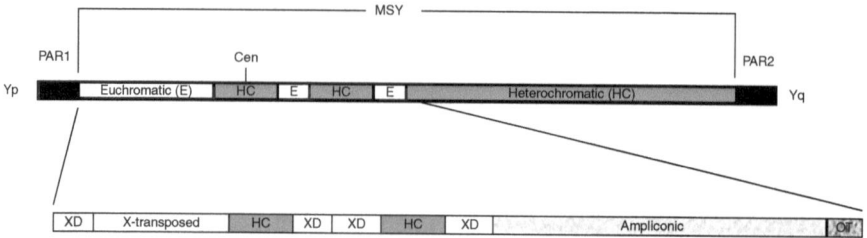

Fig. 4.2 Y chromosome: MSY, Yq, Yp, centromere (Cen), pseudoautosomal (PAR1 and PAR2), and heterochromatic (HC) regions followed by the enlarged view of euchromatic (E) region extending from boundary between PAR1 and Yp to the heterochromatic region of Yq. *XD* X-degenerate, *OT* other (From Li et al. [72], with permission)

(q10;q10) [47]. Of those sperm produced, most have a normal balanced chromosomal complement, but an unbalanced karyotype can be present in 4–40% of sperm [66, 67]. Therefore, there is increased risk of trisomies or uniparental disomy. Since the carriers of Robertsonian translocations may pass translocation of imbalanced chromosomal abnormalities to the offspring, genetic counseling and PGD is recommended if sperm from ejaculate or testis is used for ICSI.

Reciprocal translocations are due to the exchange of material between autosomes or between the X or Y chromosome and an autosome and occur in 0.7% of severely oligospermic or azoospermic men [68]. The chromosomal number is normal, and the chromosomes and the break points may be unique to that particular family involved. Depending on the chromosomal material lost, the phenotype may vary. When the sperm is produced, more than 50% are chromosomally unbalanced [66, 69], making genetic counseling even more important.

Chromosomal inversions may involve the centromere (pericentric) or a peripheral segment of the chromosome (paracentric). Although many inversions are harmless, they may have pathological implications according to the chromosome and the site involved. For example, inversion of chromosome 9 is more frequently observed in infertile men. Due to formation of abnormal loops during chromosomal pairing, chromosomal unbalance can occur effecting spermatogenesis or the resulting embryo [66, 70].

Y Chromosome

The human Y chromosome is 60 megabases (Mb) in length with the least number of genes but the highest copy number of the repetitive sequences as compared to autosomal chromosomes [71]. About 104 coding genes encode about 48 proteins. Among these proteins, 16 proteins have been discovered in the azoospermia factor (AZF) region [72]. The much smaller pseudoautosomal regions (PAR1 2.6 Mb and PAR2 320 bp) (Fig. 4.2) which pair with X chromosome during meiosis are located at both ends of the Y chromosome. The region outside of PARs previously known as the non-recombining region of Y chromosome (NRY) is now called male-specific

Y (MSY) which compromises of 95% of the chromosome's length. It has also been shown that MSY may also be somewhat involved in X–Y crossing-over during male meiosis while MSY is flanked on both sides by PARs [73]. But again, the vast majority of the Y chromosome, including MSY, is less recombining and transmitted as a single block from generation to generation with functional variants and neutral polymorphisms being linked [72].

MSY is made up of a combination of three classes of gene-rich euchromatic (X-transposed, X-degenerate, and ampliconic) and heterochromatic sequences (Fig. 4.2). MSY encodes about 27 proteins, and within MSY, the X-transposed sequences which only encode for two genes (3.4 Mb) are 99% identical to the DNA sequences in Xq21 [72]. X-degenerate sequences are surviving relics of ancient autosomes and encode 16 proteins of MSY. Amplicons which encode nine proteins are sequence of nucleotides that are nearly identical large repeats reading in the same (direct) or opposite (inverted) directions. Genes in ampliconic segments may be replicated by recombination between the repetitive sequences. Most Y-chromosome genes expressed in the testes are located in the ampliconic regions. The Yp (Yp11) and the proximal part of the Yq (Yq11 subdivided into Yq11.1, 11.21, 11.22, 11.23) consist of euchromatin, while the distal part of Yq is made up of heterochromatin which is one-half to two-thirds of the Yq (Yq12) [73, 74] (see Fig. 4.2). Loci identified in Y chromosome are thought to be involved in the production and differentiation of the sperm since microdeletions of these loci are associated with severe oligospermia or nonobstructive azoospermia. Accordingly, seven deletion intervals were described both on Yp and Yq [75].

Male infertility affects 1 in 20 men, and primary spermatogenic failure accounts for about 50% of the cases [72]. Yq microdeletions were detected in 5–15% of males with spermatogenic failure. More specifically, these deletions occur in 6–8% of severely azoospermic men and in 3–15% of azoospermic men [76]. These deletions include the total Yq12 heterochromatin block and the part of Yq at Yq11.23. Consequently, it was suggested that at least one genetic Y factor essential for spermatogenesis is located in the distal Yq11 called as azoospermia factor (AZF), although about 6% of severe oligospermia cases occur with deletions outside the AZF region [74].

AZF Region

AZF region on Yq is most thoroughly studied male fertility locus in humans [77]. AZF region is further divided into three regions defined as AZFa, AZFb, and AZFc [78] (Fig. 4.3). While AZFa region is truly separate and distinct, the AZFb and AZFc regions actually overlap one another and are simply different stretches of Yq within one much longer, encompassing expanse [79]. It is thought that AZF microdeletions result from intrachromosomal recombination events between homologous repetitive sequence blocks in Yq11 [79]. As there is no counterpart in the genome for mitotic pairing and meiotic recombination of the MSY, this repetitive palindromic sequence structure might have evolved to protect the long-term genetic integrity of Y chromosome by allowing MSY to pair with and to repair itself. However, on rare occasions, this nonallelic homologous recombination may go wrong when two spatially separate

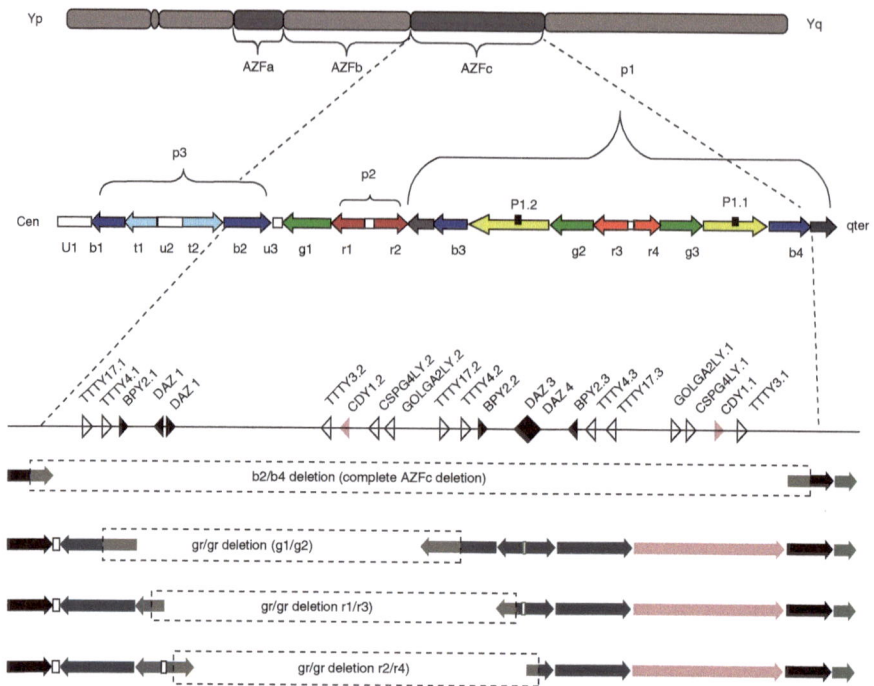

Fig. 4.3 AZFc is compromised of distinct families of nearly identical amplicons. Amplicon b, g, u, r, and t have 4, 3, 3, 4, and 2 repeats, respectively, in the haplotype. Palindromes are indicated as P1, P2, and P3. Repetitive sequences are direct repeats and inverted repeats as the direction of the *arrows* show. AZFc contains 12 families of transcription units which are all expressed in testis such as BPY2, DAZ, CDY1, and others. AZFc microdeletion subtypes include complete deletion b2/b4 and partial deletion g1/g2, r1/r3, and r2/r4 (From Li et al. [72], with permission)

ampliconic regions permanently stick together during Y-chromosome replication, resulting in loss of all chromosomal material in the intervening portion. In some cases, this may occur due to the deficiency of enzymes necessary for DNA repair. P8–P1 represents eight palindromes ordered nearest to farthest from the centromere within the euchromatic region of Yq. P5–P1 region is statistically more prone to nonallelic homologous recombination due to its unique molecular structure [80].

- AZFa: AZFa microdeletion is responsible for azoospermia in 1% of males with nonobstructive azoospermia. AZFa region is not palindromic, 792 kb in length, and is located in proximal Yq. AZFa region's candidate genes include USP9Y (ubiquitin-specific protease 9, Y chromosome), or DFFRY (Drosophila fat facets-related Y), DBY (DEAD box on the Y), and UTY (ubiquitous TPR motif on the Y) [78, 81–84]. USPY9 occupies less than half of the AZFa interval and is mostly involved with microdeletions. However, minority of patients may have a de novo point mutation in this region [83, 85]. DBY consists of 17 exons and encodes for a putative ATP-dependent RNA helicase that shuttles between nucleus and cytoplasm whose specific function in spermatogenesis remains elusive. In AZFa deletions, most frequent presentation is Sertoli cell-only syndrome (SCO). In SCO I cases, there are no germ cells in the seminiferous tubules. In SCO II associated with partial AZFa deletion, some germ cells with incomplete differentiation and maturation and degeneration can be seen.

- AZFb: An AZFb microdeletion is 6.2 Mb long and begins in P5 palindrome and ends in the proximal portion of P1, hence the name P5/proximal P1 microdeletion. The so-called AZFb/AZFc microdeletion is also named as P5/distal P1 microdeletion since it also starts in P5 but spans a larger area of 7.7 Mb and ends in distal P1. AZFb or AZFb/AZFc microdeletions are observed in 1–2% of males with nonobstructive azoospermia. AZFb candidate genes include EIF1AY (translation-initiation factor 1A, Y isoforms) and RBMY (RNA-binding motif on the Y). For the former, no deletion specifically removing EIF1AY has been reported. Complete AZFb deletions are associated with maturation arrest at the primary spermatocyte or spermatid stages.

- AZFc: AZFc region stretches from the distal portion of the P3 palindrome to the distal portion of P1 and is 3.5 Mb in length (Fig. 4.3). Initially, it was believed that AZFb and AZFc were non-overlapping areas, but subsequent studies demonstrated that both the AZFb and AZFb/AZFc regions overlap AZFc region. AZFc microdeletion is also called as b2/b4 (Fig. 4.3) since it occurs when nonallelic homologous recombination happens between the b2 and b4 amplicons in P3–P1 with loss of all intervening material [79]. AZFc microdeletions are the most common microdeletions found in men with nonobstructive azoospermia, occurring in up to 13% of cases with azoospermia and 6% of men with severe oligospermia. Deleted in azoospermia (DAZ) cluster is the primary candidate gene in the AZFc region. Several other genes in addition to DAZ were mapped in this region including CDY1 (chromodomain Y1), BPY2 (basic protein Y2), PRY (PTA-BL related Y), and TTY2 (testis transcript Y2). AZFc deletions are associated with a wide range of conditions from azoospermia to mild to severe oligospermia. This is reflected in testicular histology being consistent with hypospermatogenesis or SCO II in which there is a better chance of finding focal areas of spermatogenesis.

Among all cases with Yq microdeletions, deletions involving DAZ seem to be the most frequent one. Some reports suggest that DAZ deletions may be encountered up to 13% of cases of male infertility [77]. DAZ was thought to be acquired by Y chromosome from an autosomal homologue DAZL (DAZ-like) on chromosome 3p24 which shows a single DAZ repeat. DAZ gene cluster on Y chromosome consists of seven copies of DAZ of which four copies are located relatively close together within a deletion interval on Yq11. DAZ encodes an RNA-binding protein exclusively expressed in early germ cells and is thought to be responsible for activation of silent mRNAs during pre-meiosis stages. It was reported that AZFc may not be critical for meiotic recombination, whereas absence of AZFc regions results in extension of the zygotene stage and reduction of chromosomal condensation [86]. Although most deletions involve all four DAZ genes, an absence of only two is also associated with defective spermatogenesis [33].

Some other partial microdeletions detected in AZFc region such as b2/b3, b1/
b3, and gr/gr do not seem to have any clinical significance, although race-specific
various phenotypic outcomes were reported [87, 88]. Actually, microdeletions of
the AZFc may present with spermatogenic failure in Dutch, Spanish, Chinese, and
Italians. However, the presence of AZFc deletion in healthy French, Germans, and
Han Chinese questions its importance in male infertility [89, 90]. A partial AZFc
microdeletion such as gr/gr can be passed from father to son, but again, its clinical
significance is still debated [91, 92]. Whereas frequent deletion of DAZ gene cluster in male infertility cases suggests its importance in spermatogenesis, the variable penetration of AZFc deletions in general suggests some functional
redundancies in its function. Perhaps microdeletion is not an independent event but
is compensated by the activation of other genes by gene replication or dosage com-
pensation [72].

Yq Microdeletions in Clinical Practice

In infertile men with nonobstructive azoospermia or severe oligospermia, it is critical that the patients know the results of Y-chromosomal microdeletion analysis
before TESE and ICSI. Briefly, complete AZFa, AZFb, and AZFb/AZFc microdeletions predict that TESE will be unsuccessful since sperm will not be found and
presently there is no available treatment [93]. Men with Y-chromosomal microdeletions rarely have a sperm density above five million per milliliter. Although vast
majority of AZFc microdeletions are de novo which means that the father of the
patient is not affected, rare cases of natural transmission were also reported [79].
    As noted above, it is thought that finding of ejaculated sperm in complete AZFa
and AZFb deletions is highly unusual [35]. Combined deletions of two or more
regions that include AZFb are associated with SCO or maturation arrest histology.
Patients with AZFc deletions have the best prognosis for finding testicular sperm
during TESE. Many reports suggest that 50–60% of azoospermic AZFc-deleted
men will have testicular sperm enough for ICSI [35]. In patients with complete
AZFa or AZFb microdeletions, the probability of finding sperm during TESE
attempts is extremely low if not impossible. Successful TESE is often not possible
in cases with deletions involving one or more regions that include AZFa or AZFb
as well.
    Small studies are not clear for the outcome of ICSI when testicular sperm is used
in men with AZF deletions. Some reported normal fertilization rates but poorer
embryo quality as compared to those without AZF deletion and other demonstrated
comparable fertilization and pregnancy rates [52]. There is also evidence that men
harboring AZFc microdeletions may show time-dependent decline in sperm production. Therefore, counseling patients for sperm cryopreservation for future use is
essential.
    Men with AZF deletions who conceive via assisted reproduction are likely to
pass on the Yq deletion to male offspring [94, 95]. However, the children conceived
by testicular sperm seem to be somatically healthy, and their AZFc deletion has not

been shown to be altered, although it is expected that male offspring will suffer from similar deficiencies of spermatogenesis.

Since microdeletions cannot be detected by conventional cytogenetic methods, Yq analysis is performed on peripheral blood lymphocytes via polymerase chain reaction (PCR) where various center-specific primers were used to amplify sequence-tagged sites (STSs) of DNA which makes evaluation of data challenging. By PCR amplification of STSs which are specific to each of the AZF regions under review, deletions are identified by the absence of one or more ampliconic products. This multiplex PCR is restricted to the analysis of a set number of loci and cannot detect novel Yq microdeletions or mutations. To minimize such limitations of PCR, other genomic techniques such as array comparative genomic hybridization has been proposed although the cost of this technology limits its introduction to clinical medicine [96]. Difficulties in reporting may occur due to the fact that euchromatic Yq consists of large, nearly identical amplicon repeats and palindromes, and furthermore, the description of microdeleted regions has not always correlated with known gene deletions. It is also possible that some cases may show mosaicism when comparing to Yq deletions in leukocytes to sperm [97].

Other Y-Chromosome Conditions

Massive palindromes in the human Y chromosome harbor mirror-image gene pairs essential for spermatogenesis. These gene pairs have been maintained by intrapalindrome, arm-to-arm recombination. Isodicentric Y (idicY) chromosomes may be formed by homologous crossing-over between the opposing arms of palindromes in sister chromatids. This event is usually associated in mosaic event with 45X cell line giving a karyotype of 45X/46XidicY. These patients retain two Yps and two SRYs although the latter may not be functional due to mitotic instability leading to female phenotype. In cases with male phenotype, the end result would be azoospermia possibly due to Yq segment loss at break points [98]. It remains elusive if successful TESE and ICSI with PGD can be performed in these cases.

Short arm of Y chromosome also harbors genes related to spermatogenesis. TSPY gene is one of these genes with copies on Yq as well [99]. A study of copy number variation of TSPY demonstrated that more copies were found in infertile men [100].

X Chromosome

Many X-chromosome genes influence male infertility. From rodent studies, it was suggested that X chromosome may play an important role in premeiotic stages of mammalian spermatogenesis [101]. Deletions, translocations, and inversions of X chromosome may result in severe infertility and azoospermia [102–104]. For example, paracentric inversion involving Xq12–25 or deletion of a portion of Xp may result in a phenotype consistent with Klinefelter syndrome. Several X-linked gene mutations were reported in infertile men with oligospermia or azoospermia. These genes include SOX3 (sex-determining region Y box 3), FATE, and ZFX [105–108].

Androgen receptor (AR) gene is located on Xq11–12. Knockout mice studies have suggested that AR signaling in Sertoli cells plays an important role in meiosis I during spermatogenesis [109]. Lack of AR in Leydig cells may lead to spermatogenic arrest at the round spermatid stage [110]. The functional AR in germ cells however was not found to be essential in spermatogenesis [111]. Therefore, androgens control spermatogenesis, but germ cells themselves do not express a functional AR. Androgen regulation is thought to be mediated by Sertoli and peritubular myoid cells. Studies in mice with selective AR knockout in Sertoli cells have suggested that AR plays an important role in meiosis and progression of spermatocytes to round spermatids [112]. While complete AR gene mutations are associated with androgen insensitivity syndrome with a female phenotype, incomplete forms of AR gene mutations were detected in more frequently in infertile men [113].

X-linked spinal and bulbar muscular atrophy or Kennedy's disease is caused by expansion of a CAG repeat in the first exon of AR gene. The CAG repeat encodes a polyglutamine tract in AR protein. The greater the expansion of the CAG repeat, the greater the polyglutamine repeat expansion and the earlier the disease onset and the more severe the disease manifestations [114]. Glutamine repeat motif in the first exon of AR gene (polyQ region) is polymorphic in general population numbering between 10 and 36 repeats. In Kennedy's disease, polyQ region is expanded between 40 and 62 repeats [114].

The CAG repeat expansion mutation in AR gene does not affect sexual differentiation. The repeat expansion likely causes a toxic accumulation of mutated AR in nuclei and cytoplasm of motor neurons, resulting in their degeneration and loss [115]. Patients present with amyotrophic, proximal, or distal weakness and wasting of the facial, bulbar (dysphagia and dysarthria), and limb muscles; occasionally sensory disturbances; and endocrinologic disturbances, such as androgen resistance, gynecomastia, elevated testosterone, and reduced fertility, due to defects in spermatogenesis and testicular atrophy. The onset of neurological symptoms is between the ages of 30 and 50 years. In parallel to those observations, CAG repeat polymorphism has been investigated as possible as a possible cause for male infertility [116]. However, it is still controversial if longer or shorter CAG repeats are associated with higher or lower sperm quality [117–119].

USP26 (Xq26.2) and TAF7L (Xq22.1) genes are expressed in testis, and single-nucleotide polymorphisms (SNPs) for both genes were investigated for potential association with male factor infertility [120, 121]. Although some studies have suggested potential associations between these SNPs and abnormal spermatogenesis, since the effects of SNPs are largely influenced by ethnicity, the precise roles of these findings in relation to male infertility remain elusive [122–124].

X-linked forms of Kallmann syndrome are related to the deletions in KAL-1 gene located in the short arm of X chromosome (Xp22.32). This gene codes for a cell adhesion protein, anosmin-1, which is involved in the migration of gonadotropin-releasing hormone (GnRH) neurons during embryonic development. The condition is associated with hypogonadotropic hypogonadism with sexual infantilism due to

Table 4.1 Clinical detection of CFTR mutation-related CBAVD

Azoospermia
Low seminal fluid volume (<2.0 ml)
Biochemical features of the semen: pH < 7.2, absent or decreased fructose, and α1–4 glucosidase (markers of properly functioning seminal vesicles and epididymis, respectively)
Absence of palpable vas deferens
On transrectal ultrasound: absence of the intra-abdominal tract of the vas deferens, globus major, and different degrees of hypoplasia of the seminal vesicles
Normal plasma follicle-stimulating hormone (FSH), luteinizing hormone (LH), and testosterone levels
Normal karyotype
Normal testicular size

From Dequeker et al. [134], with permission

the deficiency of GnRH, anosmia, or hyposmia due to the absence or hypoplasia of olfactory bulbs and tracts, cognitive and ocular abnormalities, and even with mid-facial clefts and renal agenesis [125]. While X-linked KAL-1 mutations are responsible for 30–70% of the condition, the remaining cases are related to the deletions in fibroblast growth factor receptor 1 (FGFR1) gene on chromosome 8 which shows autosomal-dominant inheritance [126]. With treatment, favorable reproductive outcomes can be attained in addition to maturation of secondary sex characteristics.

Congenital Bilateral Absence of the Vas Deferens and Cystic Fibrosis

Congenital bilateral absence of the vas deferens (CBAVD) is estimated to occur in 1/1,000 to 1:10,000 and may be encountered in 1–2% of cases with male infertility. It is detected in 9.6% of cases with obstructive azoospermia [127]. It is thought to result from abnormal development of WD although it is not clear if absence of vas deferens is always congenital. Absence of distal WD derivates has been related to the early obstruction of these ducts by viscous secretions rather than an embryonic developmental defect. Approximately 80% of CBAVD cases are caused by mutations on both alleles of the cystic fibrosis transmembrane conductance regulator (CFTR) gene. CBAVD is usually associated with absence of body and tail of epididymis, vas deferens, and seminal vesicles, but the head of epididymis is intact (Table 4.1).

Given the fact that almost all CF male patients are infertile due to CBAVD, it was investigated if CFTR was also involved in infertility because of CBAVD alone. In an earlier small study, it was reported that 41% of azoospermic men with CBAVD was found to be heterozygous for F508del CFTR mutation as compared to the population risk of 2.8% [128]. Later, R117H mutation was also found at a higher frequency in CBAVD cases [129]. In more recent large study, analyzing 7,420 alleles

Table 4.2 Cystic fibrosis detection and carrier rates before and after testing

Ethnic group	Detection rate (%)	Carrier rate before testing	Carrier risk after negative test result
Ashkenazi Jewish	94	1/24	1/400
Non-Hispanic Caucasian	88	1/25	1/208
Hispanic American	72	1/46	1/164
African American	65	1/65	1/186
Asian American	49	1/94	1/184

Modified from American College of Obstetricians and Gynecologists [138], with permission of Lippincott Williams & Wilkins

of CFTR gene showed that a CFTR mutation can be identified in 78.9% of patients with CBAVD. In French men with CBAVD, about 71% of the CBAVD patients had a mutation on both CFTR genes and about 16% had a mutation on one CFTR genes and the remaining 13% of CBAVD patients had no mutation [130].

In 20% of CBAVD patients, the absence of vas deferens is associated with renal malformations [131]. Although a minority of CBAVD patients may have a mild lung disease or a positive sweat test, most CBAVD patients do not have lung disease. It is possible that a mild mutant of CFTR protein with partial chloride channel activity can sustain a normal non-diseased phenotype except for proper functioning and maintenance of vas deferens after its development [132].

The CFTR gene spans about 190 kb and contains 27 exons (chromosome 7q31). The CFTR protein is a glycosylated transmembrane protein which functions as a chloride channel. In the CFTR gene, currently 1,719 sequence variations have been reported in populations with various geographic location and ethnicity (http://www.genet.sickkids.on.ca/cftr/StatisticsPage.html) [133]. These are found in both CF and related phenotypes called as CFTR-related disorders (CFTR-RD). These are clinical disorders with CFTR dysfunction where the diagnosis of CF cannot be established. These entities include CBAVD, disseminated bronchiectasis, chronic pancreatitis, and chronic rhinosinusitis [134]. As CF is inherited in a recessive way, CF will develop when deleterious mutations are found on both CFTR alleles. If the mutation is only on one allele, the individual is a CF carrier. 1 in 2,500 newborns have CF, and 1 in 25 Caucasians is a CF carrier [132] (Table 4.2).

More than 1,200 CF-causing CFTR mutations have been identified. A CF patient may carry two identical or different mutations; the latter condition is called compound heterozygosity for two CFTR mutations. Most mutations are point mutations. The distribution of these mutations varies according to ethnicity. The most common mutation F508del is seen in 70% of Northern European populations, but it is seen in lower frequencies in Southern Europeans [132]. About 1–5% of mutations remain undetermined in CF patients and even more in patients with atypical presentations. Frequency of undetected mutations increases from Northern to Southern European populations [134]. Undetected mutations may lie within the introns or regulatory regions which are not routinely analyzed. Besides F508del, other mutations exist in most populations each reaching frequencies of about 1–2% such as

G5542X, G551D, R553X, W1282X, and N1303K. Therefore, in most populations, these mutations and some ethnic-specific mutations compromise 85–95% of all CFTR mutations. The remaining mutations are rare and sometimes can be found in a single family or particular population. Depending on the effect at protein level which predicts the severity of the clinical condition, CF mutations are divided in several arbitrary classes [132]. One large study reported that CF patients had two severe mutations (88%) or one severe and one mild/variable mutation (12%), whereas CBAVD men had either a severe and a mild/variable (88%) or two mild/variable (12%) mutations [130].

Most commercial genetic tests for CFTR mutations screen only for the most frequent CF-causing mutations and not the milder mutations, therefore resulting in a CFTR mutation detection rate of only about 60% in CBAVD patients [130]. The most common CFTR mutation presenting with a mild phenotype found in CBAVD patients is the 5T polymorphism (variant) [135].

The 5T splicing variant of the intron 8 acceptor splice site is not considered a CF-causing mutation, but it may be associated with CFTR-RD [134]. At the polypyrimidine tract of intron 8 acceptor splice site, the variants are named according to the number of thymidines as 5T, 7T, and 9T. The lower the number, the lower the efficiency of exon 9 splicing. The extent of splicing is further related to the number of adjacent TG repeats; the higher the number of TGs, the lower the efficiency of splicing. Patients with (TG)13/5T in trans with a CF-causing mutation may have mild CF. R117H CFTR-RD mutation can be found in cis with 5T or 7T. R117H;5T is considered a mild CF mutation, but R117H;7T is considered as a CFTR-RD mutation. If R117H;5T is trans with a F508del severe CF mutation, the signs of CF may be present. The presence of R117H;7T in the same configuration have been shown to be symptom-free [136].

When 5T is found in compound heterozygosity with a severe CFTR mutation, or even with another 5T, CBAVD can be observed. However, not all men compound heterozygous for a severe CFTR mutation and 5T develop CBAVD, such as fathers of some CF children [132]. Hence, 5T polymorphism is a mutation with partial penetrance. Again, the R117H mutation can either result in CF or CBAVD by being associated by either 5T or 7T allele [137]. Its association with 7T allele may result in CBAVD, and R117H;5T may result in CF. F508del mutation is found at a higher frequency in CF patients as compared with those with CBAVD, while R117H is more frequently observed in patients with CBAVD.

Initial CF screening guidelines included 25 pan-ethnic mutations that were present in at least 0.1% of patients with CF. The commercially automated methodology uses PCR with allele-specific oligonucleotide primers. After evaluation of the data, two mutations 1078delT and I148T were removed from the panel since they were not increasing the sensitivity for CF carrier state or diagnosis [138]. Some screening panels may identify 5T, 7T, and 9T variants, although they are not offered in routine CF carrier screening. As detailed above, the presence of 5T allele may decrease mRNA stability affecting exon 9 [70]. Since CF may occur when 5T is on the same chromosome (cis) with R117H missense mutation along with a CFTR mutation on the other chromosome, reflex 5T testing is done if R117H is detected in the screening panel.

Since males with 5T allele on both chromosomes are at increased risk for CBAVD, 5T testing should be ordered in CBAVD cases. CBAVD patients with two 5T variants and female with a R117H mutation with 5T variant in cis position need genetic counseling to discuss the risk of having an offspring with CF. It should always be remembered that the primary goal of universal CF screening test is to detect CF not CBAVD, with a reasonable sensitivity. Therefore, at times, complete analysis of CFTR gene by DNA sequencing may be necessary in patients with CF and in patients with CBAVD, tested negative with commercial CFTR screening test results.

Spermatozoa of CBAVD patients used in an ICSI program may transmit CFTR mutation to the offspring. Most CBAVD patients may carry a severe CF-causing CFTR mutation with 50% chance of transmitting that mutation. If the carrier risk of a Caucasian female is 1/25 (0.04), with herself having a 50% chance of transmitting the gene to the offspring, the risk of having a child with CF would be 1 in 100 ($0.5 \times 0.04 \times 0.5 = 0.01$) as compared with a risk of 1/2,500 in general population. Therefore, partner testing with genetic counseling would be of utmost importance. Since the commercial genetic tests have about 90% of sensitivity (see Table 4.1) when no mutation is found in the test, the partner still has a risk of 1/250 being a carrier of an untested mutation; therefore, the CBAVD couple may still run a risk of 1/1,000 of having a child with CF [132].

Genes Involved in Meiotic Recombination

Although the incidence of chromosome abnormalities is about ten times higher in infertile males than in the general population, most infertile men have normal karyotype. However, these patients may show an increased incidence of aneuploid sperm and diploid sperm in their ejaculate or in sperm obtained from testes [139, 140]. It has also been shown that the risk of aneuploidy or diploidy in sperm corre-lates with decreasing numbers of sperm and total progressive motility [141]. Many times, meiotic disturbances are the culprits in those cases.

Meiotic recombination in germ cell occurs in prophase of meiosis and involves the induction of double-strand DNA breaks, the pairing of parental homologous chromosomes, followed by the repair of double-strand breaks using the intact homologous chromosome as a template. Several studies have suggested signifi-cantly lower rates of meiotic recombination and impaired synapsis in infertile men [142–145]. Faulty meiotic recombination can also cause fertility problems especially if the meiotic errors cannot be corrected; meiotic checkpoint molecules activate apoptotic pathways leading to testicular failure. Furthermore, it was esti-mated that 5–10% of cases of nonobstructive azoospermia may be due to meiotic arrest [145]. There are many genes involved in meiotic recombination, investiga-tion of which has been mostly relevant to etiology of many cancers [146]. Among these gene products, the absence of type II topoisomerase, Spo11 (chromosome 20q13.2-13.3), and synaptonemal complex protein, SYCP3 (chromosome 12q23.2) is shown to be associated with nonobstructive azoospermia in humans [146–148].

Gene Mutations Associated with Sperm Functional Defects

The primary ciliary dyskinesia presents with immotile but viable sperm along with varying degrees of respiratory tract dysfunction, situs inversus totalis (Kartagener's syndrome), and hydrocephalus. Its frequency is 1 in 20,000–60,000 live births [149]. Most of the genetically characterized primary ciliary dyskinesia variants exhibit mutations in the genes dynein, axonemal, heavy chain 5 [DNAH5, 5p15.2]; dynein, axonemal, heavy chain 11 [DNAH11, 7p21]; dynein, axonemal, intermediate chain 1 [DNAI1, 9p13.3]; and dynein, axonemal, intermediate chain 2 [DNAI2, 17q25] that encode axonemal dynein-arm components responsible for ciliary-beat generation and sperm-specific thioredoxin domain containing 3 [TXNDC3, 7p14.1] encoding a thioredoxin [150]. Some cases may have mutations in retinitis pigmentosa GTPase regulator (RPGR) gene on Xp11.4 which is also associated with retinitis pigmentosa [151]. The patients initially may present with severe asthenospermia. In these cases, other clinical signs of primary ciliary dyskinesia should be sought. The majority of patients have sperm in the ejaculate, and ICSI has been successfully used in those cases [152].

Mutations of aurora kinase C (AURKC, serine/threonine kinase 13, 19q13) have been shown to cause male infertility in the region of Northwest Africa (Morocco, Tunisia, Algeria). In those countries, the carrier rate of the mutation can be as high as 1 in 50. Men homozygous for the mutation demonstrate sperm with a 4N chromosomal complement, large heads, and multiple tails [153]. In mice knockout studies, absence of AURKC was only associated with a high rate of teratospermia with retained fertility [154]. It remains to be elucidated if screening for AURKC mutations is needed in other populations.

Copy Number Variations

These are pieces of 1 kb or longer DNA segments that vary in number between individuals which are considered as submicroscopic duplications and/or deletions of the genome [155]. Copy number variations (CNVs) can be detectable by higher-resolution genome-wide microarray comparative genomic hybridization assays and can be further confirmed by PCR-based methods. The complexity about CNVs lies on the facts that their presence can cause overt disease, a predisposition to a disease, or may have no effects at all. In general, CNVs may affect up to 20% of human genome [70]. CNVs have been investigated in many medical disorders; however, the data on male infertility are scarce, and more investigation is needed.

Mitochondrial Genetics

Mitochondrial DNA is a double-stranded circular DNA molecule coding for 2 rRNAs, 22 tRNAs, and 13 polypeptides essential for respiratory enzyme complexes involved in oxidative phosphorylation [156]. Mitochondrial DNA has no introns, and it mutates at 10–20 times higher rates than nuclear DNA due to its unique structure and replication system [157]. Mid-piece of mammalian sperm contains about 80 mitochondria with single copy of DNA in each organelle. Spermatozoa are dependent on mitochondria for energy needed for rapid progressive motility. Mitochondrial DNA mutations caused by the oxidative damage induced by reactive oxygen species or free radicals may lead to male infertility [158]. In general, about 85% of sperm samples may contain various mitochondrial DNA deletions which may partly explain the age-related decline in fertility in males.

The presence of multiple mitochondrial mutations have been reported to be associated with oligoasthenoteratospermia [159, 160]. The key nuclear enzyme involved in the elongation and repair of mitochondrial DNA strands is DNA polymerase gamma (POLG). The catalytic subunit of POLG is encoded by POLG gene on chromosome 15q24 which includes a CAG repeat region [161]. POLG mutations are associated with mutations in mitochondrial genome which subsequently affects ATP production and sperm function. Expanded CAG repeats in the region of POLG gene are also associated with several neuromuscular disorders which may be associated with male factor infertility as well. Many of these disorders like Huntington's disease are transmitted in an autosomal-dominant fashion.

Epigenetic Alterations

Epigenetics refers to the alterations of the gene expression without any change in DNA nucleotide sequence. Epigenetic mechanisms are associated with the way in which the genome is packed affecting the ability of genes to be activated. It is involved mostly with regulation of transcription or translation.

The most established epigenetic mechanism heritable through germ line is DNA methylation. This is a post-replicative modification in which a methyl group is covalently added to CpG (cytosine–guanine) dinucleotide residues of DNA by DNA methyltransferases [162]. Other well-known epigenetic mechanisms include chromatin condensation and histone modifications. The regions of chromatin can be transiently condensed or uncondensed leading to variation in gene expression through transcriptional suppressors, functional RNAs, or interaction with various proteins [163]. Histones are subjected to modifications like phosphorylation, acetylation, methylation, ubiquitination, carbonylation, and such affecting gene expression [164]. Small noncoding RNAs like micro (mi)-RNAs or Piwi-interacting (pi) RNAs are the newest epigenetic mechanisms acting through transcriptional or translational regulation [165, 166]. In mice, the global loss of miRNAs in Dicer (RNase III endonuclease playing central role in miRNA biogenesis) knockout mice has detrimental effects on spermatogenesis [166].

Reprogramming of methylation patterns in mammals occurs usually after fertilization (preimplantation stage) and during fetal development of the germ line (gametogenesis) especially during germ line differentiation [167]. Allelic differences in methylation which is characteristics of imprinted genes are also delineated during the germ-cell line establishment [168]. Imprinted genes conserve their methylation patterns through generations. Therefore, if methylation changes are induced in imprinted genes or new methylation sites are established during germ-cell differentiation or after fertilization, heritable factors can either diminish or persist affecting the ultimate phenotype in the offspring [169]. Most endocrine disruptors or environmental factors do not promote DNA sequence mutation but induce modifications of DNA without altering nucleotide composition, i.e., epigenetic changes [170, 171].

Imprinting abnormalities associated with Angelman, Prader–Willi, Beckwith–Wiedemann, and Silver–Russell syndromes have been associated with assisted reproductive technologies (ART), whereas correlations have been found to be weak. It seems that these imprinting syndromes may be associated with infertility factors associated with preexisting methylation aberrations rather than ART itself [172]. Favoring this assumption, it has been reported that epigenetic abnormalities are common in sperm of men with severe oligospermia [173, 174]. Rodent studies also revealed that perturbation of DNA methyltransferases or DNA methylation in male germ cells can affect fertility and sperm function [175]. Abnormal sperm chromatin packaging may have a role in proper establishment of methylation patterns and abnormal protamine 1 and protamine 2 ratios (P1:P2 equals to unity in fertile men), which were detected in infertile men [176–178], and may lead to changes in imprinted genes [179]. One recent study has reported aberrant imprinting patterns of paternally demethylated genes in frozen sperm specimens of men with oligospermia and in those specimens showing normal sperm concentration but abnormal P1:P2 ratios [180]. It is proposed that the erasure and resetting of DNA methylation that takes place in primordial germ cells is an important stage to prevent DNA methylation defects; however, the effectors and modulators of these steps need further investigation before the applicability of this information to clinical practice [181].

Malignancy Risks Associated with Genetic Perturbations in Infertile Men

Multiple studies have suggested an association between male infertility and testicular germ-cell tumor which is the most common malignancy in men aged 15–35 years [182, 183]. Infertility probably precedes the development of occult testicular cancer. This association suggests common genetic and environmental factors in both infertility and testicular germ cell tumors. Increased risk of these cancers have been associated with factors related with genetics and epigenetics which include cryptorchidism, chromosome 12 aneuploidy, DNA mismatch repair gene defects, Y-chromosome instability, and stem cell dysregulation via abnormal RNA interference [182, 184, 185]. Cryptorchidism itself may be associated with mutations in HOXA10, INSL3 and INSL3 receptor LGR8/GREAT, AR, estrogen receptor (ER) α, and SF-1 gene mutations [186]. While elucidation of all these factors and pathways are required, all men evaluated for infertility needs to be adequately assessed and screened for testicular tumors.

Male Genetic Testing in Clinical Practice

Many genetic potential causes of both spermatogenic failure and obstructive azoospermia have been demonstrated, but despite much progress in animal data [187], the validation of the proposed genetic tests have been slow [188]. Therefore, only a limited number of tests are currently recommended in the evaluation of infertile men. Arbitrarily defining severe oligospermia as sperm concentration less than five million per milliliter and azoospermia as the sperm density below the detection limit, infertile men with those two conditions are recommended to undergo genetic testing.

Men with congenital unilateral or bilateral absence of vas deferens should be tested for a CFTR mutation which also includes 5T variant. Almost all men with clinical CF have CBAVD. At least two-thirds of men with CBAVD have mutations of the CFTR gene. However, failure to identify a CFTR mutation by commercial tests in a man with CBAVD does not rule out a mutation, since they may still harbor a mutation undetectable with the currently recommended screening panel. Even, it has been recommended that patients with CBAVD should be assumed to have a CFTR mutation [51]. Although most men with CBAVD have normal spermatogenesis, coexisting spermatogenesis defects should always be ruled out before harvesting sperm for ICSI [189]. Furthermore, since about 25% of men with unilateral absence of vas deferens and 10% of men with CBAVD may have unilateral renal agenesis, an abdominal ultrasound is also required [190].

There is a need to routinely karyotype infertile men with persistent or severe oligospermia (<10 million depending on the male phenotype or <5 million per ml for all) or nonobstructive azoospermia [66] (Fig. 4.3). Yq deletions are more frequent in azoospermia cases than men with severe oligospermia. Nevertheless, routine Yq microdeletion STS-PCR testing is required before testicular sperm harvesting or before ART in men with nonobstructive azoospermia or severe oligospermia. Chromosomal abnormalities may result in impaired testicular function, while Y-chromosome microdeletions result in isolated spermatogenic failure.

At present, testing sperm for aneuploidies or inversions in men with abnormal sperm analysis or men with abnormal karyotype is not recommended since the exact data set establishing threshold levels for the percentage of sperm with abnormal karyotype to assist in clinical and PGD decision making is lacking [70]. Currently, routine assessment of CNVs, epigenetic assessment of infertile men, or their sperm do not find any support in the clinical practice.

Gene Therapy for Male Infertility

Around 15% of the male infertility patients are azoospermic, and normal sperm production with obstructive cause accounts for 40% of these cases. In the remaining 60% of the cases with spermatogenesis defects, approximately half of them may have low levels of sperm which may be obtained through TESE techniques to be used for ICSI [191, 192]. Only for cases without any viable sperm in the testes gene therapy may be considered.

There are many challenges to gene therapy for male infertility. Karyotypic abnormalities like Klinefelter syndrome and Y-chromosome deletions involve additions or deletions of large amounts of DNA. Currently, there is no technology to manipulate large amounts of DNA for gene therapy. Furthermore, although we mentioned some genetic causes of male infertility in this article, many men with severe infertility do not have any identifiable genetic defects even if the genetic cause is likely. Knowledge of the exact gene(s) involved is essential to proceed with any gene therapy. In humans, at least 178 genes may be involved with spermatogenesis only [32], and mice models for male infertility suggests over 150 single gene defects leading to male infertility [193, 194].

Another obstacle is that gene therapy for male infertility may involve both somatic (Sertoli, Leydig cells) and germ cells needing more complex approaches. Serious ethical and safety concerns exist regarding inducing genetic alterations in the germ line, and currently, germ line genetic therapy is prohibited. There are suggested approaches like using episomes which are not integrated into the genome to be used in that respect [195]. For somatic cells, using viral vectors to integrate wild type of gene carries the risk of insertional mutagenesis or carcinogenesis since technology does not allow selected site insertion [196]. There are trials on non-viral approaches to gene therapy like cationic lipids, gold, nanoparticles, and electroporation of naked DNA, although like viral vectors, these methods may still induce immune response in the host and their efficiency is currently lower than the viral vectors [197].

New suggested approaches to deal with the obstacles include the use of embryonic stem cells, transplantation, and xenotransplantation [198–201]. Enucleated oocyte can be combined with patient's somatic cell nucleus, nucleus can be reprogrammed, and oocyte is stimulated to become blastocyst since it contains diploid chromosomes. Then stem cells can be differentiated into germ cell lineage, and these cells can be transplanted back to patient's seminiferous tubules or further development of germ cells can be achieved in vitro to be used for ICSI. In xenotransplantation, spermatogonia can be harvested from patient's testis and genetically corrected in vitro and then transferred into the testes of nonhuman primate whose seminiferous tubules are devoid of primate germ cells, to achieve spermatogenesis. Sperm obtained from xenograft can be used for ICSI. There are many safety and ethical concerns about these procedures as well.

Five-Year View and Key Issues

Primary spermatogenic failure accounts for about 50% of the cases of male infertility. Utilizing the clinically applicable tests, in only a minority of these men, the condition may be explained by genetic perturbations and the rest is called as "idiopathic" many of which may have yet unknown genetic mechanisms playing a role. Progress in the knowledge of genetics, epigenetics, and gene regulation should result in a greater understanding of male infertility. Considering the fact that the majority of infertile men may have an underlying genetic perturbation of some sort, general health surveillance of the male should become a priority before any specific treatment or assisted reproduction is attempted. The health of the offspring resulting from assisted reproductive technologies should also be followed to detect any clinical picture associated with genetic or epigenetic dysregulation. Finding a cure for spermatogenic failure will continue to be a challenge. It is fortunate that there are many new and evolving technologies to help identify the etiology of male infertility which may lead to targeted therapeutics. Although emerging animal studies offer some hope, the investigation should be directed toward how this data can find application in humans while avoiding any adverse effects. For the reasons above, male factor infertility research and treatment should incorporate a multidisciplinary approach. In this regard, collaboration between the reproductive endocrinologists, assisted reproduction laboratory staff, urologists, clinical geneticists, pediatricians, research scientists, and other members of the infertility team is essential.

Future Directions

Approaches such as microarray profiling, comparative genomic hybridization, and mutagenesis screening will have important roles in efforts to understand genetic origins of male infertility. Incorporating genomics, proteomics, and metabolomics into male infertility research may help to identify the population-specific complete role of genes involved with fertility [202–205]. These technologies provide vast amount of data with plenty of background "noise" at times. Therefore, the results from advanced genomic, proteomic, and metabolomic techniques should be confirmed by PCR, Western blot, flow cytometry, mass spectroscopy and chromatography, and protein function assays. These approaches will lead to better preconceptional counseling and more directed approaches for PGD. Future directions should also involve identifications of single gene defects associated with male infertility and advancing the field of gene therapy further to address safety and ethical concerns before these technologies could be applied in humans.

References

1. Ferlin A, Raicu F, Gatta V, Zuccarello D, Palka G, Foresta C. Male infertility: role of genetic background. Reprod Biomed Online. 2007;14:734–45.
2. Wilhelm D, Koopman P. The makings of maleness: towards an integrated view of male sexual development. Nat Rev Genet. 2006;7:620–31.
3. Miyamoto N, Yoshida M, Kuratani S, Matsuo I, Aizawa S. Defects of urogenital development in mice lacking Emx2. Development. 1997;124:1653–64.
4. Tevosian SG, Albrecht KH, Crispino JD, Fujiwara Y, Eicher EM, Orkin SH. Gonadal differentiation, sex determination and normal Sry expression in mice require direct interaction between transcription partners GATA4 and FOG2. Development. 2002;129: 4627–34.

5. Birk OS, Casiano DE, Wassif CA, Cogliati T, Zhao L, Zhao Y, et al. The LIM homeobox gene Lhx9 is essential for mouse gonad formation. Nature. 2000;403:909–13.
6. Achermann JC, Ito M, Hindmarsh PC, Jameson JL. A mutation in the gene encoding steroido-genic factor-1 causes XY sex reversal and adrenal failure in humans. Nat Genet. 1999;22:125–6.
7. Achermann JC, Ozisik G, Ito M, Orun UA, Harmanci K, Gurakan B, et al. Gonadal determina-tion and adrenal development are regulated by the orphan nuclear receptor steroidogenic fac-tor-1, in a dose-dependent manner. J Clin Endocrinol Metab. 2002;87: 1829–33.
8. Ludbrook LM, Harley VR. Sex determination: a 'window' of DAX1 activity. Trends Endocrinol Metab. 2004;15:116–21.
9. Ozisik G, Achermann JC, Jameson JL. The role of SF1 in adrenal and reproductive function: insight from naturally occurring mutations in humans. Mol Genet Metab. 2002;76:85–91.
10. Englert C. WT1—more than a transcription factor? Trends Biochem Sci. 1998;23:389–93.
11. Sinclair AH, Berta P, Palmer MS, Hawkins JR, Griffiths BL, Smith MJ, et al. A gene from the human sex-determining region encodes a protein with homology to a conserved DNA-binding motif. Nature. 1990;346:240–4.
12. Wilhelm D, Martinson F, Bradford S, Wilson MJ, Combes AN, Beverdam A, et al. Sertoli cell differentiation is induced both cell-autonomously and through prostaglandin signaling during mammalian sex determination. Dev Biol. 2005;287:111–24.
13. Bullejos M, Koopman P. Spatially dynamic expression of Sry in mouse genital ridges. Dev Dyn. 2001;221:201–5.
14. Hammes A, Guo JK, Lutsch G, Leheste JR, Landrock D, Ziegler U, et al. Two splice variants of the Wilms' tumor 1 gene have distinct functions during sex determination and nephron formation. Cell. 2001;106:319–29.
15. Nef S, Verma-Kurvari S, Merenmies J, Vassalli JD, Efstratiadis A, Accili D, et al. Testis deter-mination requires insulin receptor family function in mice. Nature. 2003;426:291–5.
16. Bullejos M, Koopman P. Delayed Sry and Sox9 expression in developing mouse gonads under-lies B6-Y(DOM) sex reversal. Dev Biol. 2005;278:473–81.
17. Taketo T, Lee CH, Zhang J, Li Y, Lee CY, Lau YF. Expression of SRY proteins in both normal and sex-reversed XY fetal mouse gonads. Dev Dyn. 2005;233:612–22.
18. Clark AM, Garland KK, Russell LD. Desert hedgehog (Dhh) gene is required in the mouse testis for formation of adult-type Leydig cells and normal development of peritubular cells and seminiferous tubules. Biol Reprod. 2000;63:1825–38.
19. Bitgood MJ, Shen L, McMahon AP. Sertoli cell signaling by desert hedgehog regulates the male germ line. Curr Biol. 1996;6: 298–304.
20. Canto P, Vilchis F, Soderlund D, Reyes E, Mendez JP. A heterozygous mutation in the desert hedgehog gene in patients with mixed gonadal dysgenesis. Mol Hum Reprod. 2005;11: 833–6.
21. Canto P, Soderlund D, Reyes E, Mendez JP. Mutations in the desert hedgehog (DHH) gene in patients with 46, XY complete pure gonadal dysgenesis. J Clin Endocrinol Metab. 2004;89: 4480–3.
22. Kitamura K, Yanazawa M, Sugiyama N, Miura H, Iizuka-Kogo A, Kusaka M, et al. Mutation of ARX causes abnormal development of forebrain and testes in mice and X-linked lissen-cephaly with abnormal genitalia in humans. Nat Genet. 2002;32:359–69.
23. Tang P, Park DJ, Marshall Graves JA, Harley VR. ATRX and sex differentiation. Trends Endocrinol Metab. 2004;15: 339–44.
24. Brennan J, Tilmann C, Capel B. Pdgfr-alpha mediates testis cord organization and fetal Leydig cell development in the XY gonad. Genes Dev. 2003;17:800–10.
25. Tanaka SS, Yamaguchi YL, Tsoi B, Lickert H, Tam PP. IFITM/Mil/fragilis family proteins IFITM1 and IFITM3 play distinct roles in mouse primordial germ cell homing and repulsion. Dev Cell. 2005;9:745–56.
26. Molyneaux KA, Zinszner H, Kunwar PS, Schaible K, Stebler J, Sunshine MJ, et al. The che-mokine SDF1/CXCL12 and its receptor CXCR4 regulate mouse germ cell migration and sur-vival. Development. 2003;130:4279–86.
27. Adham IM, Agoulnik AI. Insulin-like 3 signalling in testicular descent. Int J Androl. 2004;27:257–65.

28. Ivell R, Hartung S. The molecular basis of cryptorchidism. Mol Hum Reprod. 2003;9:175–81.
29. Quill TA, Ren D, Clapham DE, Garbers DL. A voltage-gated ion channel expressed specifically in spermatozoa. Proc Natl Acad Sci USA. 2001;98:12527–31.
30. Sha J, Zhou Z, Li J, Yin L, Yang H, Hu G, et al. Identification of testis development and spermatogenesis-related genes in human and mouse testes using cDNA arrays. Mol Hum Reprod. 2002;8: 511–7.
31. Schultz N, Hamra FK, Garbers DL. A multitude of genes expressed solely in meiotic or postmeiotic spermatogenic cells offers a myriad of contraceptive targets. Proc Natl Acad Sci USA. 2003;100: 12201–6.
32. Hermo L, Pelletier RM, Cyr DG, Smith CE. Surfing the wave, cycle, life history, and genes/proteins expressed by testicular germ cells. Part 1: background to spermatogenesis, spermatogonia, and spermatocytes. Microsc Res Tech. 2010;73(4):241–78.
33. Saxena R, de Vries JW, Repping S, Alagappan RK, Skaletsky H, Brown LG, et al. Four DAZ genes in two clusters found in the AZFc region of the human Y chromosome. Genomics. 2000;67: 256–67.
34. Yen PH. Putative biological functions of the DAZ family. Int J Androl. 2004;27:125–9.
35. Hopps CV, Mielnik A, Goldstein M, Palermo GD, Rosenwaks Z, Schlegel PN. Detection of sperm in men with Y chromosome microdeletions of the AZFa, AZFb and AZFc regions. Hum Reprod. 2003;18:1660–5.
36. Silber SJ, Repping S. Transmission of male infertility to future generations: lessons from the Y chromosome. Hum Reprod Update. 2002;8:217–29.
37. Nishimune Y, Tanaka H. Infertility caused by polymorphisms or mutations in spermatogenesis-specific genes. J Androl. 2006;27:326–34.
38. Mueller JL, Mahadevaiah SK, Park PJ, Warburton PE, Page DC, Turner JM. The mouse X chromosome is enriched for multicopy testis genes showing postmeiotic expression. Nat Genet. 2008;40:794–9.
39. Roberts LM, Visser JA, Ingraham HA. Involvement of a matrix metalloproteinase in MIS-induced cell death during urogenital development. Development. 2002;129:1487–96.
40. Belville C, Marechal JD, Pennetier S, Carmillo P, Masgrau L, Messika-Zeitoun L, et al. Natural mutations of the anti-Mullerian hormone type II receptor found in persistent Mullerian duct syndrome affect ligand binding, signal transduction and cellular transport. Hum Mol Genet. 2009;18:3002–13.
41. Belville C, Van Vlijmen H, Ehrenfels C, Pepinsky B, Rezaie AR, Picard JY, et al. Mutations of the anti-Mullerian hormone gene in patients with persistent Mullerian duct syndrome: biosynthesis, secretion, and processing of the abnormal proteins and analysis using a three-dimensional model. Mol Endocrinol. 2004;18: 708–21.
42. Hannema SE, Hughes IA. Regulation of Wolffian duct development. Horm Res. 2007;67: 142–51.
43. Dravis C, Yokoyama N, Chumley MJ, Cowan CA, Silvany RE, Shay J, et al. Bidirectional signaling mediated by ephrin-B2 and EphB2 controls urorectal development. Dev Biol. 2004;271: 272–90.
44. Goodman FR, Bacchelli C, Brady AF, Brueton LA, Fryns JP, Mortlock DP, et al. Novel HOXA13 mutations and the phenotypic spectrum of hand-foot-genital syndrome. Am J Hum Genet. 2000;67:197–202.
45. Chandley AC. Genetic contribution to male infertility. Hum Reprod. 1998;13 Suppl 3:76–83. discussion 4-8.
46. Johnson MD. Genetic risks of intracytoplasmic sperm injection in the treatment of male infertility: recommendations for genetic counseling and screening. Fertil Steril. 1998;70:397–411.
47. Ravel C, Berthaut I, Bresson JL, Siffroi JP. Prevalence of chromosomal abnormalities in phenotypically normal and fertile adult males: large-scale survey of over 10,000 sperm donor karyotypes. Hum Reprod. 2006;21:1484–9.
48. O'Flynn O'Brien KL, Varghese AC, Agarwal A. The genetic causes of male factor infertility: a review. Fertil Steril. 2010;93:1–12.

49. Palermo GD, Colombero LT, Hariprashad JJ, Schlegel PN, Rosenwaks Z. Chromosome analysis of epididymal and testicular sperm in azoospermic patients undergoing ICSI. Hum Reprod. 2002;17:570–5.
50. Van Assche E, Bonduelle M, Tournaye H, Joris H, Verheyen G, Devroey P, et al. Cytogenetics of infertile men. Hum Reprod. 1996;11 Suppl 4:1–24. discussion 5-6.
51. American Society for Reproductive Medicine. Evaluation of the azoospermic male. Fertil Steril. 2008;90:S74–7.
52. Walsh TJ, Pera RR, Turek PJ. The genetics of male infertility. Semin Reprod Med. 2009;27:124–36.
53. Friedler S, Raziel A, Strassburger D, Schachter M, Bern O, Ron-El R. Outcome of ICSI using fresh and cryopreserved-thawed testicular spermatozoa in patients with non-mosaic Klinefelter's syndrome. Hum Reprod. 2001;16:2616–20.
54. Schiff JD, Palermo GD, Veeck LL, Goldstein M, Rosenwaks Z, Schlegel PN. Success of testicular sperm extraction [corrected] and intracytoplasmic sperm injection in men with Klinefelter syndrome. J Clin Endocrinol Metab. 2005;90:6263–7.
55. Denschlag D, Tempfer C, Kunze M, Wolff G, Keck C. Assisted reproductive techniques in patients with Klinefelter syndrome: a critical review. Fertil Steril. 2004;82:775–9.
56. Blanco J, Egozcue J, Vidal F. Meiotic behaviour of the sex chromosomes in three patients with sex chromosome anomalies (47, XXY, mosaic 46, XY/47, XXY and 47, XYY) assessed by fluorescence in-situ hybridization. Hum Reprod. 2001;16:887–92.
57. Bergere M, Wainer R, Nataf V, Bailly M, Gombault M, Ville Y, et al. Biopsied testis cells of four 47, XXY patients: fluorescence in-situ hybridization and ICSI results. Hum Reprod. 2002;17: 32–7.
58. Levron J, Aviram-Goldring A, Madgar I, Raviv G, Barkai G, Dor J. Sperm chromosome analysis and outcome of IVF in patients with non-mosaic Klinefelter's syndrome. Fertil Steril. 2000;74: 925–9.
59. Staessen C, Tournaye H, Van Assche E, Michiels A, Van Landuyt L, Devroey P, et al. PGD in 47, XXY Klinefelter's syndrome patients. Hum Reprod Update. 2003;9:319–30.
60. Tournaye H, Staessen C, Liebaers I, Van Assche E, Devroey P, Bonduelle M, et al. Testicular sperm recovery in nine 47, XXY Klinefelter patients. Hum Reprod. 1996;11:1644–9.
61. Shi Q, Martin RH. Multicolor fluorescence in situ hybridization analysis of meiotic chromosome segregation in a 47, XYY male and a review of the literature. Am J Med Genet. 2000;93:40–6.
62. Gonzalez-Merino E, Hans C, Abramowicz M, Englert Y, Emiliani S. Aneuploidy study in sperm and preimplantation embryos from nonmosaic 47, XYY men. Fertil Steril. 2007;88:600–6.
63. Van der Auwera B, Van Roy N, De Paepe A, Hawkins JR, Liebaers I, Castedo S, et al. Molecular cytogenetic analysis of XX males using Y-specific DNA sequences, including SRY. Hum Genet. 1992;89:23–8.
64. De Braekeleer M, Dao TN. Cytogenetic studies in male infertility: a review. Hum Reprod. 1991;6:245–50.
65. Chantot-Bastaraud S, Ravel C, Siffroi JP. Underlying karyotype abnormalities in IVF/ICSI patients. Reprod Biomed Online. 2008;16:514–22.
66. Martin RH. Cytogenetic determinants of male fertility. Hum Reprod Update. 2008;14:379–90.
67. Ogur G, Van Assche E, Vegetti W, Verheyen G, Tournaye H, Bonduelle M, et al. Chromosomal segregation in spermatozoa of 14 Robertsonian translocation carriers. Mol Hum Reprod. 2006;12:209–15.
68. Mau-Holzmann UA. Somatic chromosomal abnormalities in infertile men and women. Cytogenet Genome Res. 2005;111:317–36.
69. Estop AM, Van Kirk V, Cieply K. Segregation analysis of four translocations, t(2;18), t(3;15), t(5;7), and t(10;12), by sperm chromosome studies and a review of the literature. Cytogenet Cell Genet. 1995;70:80–7.
70. McLachlan RI, O'Bryan MK. Clinical review#: state of the art for genetic testing of infertile men. J Clin Endocrinol Metab. 2010;95:1013–24.

71. Rozen S, Skaletsky H, Marszalek JD, Minx PJ, Cordum HS, Waterston RH, et al. Abundant gene conversion between arms of palindromes in human and ape Y chromosomes. Nature. 2003;423:873–6.
72. Li Z, Haines CJ, Han Y. "Micro-deletions" of the human Y chromosome and their relationship with male infertility. J Genet Genomics. 2008;35:193–9.
73. Skaletsky H, Kuroda-Kawaguchi T, Minx PJ, Cordum HS, Hillier L, Brown LG, et al. The male-specific region of the human Y chromosome is a mosaic of discrete sequence classes. Nature. 2003;423:825–37.
74. Foresta C, Moro E, Ferlin A. Y chromosome microdeletions and alterations of spermatogenesis. Endocr Rev. 2001;22:226–39.
75. Vollrath D, Foote S, Hilton A, Brown LG, Beer-Romero P, Bogan JS, et al. The human Y chromosome: a 43-interval map based on naturally occurring deletions. Science. 1992;258:52–9.
76. Kleiman SE, Bar-Shira Maymon B, Yogev L, Paz G, Yavetz H. The prognostic role of the extent of Y microdeletion on spermatogenesis and maturity of Sertoli cells. Hum Reprod. 2001;16: 399–402.
77. Poongothai J, Gopenath TS, Manonayaki S. Genetics of human male infertility. Singapore Med J. 2009;50:336–47.
78. Vogt PH. Genetics of idiopathic male infertility: Y chromosomal azoospermia factors (AZFa, AZFb, AZFc). Baillieres Clin Obstet Gynaecol. 1997;11:773–95.
79. Sadeghi-Nejad H, Oates RD. The Y chromosome and male infertility. Curr Opin Urol. 2008;18:628–32.
80. Repping S, Skaletsky H, Lange J, Silber S, Van Der Veen F, Oates RD, et al. Recombination between palindromes P5 and P1 on the human Y chromosome causes massive deletions and spermatogenic failure. Am J Hum Genet. 2002;71:906–22.
81. Brown GM, Furlong RA, Sargent CA, Erickson RP, Longepied G, Mitchell M, et al. Characterisation of the coding sequence and fine mapping of the human DFFRY gene and comparative expression analysis and mapping to the Sxrb interval of the mouse Y chromosome of the Dffry gene. Hum Mol Genet. 1998;7:97–107.
82. Chuang RY, Weaver PL, Liu Z, Chang TH. Requirement of the DEAD-Box protein ded1p for messenger RNA translation. Science. 1997;275:1468–71.
83. Foresta C, Ferlin A, Moro E. Deletion and expression analysis of AZFa genes on the human Y chromosome revealed a major role for DBY in male infertility. Hum Mol Genet. 2000;9:1161–9.
84. Moro E, Ferlin A, Yen PH, Franchi PG, Palka G, Foresta C. Male infertility caused by a de novo partial deletion of the DAZ cluster on the Y chromosome. J Clin Endocrinol Metab. 2000;85: 4069–73.
85. Sun C, Skaletsky H, Birren B, Devon K, Tang Z, Silber S, et al. An azoospermic man with a de novo point mutation in the Y-chromosomal gene USP9Y. Nat Genet. 1999;23:429–32.
86. Geoffroy-Siraudin C, Aknin-Seiffer I, Metzler-Guillemain C, Ghalamoun-Slaimi R, Bonzi MF, Levy R, et al. Meiotic abnormalities in patients bearing complete AZFc deletion of Y chromosome. Hum Reprod. 2007;22:1567–72.
87. Navarro-Costa P, Pereira L, Alves C, Gusmao L, Proenca C, Marques-Vidal P, et al. Characterizing partial AZFc deletions of the Y chromosome with amplicon-specific sequence markers. BMC Genomics. 2007;8:342.
88. Wu B, Lu NX, Xia YK, Gu AH, Lu CC, Wang W, et al. A frequent Y chromosome b2/b3 subdeletion shows strong association with male infertility in Han-Chinese population. Hum Reprod. 2007;22:1107–13.
89. Zhang F, Li Z, Wen B, Jiang J, Shao M, Zhao Y, et al. A frequent partial AZFc deletion does not render an increased risk of spermatogenic impairment in East Asians. Ann Hum Genet. 2006;70:304–13.
90. Zhu XB, Liu YL, Zhang W, Ping P, Cao XR, Liu Y, et al. Vertical transmission of the Yq AZFc microdeletion from father to son over two or three generations in infertile Han Chinese families. Asian J Androl. 2010;12:240–6.
91. Giachini C, Nuti F, Marinari E, Forti G, Krausz C. Partial AZFc deletions in infertile men with cryptorchidism. Hum Reprod. 2007;22:2398–403.

92. Zhang F, Lu C, Li Z, Xie P, Xia Y, Zhu X, et al. Partial deletions are associated with an increased risk of complete deletion in AZFc: a new insight into the role of partial AZFc deletions in male infertility. J Med Genet. 2007;44:437–44.
93. Ferlin A, Arredi B, Speltra E, Cazzadore C, Selice R, Garolla A, et al. Molecular and clinical characterization of Y chromosome microdeletions in infertile men: a 10-year experience in Italy. J Clin Endocrinol Metab. 2007;92:762–70.
94. Mulhall JP, Reijo R, Alagappan R, Brown L, Page D, Carson R, et al. Azoospermic men with deletion of the DAZ gene cluster are capable of completing spermatogenesis: fertilization, normal embryonic development and pregnancy occur when retrieved testicular spermatozoa are used for intracytoplasmic sperm injection. Hum Reprod. 1997;12:503–8.
95. Oates RD, Silber S, Brown LG, Page DC. Clinical characterization of 42 oligospermic or azoospermic men with microdeletion of the AZFc region of the Y chromosome, and of 18 children conceived via ICSI. Hum Reprod. 2002;17:2813–24.
96. Osborne EC, Lynch M, McLachlan R, Trounson AO, Cram DS. Microarray detection of Y chromosome deletions associated with male infertility. Reprod Biomed Online. 2007;15: 673–80.
97. Ferlin A, Moro E, Onisto M, Toscano E, Bettella A, Foresta C. Absence of testicular DAZ gene expression in idiopathic severe testiculopathies. Hum Reprod. 1999;14:2286–92.
98. Lange J, Skaletsky H, van Daalen SK, Embry SL, Korver CM, Brown LG, et al. Isodicentric Y chromosomes and sex disorders as byproducts of homologous recombination that maintains palindromes. Cell. 2009;138:855–69.
99. Lardone MC, Parodi DA, Valdevenito R, Ebensperger M, Piottante A, Madariaga M, et al. Quantification of DDX3Y, RBMY1, DAZ and TSPY mRNAs in testes of patients with severe impairment of spermatogenesis. Mol Hum Reprod. 2007;13:705–12.
100. Vodicka R, Vrtel R, Dusek L, Singh AR, Krizova K, Svacinova V, et al. TSPY gene copy number as a potential new risk factor for male infertility. Reprod Biomed Online. 2007;14:579–87.
101. Wang PJ, McCarrey JR, Yang F, Page DC. An abundance of X-linked genes expressed in spermatogonia. Nat Genet. 2001;27: 422–6.
102. Cantu JM, Diaz M, Moller M, Jimenez-Sainz M, Sandoval L, Vaca G, et al. Azoospermia and duplication 3qter as distinct consequences of a familial t(X;3) (q26;q13.2). Am J Med Genet. 1985;20:677–84.
103. Lee S, Lee SH, Chung TG, Kim HJ, Yoon TK, Kwak IP, et al. Molecular and cytogenetic characterization of two azoospermic patients with X-autosome translocation. J Assist Reprod Genet. 2003;20:385–9.
104. Nemeth AH, Gallen IW, Crocker M, Levy E, Maher E. Klinefelter-like phenotype and primary infertility in a male with a paracentric Xq inversion. J Med Genet. 2002;39:E28.
105. Olesen C, Silber J, Eiberg H, Ernst E, Petersen K, Lindenberg S, et al. Mutational analysis of the human FATE gene in 144 infertile men. Hum Genet. 2003;113:195–201.
106. Raverot G, Lejeune H, Kotlar T, Pugeat M, Jameson JL. X-linked sex-determining region Y box 3 (SOX3) gene mutations are uncommon in men with idiopathic oligoazoospermic infertility. J Clin Endocrinol Metab. 2004;89:4146–8.
107. Schneider-Gadicke A, Beer-Romero P, Brown LG, Mardon G, Luoh SW, Page DC. Putative transcription activator with alternative isoforms encoded by human ZFX gene. Nature. 1989;342: 708–11.
108. Schneider-Gadicke A, Beer-Romero P, Brown LG, Nussbaum R, Page DC. ZFX has a gene structure similar to ZFY, the putative human sex determinant, and escapes X inactivation. Cell. 1989;57:1247–58.
109. Wang RS, Yeh S, Tzeng CR, Chang C. Androgen receptor roles in spermatogenesis and fertility: lessons from testicular cell-specific androgen receptor knockout mice. Endocr Rev. 2009;30:119–32.
110. Xu Q, Lin HY, Yeh SD, Yu IC, Wang RS, Chen YT, et al. Infertility with defective spermatogenesis and steroidogenesis in male mice lacking androgen receptor in Leydig cells. Endocrine. 2007;32: 96–106.

111. Tsai MY, Yeh SD, Wang RS, Yeh S, Zhang C, Lin HY, et al. Differential effects of spermatogenesis and fertility in mice lacking androgen receptor in individual testis cells. Proc Natl Acad Sci USA. 2006;103:18975–80.
112. De Gendt K, Swinnen JV, Saunders PT, Schoonjans L, Dewerchin M, Devos A, et al. A Sertoli cell-selective knockout of the androgen receptor causes spermatogenic arrest in meiosis. Proc Natl Acad Sci USA. 2004;101:1327–32.
113. Ferlin A, Vinanzi C, Garolla A, Selice R, Zuccarello D, Cazzadore C, et al. Male infertility and androgen receptor gene mutations: clinical features and identification of seven novel mutations. Clin Endocrinol (Oxf). 2006;65:606–10.
114. Greenland KJ, Zajac JD. Kennedy's disease: pathogenesis and clinical approaches. Intern Med J. 2004;34:279–86.
115. Finsterer J. Bulbar and spinal muscular atrophy (Kennedy's disease): a review. Eur J Neurol. 2009;16:556–61.
116. Lazaros L, Xita N, Kaponis A, Zikopoulos K, Sofikitis N, Georgiou I. Evidence for association of sex hormone-binding globulin and androgen receptor genes with semen quality. Andrologia. 2008;40:186–91.
117. Rajpert-De Meyts E, Leffers H, Petersen JH, Andersen AG, Carlsen E, Jorgensen N, et al. CAG repeat length in androgen-receptor gene and reproductive variables in fertile and infertile men. Lancet. 2002;359:44–6.
118. Yong EL, Loy CJ, Sim KS. Androgen receptor gene and male infertility. Hum Reprod Update. 2003;9:1–7.
119. Dowsing AT, Yong EL, Clark M, McLachlan RI, de Kretser DM, Trounson AO. Linkage between male infertility and trinucleotide repeat expansion in the androgen-receptor gene. Lancet. 1999;354:640–3.
120. Stouffs K, Lissens W, Tournaye H, Van Steirteghem A, Liebaers I. Possible role of USP26 in patients with severely impaired spermatogenesis. Eur J Hum Genet. 2005;13:336–40.
121. Nuti F, Krausz C. Gene polymorphisms/mutations relevant to abnormal spermatogenesis. Reprod Biomed Online. 2008;16: 504–13.
122. Akinloye O, Gromoll J, Callies C, Nieschlag E, Simoni M. Mutation analysis of the X-chromosome linked, testis-specific TAF7L gene in spermatogenic failure. Andrologia. 2007;39: 190–5.
123. Ravel C, El Houate B, Chantot S, Lourenco D, Dumaine A, Rouba H, et al. Haplotypes, mutations and male fertility: the story of the testis-specific ubiquitin protease USP26. Mol Hum Reprod. 2006;12:643–6.
124. Stouffs K, Willems A, Lissens W, Tournaye H, Van Steirteghem A, Liebaers I. The role of the testis-specific gene hTAF7L in the aetiology of male infertility. Mol Hum Reprod. 2006;12:263–7.
125. Fechner A, Fong S, McGovern P. A review of Kallmann syndrome: genetics, pathophysiology, and clinical management. Obstet Gynecol Surv. 2008;63:189–94.
126. Kim SH, Hu Y, Cadman S, Bouloux P. Diversity in fibroblast growth factor receptor 1 regulation: learning from the investigation of Kallmann syndrome. J Neuroendocrinol. 2008;20: 141–63.
127. Stuhrmann M, Dork T. CFTR gene mutations and male infertility. Andrologia. 2000;32: 71–83.
128. Dumur V, Gervais R, Rigot JM, Lafitte JJ, Manouvrier S, Biserte J, et al. Abnormal distribution of CF delta F508 allele in azoospermic men with congenital aplasia of epididymis and vas deferens. Lancet. 1990;336:512.
129. Gervais R, Dumur V, Rigot JM, Lafitte JJ, Roussel P, Claustres M, et al. High frequency of the R117H cystic fibrosis mutation in patients with congenital absence of the vas deferens. N Engl J Med. 1993;328:446–7.
130. Claustres M, Guittard C, Bozon D, Chevalier F, Verlingue C, Ferec C, et al. Spectrum of CFTR mutations in cystic fibrosis and in congenital absence of the vas deferens in France. Hum Mutat. 2000;16:143–56.

131. Daudin M, Bieth E, Bujan L, Massat G, Pontonnier F, Mieusset R. Congenital bilateral absence of the vas deferens: clinical characteristics, biological parameters, cystic fibrosis transmembrane conductance regulator gene mutations, and implications for genetic counseling. Fertil Steril. 2000;74:1164–74.
132. Cuppens H, Cassiman JJ. CFTR mutations and polymorphisms in male infertility. Int J Androl. 2004;27:251–6.
133. Cystic fibrosis mutation database. http://www.genet.sickkids.on.ca/cftr/StatisticsPage.html. Last updated 1 Apr 2010.
134. Dequeker E, Stuhrmann M, Morris MA, Casals T, Castellani C, Claustres M, et al. Best practice guidelines for molecular genetic diagnosis of cystic fibrosis and CFTR-related disorders—updated European recommendations. Eur J Hum Genet. 2009;17:51–65.
135. Chillon M, Casals T, Mercier B, Bassas L, Lissens W, Silber S, et al. Mutations in the cystic fibrosis gene in patients with congenital absence of the vas deferens. N Engl J Med. 1995;332: 1475–80.
136. Scotet V, Audrezet MP, Roussey M, Rault G, Dirou-Prigent A, Journel H, et al. Immunoreactive trypsin/DNA newborn screening for cystic fibrosis: should the R117H variant be included in CFTR mutation panels? Pediatrics. 2006;118:e1523–9.
137. Kiesewetter S, Macek Jr M, Davis C, Curristin SM, Chu CS, Graham C, et al. A mutation in CFTR produces different phenotypes depending on chromosomal background. Nat Genet. 1993;5: 274–8.
138. American College of Obstetricians and Gynecologists. Update on carrier screening for cystic fibrosis. ACOG Committee Opinion Number 325, December 2005. Obstet Gynecol. 2005; 106:1465–8.
139. Egozcue J, Blanco J, Anton E, Egozcue S, Sarrate Z, Vidal F. Genetic analysis of sperm and implications of severe male infertility—a review. Placenta. 2003;24(Suppl B):S62–5.
140. Bernardini L, Gianaroli L, Fortini D, Conte N, Magli C, Cavani S, et al. Frequency of hyper-, hypohaploidy and diploidy in ejaculate, epididymal and testicular germ cells of infertile patients. Hum Reprod. 2000;15:2165–72.
141. Vegetti W, Van Assche E, Frias A, Verheyen G, Bianchi MM, Bonduelle M, et al. Correlation between semen parameters and sperm aneuploidy rates investigated by fluorescence in-situ hybridization in infertile men. Hum Reprod. 2000;15:351–65.
142. Gonsalves J, Sun F, Schlegel PN, Turek PJ, Hopps CV, Greene C, et al. Defective recombination in infertile men. Hum Mol Genet. 2004;13:2875–83.
143. Sun F, Greene C, Turek PJ, Ko E, Rademaker A, Martin RH. Immunofluorescent synaptonemal complex analysis in azoospermic men. Cytogenet Genome Res. 2005;111:366–70.
144. Sun F, Turek P, Greene C, Ko E, Rademaker A, Martin RH. Abnormal progression through meiosis in men with nonobstructive azoospermia. Fertil Steril. 2007;87:565–71.
145. Topping D, Brown P, Judis L, Schwartz S, Seftel A, Thomas A, et al. Synaptic defects at meiosis I and non-obstructive azoospermia. Hum Reprod. 2006;21:3171–7.
146. Sanderson ML, Hassold TJ, Carrell DT. Proteins involved in meiotic recombination: a role in male infertility? Syst Biol Reprod Med. 2008;54:57–74.
147. Miyamoto T, Hasuike S, Yogev L, Maduro MR, Ishikawa M, Westphal H, et al. Azoospermia in patients heterozygous for a mutation in SYCP3. Lancet. 2003;362:1714–9.
148. Aarabi M, Modarressi MH, Soltanghoraee H, Behjati R, Amirjannati N, Akhondi MM. Testicular expression of synaptonemal complex protein 3 (SYCP3) messenger ribonucleic acid in 110 patients with nonobstructive azoospermia. Fertil Steril. 2006;86:325–31.
149. Meeks M, Bush A. Primary ciliary dyskinesia (PCD). Pediatr Pulmonol. 2000;29:307–16.
150. Loges NT, Olbrich H, Becker-Heck A, Haffner K, Heer A, Reinhard C, et al. Deletions and point mutations of LRRC50 cause primary ciliary dyskinesia due to dynein arm defects. Am J Hum Genet. 2009;85:883–9.
151. Moore A, Escudier E, Roger G, Tamalet A, Pelosse B, Marlin S, et al. RPGR is mutated in patients with a complex X linked phenotype combining primary ciliary dyskinesia and retinitis pigmentosa. J Med Genet. 2006;43:326–33.

152. Gerber PA, Kruse R, Hirchenhain J, Krussel JS, Neumann NJ. Pregnancy after laser-assisted selection of viable spermatozoa before intracytoplasmatic sperm injection in a couple with male primary cilia dyskinesia. Fertil Steril. 1826;2008(89):e9–12.

153. Dieterich K, Zouari R, Harbuz R, Vialard F, Martinez D, Bellayou H, et al. The Aurora Kinase C c.144delC mutation causes meiosis I arrest in men and is frequent in the North African population. Hum Mol Genet. 2009;18:1301–9.

154. Kimmins S, Crosio C, Kotaja N, Hirayama J, Monaco L, Hoog C, et al. Differential functions of the Aurora-B and Aurora-C kinases in mammalian spermatogenesis. Mol Endocrinol. 2007;21:726–39.

155. Lee C, Iafrate AJ, Brothman AR. Copy number variations and clinical cytogenetic diagnosis of constitutional disorders. Nat Genet. 2007;39:S48–54.

156. Anderson S, Bankier AT, Barrell BG, de Bruijn MH, Coulson AR, Drouin J, et al. Sequence and organization of the human mitochondrial genome. Nature. 1981;290:457–65.

157. Yakes FM, Van Houten B. Mitochondrial DNA damage is more extensive and persists longer than nuclear DNA damage in human cells following oxidative stress. Proc Natl Acad Sci USA. 1997;94:514–9.

158. Wei YH, Kao SH, Lee HC. Simultaneous increase of mitochondrial DNA deletions and lipid peroxidation in human aging. Ann N Y Acad Sci. 1996;786:24–43.

159. Rovio AT, Marchington DR, Donat S, Schuppe HC, Abel J, Fritsche E, et al. Mutations at the mitochondrial DNA polymerase (POLG) locus associated with male infertility. Nat Genet. 2001;29:261–2.

160. St John JC, Jokhi RP, Barratt CL. The impact of mitochondrial genetics on male infertility. Int J Androl. 2005;28:65–73.

161. Ropp PA, Copeland WC. Cloning and characterization of the human mitochondrial DNA polymerase, DNA polymerase gamma. Genomics. 1996;36:449–58.

162. Surani MA. Reprogramming of genome function through epigenetic inheritance. Nature. 2001;414:122–8.

163. Wallace JA, Orr-Weaver TL. Replication of heterochromatin: insights into mechanisms of epigenetic inheritance. Chromosoma. 2005;114:389–402.

164. Margueron R, Trojer P, Reinberg D. The key to development: interpreting the histone code? Curr Opin Genet Dev. 2005;15: 163–76.

165. Kim VN. Small RNAs just got bigger: Piwi-interacting RNAs (piRNAs) in mammalian testes. Genes Dev. 2006;20:1993–7.

166. Papaioannou MD, Nef S. microRNAs in the testis: building up male fertility. J Androl. 2010;31:26–33.

167. Reik W, Dean W, Walter J. Epigenetic reprogramming in mammalian development. Science. 2001;293:1089–93.

168. Ferguson-Smith AC, Surani MA. Imprinting and the epigenetic asymmetry between parental genomes. Science. 2001;293: 1086–9.

169. Guerrero-Bosagna C, Sabat P, Valladares L. Environmental signaling and evolutionary change: can exposure of pregnant mammals to environmental estrogens lead to epigenetically induced evolutionary changes in embryos? Evol Dev. 2005;7:341–50.

170. MacPhee DG. Epigenetics and epimutagens: some new perspectives on cancer, germ line effects and endocrine disrupters. Mutat Res. 1998;400:369–79.

171. Guerrero-Bosagna CM, Skinner MK. Epigenetic transgenerational effects of endocrine disruptors on male reproduction. Semin Reprod Med. 2009;27:403–8.

172. Bukulmez O. Does assisted reproductive technology cause birth defects? Curr Opin Obstet Gynecol. 2009;21:260–4.

173. Marques CJ, Carvalho F, Sousa M, Barros A. Genomic imprinting in disruptive spermatogenesis. Lancet. 2004;363:1700–2.

174. Marques CJ, Costa P, Vaz B, Carvalho F, Fernandes S, Barros A, et al. Abnormal methylation of imprinted genes in human sperm is associated with oligozoospermia. Mol Hum Reprod. 2008;14: 67–74.

175. Trasler JM. Epigenetics in spermatogenesis. Mol Cell Endocrinol. 2009;306:33–6.

176. Aoki VW, Emery BR, Carrell DT. Global sperm deoxyribonucleic acid methylation is unaffected in protamine-deficient infertile males. Fertil Steril. 2006;86:1541–3.
177. Aoki VW, Emery BR, Liu L, Carrell DT. Protamine levels vary between individual sperm cells of infertile human males and correlate with viability and DNA integrity. J Androl. 2006;27: 890–8.
178. Aoki VW, Liu L, Carrell DT. A novel mechanism of protamine expression deregulation highlighted by abnormal protamine transcript retention in infertile human males with sperm protamine deficiency. Mol Hum Reprod. 2006;12:41–50.
179. Paldi A. Genomic imprinting: could the chromatin structure be the driving force? Curr Top Dev Biol. 2003;53:115–38.
180. Hammoud SS, Purwar J, Pflueger C, Cairns BR, Carrell DT. Alterations in sperm DNA methylation patterns at imprinted loci in two classes of infertility. Fertil Steril. 2010;94(5):1728–33.
181. Barratt CL, Aitken RJ, Bjorndahl L, Carrell DT, de Boer P, Kvist U, et al. Sperm DNA: organization, protection and vulnerability: from basic science to clinical applications—a position report. Hum Reprod. 2010;25:824–38.
182. Hotaling JM, Walsh TJ. Male infertility: a risk factor for testicular cancer. Nat Rev Urol. 2009;6:550–6.
183. Walsh TJ, Croughan MS, Schembri M, Chan JM, Turek PJ. Increased risk of testicular germ cell cancer among infertile men. Arch Intern Med. 2009;169:351–6.
184. Dieckmann KP, Pichlmeier U. Clinical epidemiology of testicular germ cell tumors. World J Urol. 2004;22:2–14.
185. Nathanson KL, Kanetsky PA, Hawes R, Vaughn DJ, Letrero R, Tucker K, et al. The Y deletion gr/gr and susceptibility to testicular germ cell tumor. Am J Hum Genet. 2005;77: 1034–43.
186. Kojima Y, Mizuno K, Kohri K, Hayashi Y. Advances in molecular genetics of cryptorchidism. Urology. 2009;74:571–8.
187. Yan W. Male infertility caused by spermiogenic defects: lessons from gene knockouts. Mol Cell Endocrinol. 2009;306:24–32.
188. Matzuk MM, Lamb DJ. The biology of infertility: research advances and clinical challenges. Nat Med. 2008;14:1197–213.
189. Meng MV, Black LD, Cha I, Ljung BM, Pera RA, Turek PJ. Impaired spermatogenesis in men with congenital absence of the vas deferens. Hum Reprod. 2001;16:529–33.
190. Schlegel PN, Shin D, Goldstein M. Urogenital anomalies in men with congenital absence of the vas deferens. J Urol. 1996;155: 1644–8.
191. Kim ED, Gilbaugh 3rd JH, Patel VR, Turek PJ, Lipshultz LI. Testis biopsies frequently demonstrate sperm in men with azoospermia and significantly elevated follicle-stimulating hormone levels. J Urol. 1997;157:144–6.
192. Schlegel PN, Palermo GD, Goldstein M, Menendez S, Zaninovic N, Veeck LL, et al. Testicular sperm extraction with intracytoplasmic sperm injection for nonobstructive azoospermia. Urology. 1997;49:435–40.
193. Brugh 3rd VM, Maduro MR, Lamb DJ. Genetic disorders and infertility. Urol Clin North Am. 2003;30:143–52.
194. O'Bryan MK, de Kretser D. Mouse models for genes involved in impaired spermatogenesis. Int J Androl. 2006;29:76–89. discussion 105-8.
195. Manzini S, Vargiolu A, Stehle IM, Bacci ML, Cerrito MG, Giovannoni R, et al. Genetically modified pigs produced with a nonviral episomal vector. Proc Natl Acad Sci USA. 2006;103: 17672–7.
196. Boekelheide K, Sigman M. Is gene therapy for the treatment of male infertility feasible? Nat Clin Pract Urol. 2008;5:590–3.
197. Lamb DJ. Would gene therapy for the treatment of male infertility be safe? Nat Clin Pract Urol. 2008;5:594–5.
198. Brinster RL. Germ line stem cell transplantation and transgenesis. Science. 2002;296: 2174–6.
199. Brinster RL. Male germ line stem cells: from mice to men. Science. 2007;316:404–5.

200. Nayernia K, Nolte J, Michelmann HW, Lee JH, Rathsack K, Drusenheimer N, et al. In vitro-differentiated embryonic stem cells give rise to male gametes that can generate offspring mice. Dev Cell. 2006;11:125–32.
201. Ryu BY, Orwig KE, Oatley JM, Lin CC, Chang LJ, Avarbock MR, et al. Efficient generation of transgenic rats through the male germ line using lentiviral transduction and transplantation of spermatogonial stem cells. J Androl. 2007;28:353–60.
202. Deepinder F, Chowdary HT, Agarwal A. Role of metabolomic analysis of biomarkers in the management of male infertility. Expert Rev Mol Diagn. 2007;7:351–8.
203. He Z, Chan WY, Dym M. Microarray technology offers a novel tool for the diagnosis and identification of therapeutic targets for male infertility. Reproduction. 2006;132:11–9.
204. Lin YH, Lin YM, Teng YN, Hsieh TY, Lin YS, Kuo PL. Identification of ten novel genes involved in human spermatogenesis by microarray analysis of testicular tissue. Fertil Steril. 2006;86:1650–8.
205. Martinez-Heredia J, de Mateo S, Vidal-Taboada JM, Ballesca JL, Oliva R. Identification of proteomic differences in asthenozoospermic sperm samples. Hum Reprod. 2008;23:783–91.

Chapter 5
Ejaculatory Dysfunction and Vasodynamics

Aleksey P. Ignatov and Paul J. Turek

Ejaculation begins approximately 12 months after the onset of puberty in the male. While its importance to reproductive fitness is clear, current knowledge of the physiology of ejaculation is limited. This chapter reviews the events of ejaculation, its anatomic and neuroanatomic underpinnings, the range of ejaculatory disorders, and clinical methods for evaluating and treating ejaculatory disorders. Our current understanding of reproductive tract physiology and function as well as ejaculatory duct obstruction (EDO) is also reviewed.

Physiology of Ejaculation

The Events

Ejaculation is two distinct processes: emission and ejaculation [1]. Although not technically considered a separate event, pre-ejaculation, occurring during foreplay, involves closure of the bladder neck that prevents retrograde ejaculation and contractions of the prostate that lubricate the urethra. Importantly, ejaculation is also distinct from orgasm, which is a purely cerebral cortical event. Most often, these two processes are coincident.

Emission combines the transport of both seminal fluid and sperm through peristalsis from the cauda epididymis, vas deferens, seminal vesicles, and prostate into the prostatic urethra. During seminal emission, the ampullary vasa deferentia contents are transported into the prostatic urethra and mixed with prostatic fluid. The expulsion of seminal vesicle contents into the prostatic urethra completes the emission

A.P. Ignatov, BS (✉) • P.J. Turek, MD, FACS, FRSM
The Turek Clinic, 55 Francisco Street, Suite 300,
San Francisco, CA 94133, USA
e-mail: apignatov@yahoo.com; drpaulturek@gmail.com

S.J. Parekattil, A. Agarwal (eds.), *Male Infertility for the Clinician*,
© Springer Science+Business Media New York 2013

phase. Subsequently, ejaculation is the forceful expulsion of the seminal mixture from the urethra. The ejaculate is expelled from the urethra in a series of spurts, 0.8 s apart, caused by the rhythmic contractions of the ischiocavernosus, bulbospongiosus, and other associated periurethral muscles [2]. The entire process is governed by the autonomic and somatic nervous systems and is considered a spinal reflex.

Neural Control

Control of the ejaculatory reflex is mediated by the sympathetic and somatic nervous systems [3]. Control of emission involves mainly the sympathetic nervous system while ejaculation is governed largely by the somatic nervous system. Efferent sympathetic nerves emerge from the thoracolumbar spine at T10–L2 and then merge to form the lumbar sympathetic ganglia that encircle the aorta. These nerves subsequently combine in the midline below the aortic bifurcation to form the superior hypogastric plexus (Fig. 5.1). Ultimately, these adrenergic nerves terminate as postganglionic fibers that innervate the bladder neck, prostate, vasa deferentia, and seminal vesicles [4]. The sympathetic outflow generated by these nerves is responsible for closure of the bladder neck and seminal emission.

The muscular expulsion of the ejaculate is mediated by somatic motor efferent nerves derived from the perineal branch of the pudendal nerve (S2–S4). Additional control is provided by relaxation of the external urethral sphincter and the urogenital diaphragm. Interruption at any point in this reflex arc may result in disordered ejaculation.

Definitions

Aspermia: Disordered ejaculation characterized by an inability to produce semen, despite the occurrence of climax.

Azoospermia: The absence of sperm in the ejaculate.

Anejaculation: The failure of ejaculation, including an absence of seminal emission and ejaculation. Climax is usually absent as well.

Premature ejaculation (*ejaculatio praecox*): Ejaculation which always or nearly always occurs prior to or within about 1 min of vaginal penetration, and inability to delay ejaculation on all or nearly all vaginal penetrations, and negative personal consequences, such as distress, bother, frustration, and/or the avoidance of sexual intimacy.

Delayed ejaculation (anorgasmia): A form of sexual dysfunction characterized by the inability to achieve climax, or an extreme delay in achieving climax and ejaculation.

Retrograde ejaculation: Ejaculation of semen in reverse direction into the bladder during climax due to failure of bladder neck closure.

Congenital anorgasmia: Failure of ejaculation as primary, lifelong event.

Ejaculatory anhedonia: Ejaculation associated with a lack of pleasure.

Fig. 5.1 Innervation of the
male reproductive tract
showing sympathetic and
parasympathetic nerves and
somatic innervation (From
Master and Turek [1], with
permission)

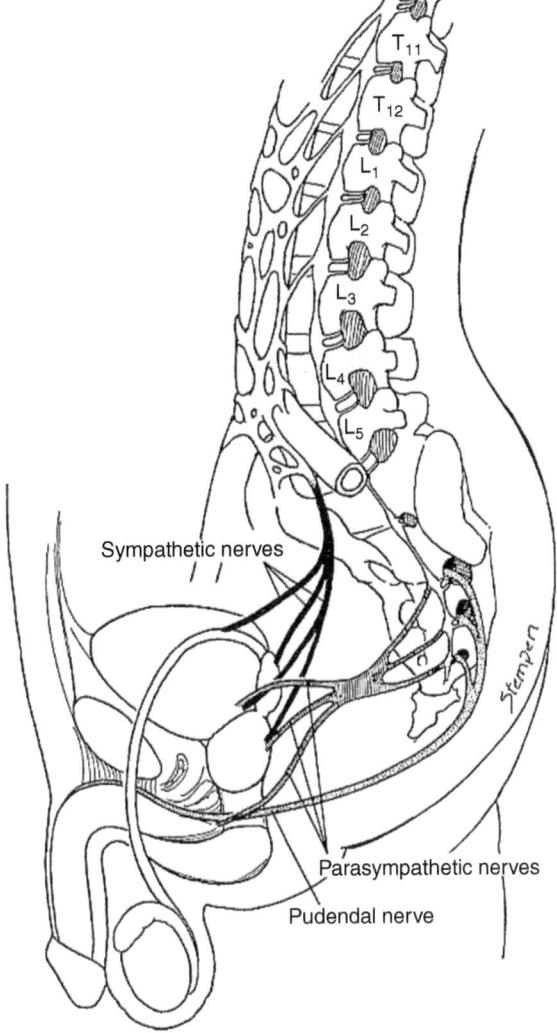

Evaluation

History

The cornerstone of evaluating ejaculatory dysfunction is a detailed patient history.
Critical information to obtain from the history is whether or not normal ejaculation
was ever present. This suggests a primary (congenital) or secondary (acquired) cause
of sexual dysfunction. In addition, a thorough review of the medical and surgical history can be informative regarding possible neurologic etiologies for disordered

ejaculation. Finally, a careful review of current medications such as alpha-blockers or antidepressants can suggest the presence of drug-induced ejaculatory dysfunction [1].

Physical Examination

A complete physical examination should include an assessment of body habitus and secondary sex characteristics, a screening neurological examination, and a thorough genital examination. Testis and epididymis size and consistency, penile length and morphology, and genital birth defects such as hypospadias, epispadias, or surgical scars suggestive of their correction should be noted. Palpation of scrotum for masses and a check for the presence of the vas deferens should also be performed. A rectal examination noting rectal tone and any masses is also important.

Laboratory Evaluation

An attempt should be made to procure a semen analysis. In cases where no ejaculate is obtained, a post-ejaculate urine sample should be retrieved and assessed for the presence of sperm, suggesting retrograde ejaculation. Blood testosterone, prolactin, and serum follicle-stimulating hormone (FSH) levels should also be assessed because low ejaculate volumes may be caused by hypoandrogenism. Further diagnostic evaluation may include imaging with transrectal ultrasonography (TRUS) to define anatomical or structural abnormalities in the prostate, seminal vesicles, or ejaculatory duct complex. If indicated, formal ejaculatory duct chromotubation, seminal vesiculography, and ejaculatory duct manometry can be performed to detect subtle ejaculatory duct abnormalities [5].

Genetic Testing

Patients with disordered ejaculation and a history of infertility or with suspected congenital abnormalities such as congenital absence of the vas deferens (CAVD) or ejaculatory duct obstruction (EDO) should be counseled on appropriate genetic testing for cystic fibrosis transmembrane regulatory (CFTR) gene mutations [6].

Management of Ejaculatory Disorders

Anatomic

Bladder Neck Incompetence

A patent bladder neck is most commonly the consequence of an incompetent internal urethral (bladder neck) sphincter. The ensuing "dry ejaculate" is due to retrograde ejaculation. It can be caused by α-blocker medication for prostate enlargement or hypertension, diabetic neuropathy, neurologic disorders such as spina bifida or multiple sclerosis, or other congenital anatomic abnormalities. It is also a common postsurgical complication of transurethral prostatectomy (TURP) [7]. Interestingly, from the patient perspective, retrograde ejaculation after TURP is often confused with anorgasmia or erectile dysfunction [8].

If retrograde ejaculation is drug induced, the offending medication should be discontinued. With neurological causes such as that associated with diabetes, alpha agonist therapy can help "close" the bladder neck and encourage antegrade ejaculation [1, 9]. Reversal after TURP is difficult. However, if fertility is sought in men after TURP, sperm in the postmasturbatory urine can be used with intrauterine insemination (IUI) or in vitro fertilization (IVF) for paternity.

Müllerian Duct Cyst

Persistence of remnants of the Müllerian ducts may exist as midline cysts associated with the prostatic utricle and ejaculatory ducts in men. If significant in size, such cysts may be occlusive and produce a low-volume ejaculate due to ejaculatory duct compression. This diagnosis is confirmed by TRUS and further investigation of ejaculatory anatomy and function with chromotubation or manometry [5, 10]. Stones, calcification, ejaculatory duct agenesis, and seminal vasculopathy resulting in acontractile, dysfunctional seminal vesicles may present similarly [11].

In patients with confirmed obstruction, transurethral unroofing of cysts, drainage of stones, or recanalizing the ejaculatory ducts effectively treats the problem [12]. In men with functional but not obstructive disorders of the reproductive tract, surgical procedures are not indicated and have no clinical value [5].

Congenital Bilateral Absence of the Vas Deferens/Cystic Fibrosis

Among men with cystic fibrosis, 99% also have Wolffian duct abnormalities that typically cause low ejaculate volume. There may be atresia or agenesis of the vas deferens, seminal vesicles, or ejaculatory ducts with this diagnosis. Low-volume ejaculation is also associated with a form fruste of cystic fibrosis, termed CAVD [11]. In this condition, there may be absence of the vas deferens but without other, systemic manifestations of cystic fibrosis.

The ejaculatory disorder associated with cystic fibrosis and CAVD is currently irreversible. Parenthood, however, can be achieved with surgical sperm retrieval procedures and assisted reproduction.

Ejaculatory Duct Obstruction

The combination of low-volume ejaculate, painful ejaculation, hematospermia, and perineal or testicular pain is highly suggestive of EDO. The diagnosis is supported by the finding of a normal physical examination and a semen analysis that shows a volume <2.0 mL, with a seminal pH < 7.2, and no sperm or fructose present. Partial EDO, a variant, is harder to diagnose, but typically presents with low normal ejaculate volume and disproportionately low sperm motility. Confirmatory diagnostic tests include TRUS that shows dilated seminal vesicles (>1.5 cm) or dilated ejaculatory ducts (>2.3 mm) in association with a cyst, calcification, or stones along the ducts [13, 14]. Recently, it has become clear that *static* imaging such as TRUS cannot reliably differentiate true physical obstruction from functional disorders of the reproductive tract. TRUS, although sensitive, is not specific for the diagnosis of EDO [10]. As such, adjunctive procedures such as seminal vesicle aspiration [15], seminal vesiculography, and chromotubation can further delineate the diagnosis. Such "functional" testing has been suggested before definitive surgery on the ejaculatory duct complex [10]. To this end, a prospective study of these three adjunctive techniques in EDO patients revealed that patency with chromotubation was the most accurate way to diagnose complete or incomplete EDO [10].

With these considerations in mind and based on the concept of bladder urodynamics to assess bladder outlet obstruction, we recently described the technique of ejaculatory duct manometry to confirm the diagnosis of EDO (Fig. 5.2) [5]. This technique stemmed from the idea that the varying flow resistance patterns encountered with antegrade chromotubation in EDO patients could be more precisely quantified. We hypothesized that measuring ED "opening pressures," defined as the pressure above which fluid enters the prostatic urethra, could distinguish among the various forms of EDO. Indeed, in a prospective, comparative study of fertile men (vasectomy reversals) and men with confirmed EDO, ejaculatory duct opening pressures were significantly higher in untreated EDO patients (mean 116 cmH_2O) compared to fertile men (mean 33 cmH_2O) (Fig. 5.3). In addition, post-TURED duct opening pressures fell to values similar to controls. The study concluded that (1) fertile patients have consistent and low ED opening pressures with a normal pressure defined as <45 cm H_2O, (2) infertile men with EDO have significantly higher ED pressures, (3) opening pressures after EDO treatment can be lowered to that of controls, and (4) patients with suspected EDO may have other kinds of underlying pathology that will not respond to ED resection, including urethral strictures. From this analysis, ED manometry currently has the most potential to differentiate complete from partial and physical from functional forms of EDO.

Men with EDO can be treated with a transurethral resection or incision of the ejaculatory ducts, which is very effective at increasing semen volume and restoring sperm flow [13]. In cases of absence of reproductive tract organs, no remedy is currently available.

Neuropathic

Spinal Cord Injury

Most patients with spinal cord injury are young men who have sustained traumatic interruption of nerve pathways that modulate ejaculation. Spinal cord lesions at or below the

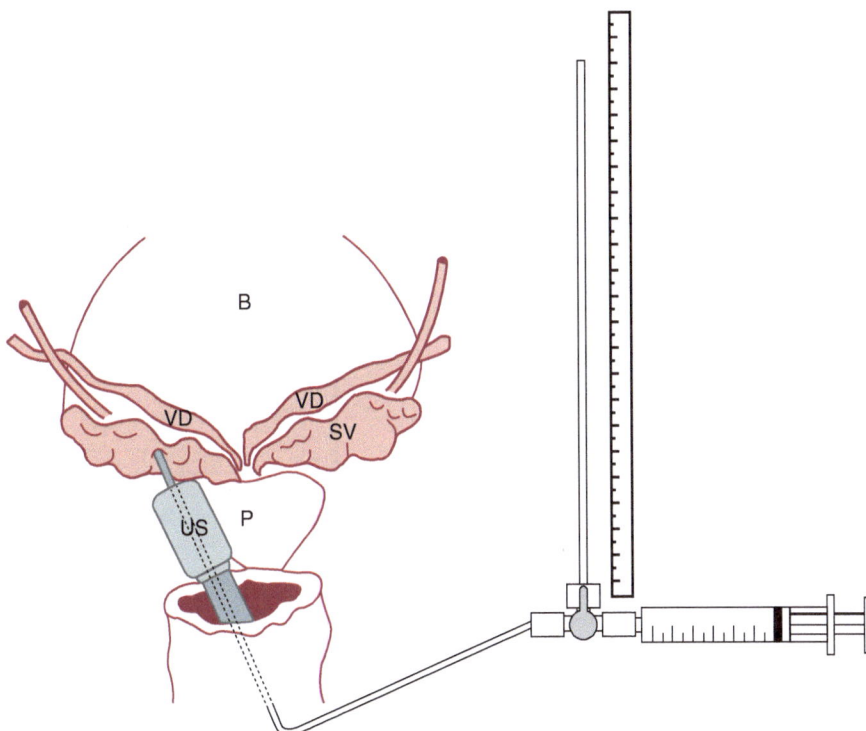

Fig. 5.2 The ejaculatory duct manometry device. Schematic representation of the intravenous tubing manometer used to measure ejaculatory duct pressure in EDO patients. After intubation of the seminal vesicle with a spinal needle attached to a three-way stopcock, the seminal vesicle is injected with saline/indigo carmine (chromotubation). The pressure at which fluid begins to traverse the ejaculatory duct orifice into the prostatic urethra cystoscopically is the "opening pressure." The pressure within the seminal vesicle is monitored by the height of the column of fluid within the IV tubing (From Eisenberg et al. [5], with permission)

level of T10–L2 level commonly lead to complete loss of ejaculation with preserved erections, whereas injuries above the T10 spinal level generally retain the ejaculatory reflex arc as the peripheral efferent nerves from T10–L2 and S2–S4 are intact. The integrity of this reflex arc can be confirmed by demonstrating an intact bulbocavernosus reflex and the ability to perform hip flexion, both of which predict successful ejaculation when sensory afferent input is increased to suprathreshold levels [16].

Fertility and paternity are commonly achieved in affected patients with the use of assisted reproductive technology in association with penile vibratory stimulation (PVS) [17] or rectal probe electroejaculation (EEJ) [18–20]. Patients with spinal cord lesions above T4 also are prone to autonomic dysreflexia from penile stimulation. Symptoms of autonomic dysreflexia include hypertension, bradycardia, sweating, chills, and headache. In some cases, autonomic dysreflexia can lead to dangerously high blood pressures and can lead to stroke, seizure, or death. Pretreatment with an oral calcium channel blocker for prophylactic management of these symptoms is advised. For patients with lower spinal cord lesions (below T10)

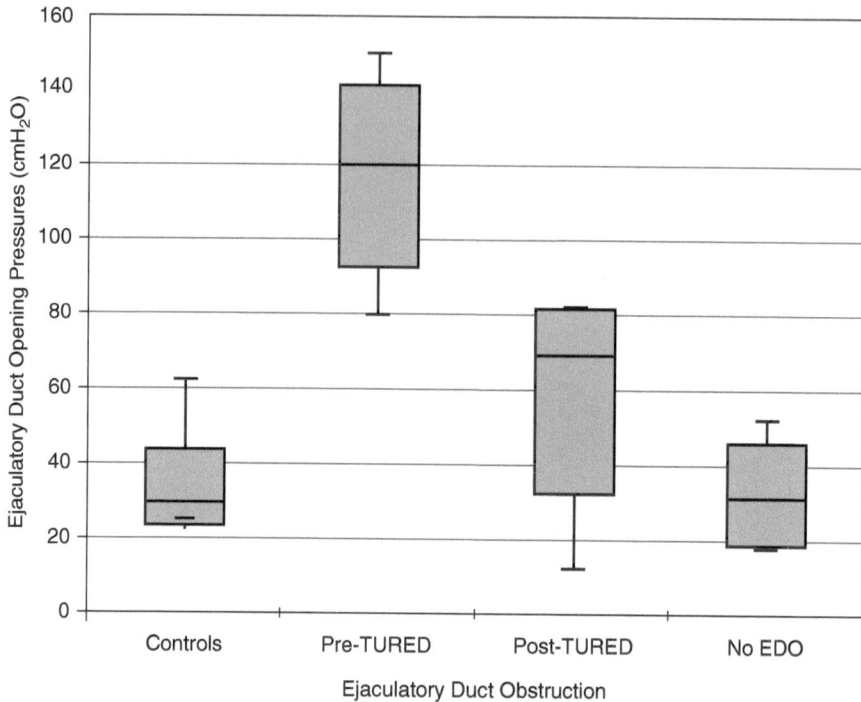

Fig. 5.3 Ejaculatory duct opening pressures in fertile men and EDO patients. *Gray boxes* represent the first to third interquartile range for measured values. *Black horizontal lines* represent the median, and whiskers represent the absolute range of values. Ejaculatory duct pressures in EDO patients were significantly higher than controls ($p < 0.001$) or post-TURED ($p < 0.001$) patients. Pressures after TURED were not significantly different from controls or the "No EDO" group. The "No EDO" group represents ejaculatory ducts evaluated and deemed clinically not to harbor EDO (From Eisenberg et al. [5], with permission)

in whom penile vibratory therapy fails, EEJ is an excellent alternative to achieve ejaculation [21]. For patients who fail electroejaculation, surgical sperm retrieval provides an excellent alternative for paternity [22].

Diabetes Mellitus

Long-standing diabetes is associated with genitourinary autonomic neuropathy. About 87% of type I diabetics have evidence of bladder dysfunction, and erectile dysfunction is observed in 35–75% of affected males [23]. The associated ejaculatory dysfunction may manifest as either retrograde ejaculation or total anejaculation depending on the degree of sympathetic autonomic neuropathy. This dysfunction results from incomplete closure of the bladder neck during ejaculation (retrograde ejaculation) or complete neurogenic "paralysis" of the reproductive tract smooth musculature (anejaculation). In cases of complete anejaculation, the postmasturbatory urine contains no sperm [24].

To aid in conception, sympathomimetic drugs may be taken to stimulate bladder neck closure in retrograde ejaculation and produce an antegrade ejaculate [9]. Because most sympathomimetics will exhibit tachyphylaxis with prolonged use, their administration should be limited to the window of timed intercourse around ovulation. Unlike with retrograde ejaculation, diabetic patients with anejaculation are more difficult to treat. If there is no conversion to retrograde or antegrade ejaculation with sympathomimetics, EEJ can be effective to induce a useful ejaculate [21]. Of note, patients with long-standing diabetes may have calcified vasa deferentia and seminal vesicles that are unable to contract and propel sperm. In such cases, surgical sperm retrieval is necessary to treat associate fertility issues [25].

Postsurgical

In general, retroperitoneal or pelvic procedures that disrupt the sympathetic nerves that course along the aorta, especially near the aortic bifurcation (hypogastric plexus), may result in ejaculatory dysfunction. The spectrum of the functional defects correlates to the degree and severity of nerve damage. Retrograde ejaculation, failure of ejaculation, or failure of ejaculation along with failure of seminal emission are all possible, depending on the degree of injury [1].

Approximately two-thirds of men will have retrograde ejaculation following TURP, and one quarter to one-third of patients will have a similar issue after bladder neck incision due to incomplete bladder neck closure. Major abdominopelvic surgery, such as colorectal resection for malignancy, ileoanal anastomosis for inflammatory bowel disease, repair of abdominal aortic aneurysm, aortoiliac bypass grafting, and retroperitoneal lymphadenectomy for testicular cancer, may lead to some damage of the lumbar sympathetic ganglia and/or the superior hypogastric plexus and result in retrograde ejaculation or anejaculation [26, 27].

The operative procedure that historically has resulted in the highest frequency of ejaculatory disorders is retroperitoneal lymph node dissection performed largely as curative treatment for metastatic testicular cancer. In its original form, the operation consisted of a bilateral suprahilar extended dissection of retroperitoneal nodes and almost uniformly resulted in ejaculatory dysfunction. Advances in surgical technique combined with newer limited surgical dissection templates have decreased the incidence of ejaculatory dysfunction [28–30].

Radical prostatectomy is another major procedure that results in functional anejaculation because the prostate and seminal vesicles are excised. Other operative procedures that can cause ejaculatory dysfunction include abdominoperineal operations for rectal cancer and spine surgeries performed anteriorly (transabdominally), which are associated with rates of ejaculatory disorders of approximately 14% [31].

Pediatric congenital anomalies of the pelvis are associated with anejaculation and retrograde ejaculation later in life. Ejaculatory disorders in these patients can be caused by the anatomic nature of the pelvic anomaly (cloacal exstrophy, imperforate anus) or the associated surgical procedure needed for its correction (exstrophy/epispadias repair, bladder neck reconstruction) [1].

The reversal of ejaculatory disorders from surgical sympathetic nerve disruption is difficult. In general, treatment with α-adrenergic stimulants can be attempted [9]. In a few instances, therapy can convert a failure of emission into simply retrograde ejaculation, or convert retrograde into antegrade ejaculation. Success with drug therapy depends on the integrity and number of residual sympathetic nerve fibers that innervate the seminal vesicles, vasa deferentia, and bladder neck areas.

If medical therapy is unsuccessful, EEJ is required to induce ejaculation and to harvest sperm for use in assisted reproductive technology. When performed under a light general anesthesia in the sensate patient, this procedure uses rhythmically applied, graded increases in voltage (0–25 V) to a rectal probe to cause contraction of the seminal vesicles and vasa ampullae directly and to induce the ejaculatory reflex. Ejaculation is obtained in virtually all men with surgically induced ejaculatory disorders through this technique [21].

Neurologic Disorders

The entire spectrum of ejaculatory disorders, ranging from premature ejaculation to anejaculation, is associated with demyelinating and inflammatory neurologic diseases including multiple sclerosis and transverse myelitis [32]. Patients with spinal dysraphism disorders (e.g., myelodysplasia, myelomeningocele, spina bifida) also harbor many of the same ejaculatory disorders. Defects above the T10–T11 cord level commonly are associated with anejaculation, whereas defects below this level allow emission without ejaculation. Patients with sacral lesions are generally spared any ejaculatory dysfunction [33].

Neurostimulatory methods may be used to induce ejaculation in men with neurogenic anejaculation. The most commonly used methods to induce ejaculation in men with neurologic disorders are PVS and EEJ [3]. PVS involves placing a vibrator on the dorsum or frenulum of the glans penis [17]. Mechanical stimulation produced by the vibrator recruits the ejaculatory reflex to induce ejaculation [34]. This method is more effective in men with an intact ejaculatory reflex, that is, men with a level of injury above the T10 cord level. Individuals who do not respond to PVS are often candidates for EEJ [35, 36]. EEJ is performed with the patient in the lateral decubitus position. A probe is placed in the rectum, and electrodes on the probe are oriented toward the prostate and seminal vesicles. Current delivered through the probe stimulates nerves that lead to emission of semen.

Pharmacologic

Antidepressants

Many common medications can cause ejaculatory dysfunction. Antidepressants, including the tricyclic antidepressants, monoamine oxidase inhibitors (MAOIs), and the newer selective serotonin reuptake inhibitors (SSRIs), are associated with sexual dysfunction and disordered ejaculation [37]. Sexual dysfunction resulting from these medications may include hypoactive sexual desire, erectile dysfunction, and delayed ejaculation. It is thought that these side effects are due to elevated central nervous system levels of serotonin (SSRIs) or catecholamines (tricyclics) [38]. In most patients, discontinuation of antidepressant therapy will restore normal sexual function.

Alpha-Adrenergic Antagonists

Both the transport of seminal fluid within the reproductive tract and bladder neck closure are controlled by α-adrenergic nerves. Therefore, α-adrenergic antagonists, given for hypertension or prostatic hypertrophy, may inhibit both seminal emission and bladder neck closure [39]. In either case, the result presents as a low-volume or dry ejaculate. In general, the sensation of orgasm is normal or nearly normal. Treatment should be directed at removal of these drugs.

Functional

Premature or Early Ejaculation

Premature ejaculation (PE) is defined as ejaculation which always or nearly always occurs prior to or within 1 min of vaginal penetration, the inability to delay ejaculation on all or nearly all vaginal penetrations and is associated with negative personal consequences, such as distress, bother, frustration, and/or the avoidance of sexual intimacy [40]. The incidence of this problem is high, affecting 35% of men between the ages of 18 and 59, and it is the most common form of male sexual dysfunction [41]. Given how commonly PE is reported, this raises the question of whether it is truly an organic, treatable disease, or merely a consequence of normal sexual function associated with abnormal expectations. Implicated etiologic factors include sexual anxiety and penile skin hypersensitivity, although there is little consensus regarding exact causes [42].

The goal of therapy for PE is to increase patient control over the ejaculation process by decreasing penile sensitivity and by adjusting the behavioral response. Treatments include oral medication, local anesthetic therapy, and sexual therapy. The most effective treatments are behavioral as drug therapy demands high compliance rates that may not be achievable with younger men who do not otherwise take medications.

Drugs that delay ejaculation are logical choices for PE treatment, and clinical trials have shown that SSRIs can effectively prolong the time to ejaculation [43–48]. However, the increase in latency time to ejaculation varies widely depending on the selected medication. Paroxetine, fluoxetine, sertraline, and clomipramine are the best tolerated medications for PE and have been observed to increase latency times to anywhere from 2 to 10 min. Treatment regimens that employ tricyclic antidepressants are generally limited by side effects such as drowsiness and insomnia.

Topical anesthetic agents such as 2% lidocaine jelly and topical 2.5% lidocaine/2.5% prilocaine cream (EMLA) [49] have been shown to decrease penile sensitivity and prolong ejaculatory latency [50]. When applied to the penile skin with a condom for 30 min before intercourse, EMLA cream has been observed to increase the time to ejaculation in 80% of men. Newer topical medications are now under investigation and include a quick-acting, local anesthetic spray and SS-cream, a herbal preparation that has been demonstrated to increase ejaculatory latency [51].

Given the frequency of PE among younger, sexually active men, durable success is an important treatment goal. Therefore, medical therapy should always be combined with behavioral modification therapy [52]. The goal of sexual therapy is to provide the patient with greater control over, and satisfaction from, sexual stimulation. Typically, the sensation of ejaculatory inevitability must be explained to patients so that they can understand, observe, and ultimately control the sensations experienced and enhance sexual pleasure. Typically, patients and their partners undergo a 6- to 20-week course of therapy in which they learn systematic relaxation techniques and acquire skills to perform prolonged self- or partner-performed sexual stimulation without the demand for erection or ejaculation. Subsequently, patients are instructed in methods of passive coitus without thrusting and, eventually, coitus with pelvic thrusting. Partner participation and cooperation with such therapy is critical for long-term success.

Seminal Megavesicles

Enlarged seminal vesicles without evidence of physical obstruction, also known as seminal megavesicles, have been reported in association with polycystic kidney disease and after surgical failure of transurethral resection of ejaculatory ducts. Dilation of the seminal vesicles may mimic obstruction of the ejaculatory ducts, and these conditions are not easily distinguishable on TRUS imaging. In a study by Hendry and coworkers, six azoospermic men with adult polycystic kidney disease had enlarged seminal vesicles. When these men were studied with seminal vesiculography, there was no obstruction found [53]. In addition, all attempts at transurethral resection of the ejaculatory ducts failed. We hypothesized that this abnormality may partly explain why 25–30% of men with presumed EDO fail to improve after TURED [54]. To demonstrate this concept, we constructed an in vivo rat model and assessed the urodynamic properties of active and resting compliance within the seminal vesicle. We found that seminal vesicles, as hollow organs lined with smooth muscle, act urodynamically like urinary bladders, thus lending credence to the concept that seminal vesicle myopathies, like bladder myopathies, can exist and result in "functional" obstruction of the reproductive tract [55]. Similar to neurogenic bladders, to date, no effective treatments have been shown to correct this type of organ dysfunction.

Retrograde Ejaculation

The true incidence of retrograde ejaculation is difficult to estimate, but approximately 14–18% of patients with ejaculatory disorders harbor this diagnosis [56]. Among 1,400 infertile couples, 0.7% of men presented with retrograde ejaculation [57]. This diagnosis is relatively straightforward and requires a history of low-volume or dry ejaculate, with a postmasturbatory voided urine sample demonstrating sperm. Systemic diseases such as diabetes mellitus, medications including alpha-blockers, neurogenic causes such as spinal cord injury, multiple sclerosis or spina bifida, and surgical treatments such as retroperitoneal lymph node dissection and transurethral prostate resection can all cause retrograde ejaculation.

Several treatment options are available for retrograde ejaculation. If the condition is drug induced, the offending medication should be discontinued if possible. In many patients without scar tissue at the bladder neck, oral therapy can be attempted with alpha-adrenergic agonists [9]. Approximately one-third of men will respond to this therapy. Sympathomimetic agents, such as imipramine, phenylpropanolamine, or pseudoephedrine, have been used with schedules ranging from interval dosing to as needed dosing immediately prior to coitus [58]. Generally, oral medical therapy is limited by side effects, including dizziness, weakness, nausea, sweating, or palpitations. If oral therapy fails, sperm-harvesting from the bladder urine obtained on post-ejaculate urination or by catheterization can be used with IUI or IVF to achieve family building goals.

Anejaculation

Congenital anorgasmia, also known as primary or psychogenic anejaculation, is a rare, well-described cause of conscious anejaculation. Despite the lack of willful orgasm, nocturnal emissions may occur [59]. The incidence of this condition is 0.14% in the general population and 0.39% among male patients seeking infertility care [60]. The cause is thought to be overly strict childhood upbringing. A classic setting includes parenting with intense performance demands and minimal physical affection. Secondary anejaculation is present in anejaculatory patients with a previous history of normal ejaculation and is generally due to neurologic disease or trauma (e.g., spinal cord injury).

Treatments that seek to reverse anejaculation are difficult. Often, affected individuals lack sensual awareness of their bodies. In addition, they often may seek a partner from a similar background and, as such, may accommodate to an asexual or minimally sexual lifestyle. Treatment is usually sought when the couple desires a pregnancy. Psychotherapy is often effective and is initiated with instruction in sex education, followed by cognitive behavioral treatment that includes systematic relaxation and sensate focus exercises [60]. At first, partners are taught to tolerate and become comfortable with touch. Later, when touch induces pleasure, sexual stimulation is encouraged as the shaping of the sexual response and orgasm occurs. Fertility issues can be managed relatively efficiently in almost all cases of anejaculation with PVS, EEJ, or/and microsurgical sperm aspiration [22, 61].

Expert Commentary

The study of disordered ejaculation remains complex since with many of these conditions an intricate web of connectivity exists between the psychosocial and neurophysiological aspects of human behavior that complicates scientific evaluation. For example, the causal etiologies ascribed to primary and secondary premature ejaculation are vastly different, yet the resultant behaviors are very similar. Likewise, the difference between normal ejaculatory latency and delayed ejaculation may simply reflect differences in learned behaviors. This complex interaction of mind and body is no more obvious than in the association between ejaculatory climax, a cerebral event, and the purely spinal reflex that defines ejaculation.

Indeed, the one physiological constant in the study of disordered ejaculation is that ejaculation is a simple spinal cord reflex. This fact makes animal models very relevant for study of the human condition, and it is precisely through model organisms that we have learned as much as we have about the neurobiology of sex. This is aptly demonstrated by the animal papers that showed that seminal vesicle physiology mimics that of the bladder as both are hollow, smooth muscular organs. This comparison led to the recent concept that seminal vesicles could be inherently dysfunctional and to the development of the "vasodynamic" study of the human reproductive tract to more accurately delineate cases of EDO.

Five-Year View

With the increasing use of animal models and surging knowledge of molecular biology and cell signaling, we look forward to improving the precision of defining many human ejaculatory disorders in the future. In addition, the continued worldwide standardization of definitions and terms used to describe ejaculatory disorders, as typified by consensus statements developed for erectile dysfunction and premature ejaculation, will further enhance our ability to work together and dissect the neurobiological from the psychosocial aspects of these conditions. This, in turn, should improve our ability to evaluate and accurately diagnose sexual disorders in the male and increase our ability to analyze response to treatment.

Although anatomical-based disorders such as EDO or spinal cord injury are fairly well understood at this point, there is ample room for an increased understanding of the effect of pharmacologic agents on ejaculation in the future. This should occur as the field of pharmacogenetics gains further traction in this field. The true value of gene and stem cell therapy has also yet to be fully realized in this discipline of medicine, especially in postsurgical, iatrogenic, or traumatic neurologically based disorders of ejaculation, but offers tremendous potential for functional restoration and cure over the next decade.

Key Issues

- A thorough history and physical examination is fundamental to defining the various behavioral and physiological bases for human ejaculatory disorders.
- There is a growing trend to develop international, consensus-based, standardized definitions of ejaculatory disorders that should help to more precisely define and study these conditions in the future.
- The anatomical and physiological basis for EDO and spinal cord injury are increasingly clear from research to date, but disorders of ejaculatory latency are currently the subject of intensive research to delineate their fundamental underlying pathophysiology.
- The psychosocial aspects of sexual and ejaculatory dysfunction are an integral part of human sexual behavior and, as such, will continue to require consideration and recognition if our understanding of these conditions is to improve in the future.

Acknowledgments The authors would like to acknowledge the contributions of Melody Lowman MA of San Francisco, California, to this chapter. As a psychotherapist with 45 years of experience, her knowledge and experience in reproductive psychology has been invaluable to us.

References

1. Master VA, Turek PJ. Ejaculatory physiology and dysfunction. Urol Clin North Am. 2001;28:363–75.
2. Yang CC, Bradley WE. Somatic innervation of the human bulbocavernosus muscle. Clin Neurophysiol. 1999;110:412.
3. Brackett NL, Ohl DA, Sønksen J, Lynne CM. Abnormalities of ejaculation. In: Lipshultz LI, Howards SS, Niederberger CS, editors. Infertility in the male. 4th ed. New York: Cambridge University Press; 2009. p. 454–73.
4. Benson GS. Erection, emission and ejaculation: physiologic mechanisms. In: Lipshultz LI, Howards SS, editors. Infertility in the male. 3rd ed. St. Louis: Mosby; 1997. p. 155.
5. Eisenberg M, Walsh TJ, Garcia M, et al. Ejaculatory duct manometry in normal men and in patients with ejaculatory duct obstruction. J Urol. 2008;180:255–60.
6. Jarvi K, Zielenski J, Wilschanski M, et al. Cystic fibrosis transmembrane conductance regulator and obstructive azoospermia. Lancet. 1995;345:1578.
7. Thorpe AC, Cleary R, Coles J, et al. Written consent about sexual function in men undergoing transurethral prostatectomy. Br J Urol. 1994;74:479.
8. Dunsmuir WD, Emberton M, Neal DE. On behalf of the steering group of the National Prostatectomy Audit. There is significant sexual dissatisfaction following TURP. Br J Urol. 1996;77:161A.
9. Lue TF, Giuliano F, Montorsi F, et al. Summary of the recommendations on sexual dysfunctions in men. J Sex Med. 2004;1:6–23.
10. Purohit RS, Wu DS, Shinohara K, Turek PJ. A prospective comparison of 3 diagnostic methods to evaluate ejaculatory duct obstruction. J Urol. 2004;171:232–5, discussion 235–36.

11. Hendry WF. Disorders of ejaculation: congenital, acquired and functional. Br J Urol. 1998;82:331.

12. Hendry WF, Pryor JP. Mullerian duct (prostatic utricle) cyst: diagnosis and treatment in sub-fertile males. Br J Urol. 1992;69:79.

13. Turek PJ. Seminal vesicle and ejaculatory duct surgery. In: Graham S, editor. Glenn's urologic surgery. 6th ed. Philadelphia: Lippincott, Williams & Wilkins; 2006. p. 439–45.

14. Nguyen HT, Etzell J, Turek PJ. Normal human ejaculatory duct anatomy: a study of cadaveric and surgical specimens [see comments]. J Urol. 1996;155:1639.

15. Jarow JP. Seminal vesicle aspiration in the management of patients with ejaculatory duct obstruction. J Urol. 1994;152:899.

16. Bird VG, Brackett NL, Lynne CM, et al. Reflexes and somatic responses as predictors of ejaculation by penile vibratory stimulation in men with spinal cord injury. Spinal Cord. 2001;39:514–9.

17. Brackett NL. Semen retrieval by penile vibratory stimulation in men with spinal cord injury. Hum Reprod Update. 1999;5:216–22.

18. Momose H, Hirao Y, Yamamoto M, et al. Electroejaculation in patients with spinal cord injury: first report of a large-scale experience from Japan. Int J Urol. 1995;2:326.

19. Brinsden PR, Avery SM, Marcus S, et al. Transrectal electroejaculation combined with in-vitro fertilization: effective treatment of anejaculatory infertility due to spinal cord injury. Hum Reprod. 1997;12:2687.

20. Schatte EC, Orejuela FJ, Lipshultz LI, et al. Treatment of infertility due to anejaculation in the male with electroejaculation and intracytoplasmic sperm injection. J Urol. 2000;163:1717.

21. Ohl DA. Electroejaculation. Urol Clin North Am. 1993;20:181.

22. Vanderschueren D, Spiessens C, Kiekens C, et al. Successful treatment of idiopathic anejaculation with electroejaculation after microsurgical vas aspiration. Hum Reprod. 1998;13:370.

23. Vinik AI, Maser RE, Mitchell BD, Freeman R. Diabetic autonomic neuropathy. Diabetes Care. 2003;26:1553–79.

24. Dunsmuir WD, Holmes SA. The aetiology and management of erectile, ejaculatory, and fertility problems in men with diabetes mellitus. Diabet Med. 1996;13:700.

25. Sexton WJ, Jarow JP. Effect of diabetes mellitus upon male reproductive function. Urology. 1997;49:508.

26. Hojo K, Vernava III AM, Sugihara K, et al. Preservation of urine voiding and sexual function after rectal cancer surgery. Dis Colon Rectum. 1991;34:532.

27. Nesbakken A, Nygaard K, Bull-Njaa T, et al. Bladder and sexual dysfunction after mesorectal excision for rectal cancer. Br J Surg. 2000;87:206.

28. Turek PJ, Lowther DN, Carroll PR. Fertility issues and their management in men with testis cancer. Urol Clin North Am. 1998;25:517.

29. Holman E, Kovacs G, Flasko T, et al. Hand-assisted laparoscopic retroperitoneal lymph node dissection for nonseminomatous testicular cancer. J Laparoendosc Adv Surg Tech A. 2007;17:16–20.

30. Neyer M, Peschel R, Akkad T, et al. Long-term results of laparoscopic retroperitoneal lymph-node dissection for clinical stage I nonseminomatous germ-cell testicular cancer. J Endourol. 2007;21:180–3.

31. Styblo K, Bossers GT, Slot GH. Osteotomy for kyphosis in ankylosing spondylitis. Acta Orthop Scand. 1985;56:294.

32. Berger Y, Blaivas JG, Oliver L. Urinary dysfunction in transverse myelitis. J Urol. 1990;144:103.

33. Decter RM, Furness III PD, Nguyen TA, et al. Reproductive understanding, sexual functioning and testosterone levels in men with spina bifida. J Urol. 1997;157:1466.

34. Sønksen J, Ohl DA. Penile vibratory stimulation and electroejaculation in the treatment of ejaculatory dysfunction. Int J Androl. 2002;25:324–32.

35. Kafetsoulis A, Brackett NL, Ibrahim E, et al. Current trends in the treatment of infertility in men with spinal cord injury. Fertil Steril. 2006;86:781–9.

36. Sønksen J. Assisted ejaculation and semen characteristics in spinal cord injured males. Scand J Urol Nephrol Suppl. 2003;213:1–31.
37. Kennedy SH, Dickens SE, Eisfeld BS, et al. Sexual dysfunction before antidepressant therapy in major depression. J Affect Disord. 1999;56:201.
38. Seidman S. Ejaculatory dysfunction and depression: pharmacological and psychobiological interactions. Int J Impot Res. 2006;18 Suppl 1:S33–8.
39. Hellstrom WJ, Sikka SC. Effects of acute treatment with tamsulosin versus alfuzosin on ejaculatory function in normal volunteers. J Urol. 2006;176:1529–33.
40. Sharlip ID, Hellstrom WJG, Broderick GA. The ISSM definition of premature ejaculation: a contemporary, evidence-based definition. J Urol. 2008;179(Suppl):340.
41. Read S, King M, Watson J. Sexual dysfunction in primary medical care: prevalence, characteristics and detection by the general practitioner. J Public Health Med. 1997;19:387.
42. Rowland DL, Haensel SM, Blom JH, et al. Penile sensitivity in men with premature ejaculation and erectile dysfunction. J Sex Marital Ther. 1993;19:189.
43. Biri H, Isen K, Sinik Z, et al. Sertraline in the treatment of premature ejaculation: a double-blind placebo controlled study. Int Urol Nephrol. 1998;30:611.
44. Haensel SM, Klem TM, Hop WC, et al. Fluoxetine and premature ejaculation: a double-blind, crossover, placebo-controlled study. J Clin Psychopharmacol. 1998;18:72.
45. Kara H, Aydin S, Yucel M, et al. The efficacy of fluoxetine in the treatment of premature ejaculation: a double-blind placebo controlled study [see comments]. J Urol. 1996;156:1631.
46. Kim SC, Seo KK. Efficacy and safety of fluoxetine, sertraline and clomipramine in patients with premature ejaculation: a double-blind, placebo controlled study. J Urol. 1998;159:425.
47. McMahon CG, Touma K. Treatment of premature ejaculation with paroxetine hydrochloride as needed: 2 single-blind placebo controlled crossover studies. J Urol. 1999;161:1826.
48. Waldinger MD, Hengeveld MW, Zwinderman AH. Ejaculation-retarding properties of paroxetine in patients with primary premature ejaculation: a double-blind, randomized, dose-response study. Br J Urol. 1997;79:592.
49. Berkovitch M, Keresteci AG, Koren G. Efficacy of prilocaine-lidocaine cream in the treatment of premature ejaculation [see comments]. J Urol. 1995;154:1360.
50. Andersen KH. A new method of analgesia for relief of circumcision pain. Anaesthesia. 1989;44:118.
51. Choi HK, Jung GW, Moon KH, et al. Clinical study of SS-cream in patients with lifelong premature ejaculation. Urology. 2000;55:257.
52. Annon J. The behavioral treatment of sexual problems, vol. 1. Honolulu: Enabling Systems; 1974.
53. Hendry WF, Rickards D, Pryor JP, et al. Seminal megavesicles with adult polycystic kidney disease. Hum Reprod. 1998;13:1567.
54. Turek PJ, Magana JO, Lipshultz LI. Semen parameters before and after transurethral surgery for ejaculatory duct obstruction. J Urol. 1996;155:1291.
55. Turek PJ, Aslam K, Younes AK, et al. Observations on seminal vesicle dynamics in an in vivo rat model. J Urol. 1998;159:1731.
56. Sandler B. Idiopathic retrograde ejaculation. Fertil Steril. 1979;32:474.
57. Van der Linden PJQ, Nan PM, te Velde ER, et al. Retrograde ejaculation: successful treatment with artificial insemination. Obstet Gynecol. 1992;79:126.
58. Kim SW, Paick JS. Short-term analysis of the effects of as needed use of sertraline at 5 PM for the treatment of premature ejaculation. Urology. 1999;54:544.
59. Hovav Y, Dan-Goor M, Yaffe H, et al. Nocturnal sperm emission in men with psychogenic anejaculation. Fertil Steril. 1999;72:364.
60. Geboes K, Steeno O, De Moor P. Primary anejaculation: diagnosis and therapy. Fertil Steril. 1975;26:1018.
61. Denil J, Kupker W, Al-Hasani S, et al. Successful combination of transrectal electroejaculation and intracytoplasmic sperm injection in the treatment of anejaculation. Hum Reprod. 1996;11:1247.

Chapter 6
Impact of Spinal Cord Injury

Viacheslav Iremashvili, Nancy L. Brackett, and Charles M. Lynne

Although medical advances have greatly improved the prognosis for people who sustain spinal cord injury, it remains a major social and health-care problem. There are estimated 10,000–12,000 spinal cord injuries every year in the USA alone. More than a quarter of a million Americans are currently living with spinal cord injury [1], with many millions more worldwide. The cost of managing the care of patients with spinal cord injury is approximately $4 billion per year. Car accidents are the most common cause of spinal cord injury followed by violent encounters, sporting and work-related accidents, and falls [1].

The majority of spinal cord injury victims are young adults. Of them, more than 80% are men. As a result, young males constitute the largest part of this patient population. Reproductive function is essential for men with spinal cord injury, but unfortunately, less than 10% of them can father children without medical assistance [2]. Infertility in male patients with spinal cord injury results from a combination of erectile dysfunction, ejaculatory dysfunction, and poor semen quality [3]. As a result of advancements in assisted ejaculation techniques

V. Iremashvili, MD, PhD
Department of Urology, University of Miami Miller School of Medicine,
016960 (M-14), Miami, FL 33101, USA
e-mail: iremashvili@hotmail.com

N.L. Brackett, PhD, HCLD (✉)
The Miami Project to Cure Paralysis,
University of Miami Miller School of Medicine,
Lois Pope Life Center, Room 2-17, 1095 NW 14th Terrace,
Miami, FL 33136, USA
e-mail: nbrackett@miami.edu

C.M. Lynne, MD
Department of Urology, University of Miami Miller School of Medicine,
Miami, FL, USA
e-mail: clynne@miami.edu

S.J. Parekattil, A. Agarwal (eds.), *Male Infertility for the Clinician,*
© Springer Science+Business Media New York 2013

including electroejaculation and high-amplitude penile vibratory stimulation, semen can be safely obtained from nearly all men with spinal cord injury without resorting to surgical procedures [4]; however, semen quality is poor in the majority of cases [5].

Semen Abnormalities in Men with Spinal Cord Injury

The origin and/or cause of low sperm quality in men with spinal cord injury has not been clearly defined. Several possible etiologies have been postulated, including hormonal dysfunction [6], elevated scrotal temperature [7], methods of bladder management [8], and alterations in sperm transport and storage due to reproductive tract stasis [9, 10], but none of these causes has been conclusively proven.

Role of Hormonal Alterations

Alterations in the hypothalamic-pituitary-gonadal axis may result in the disruption of spermatogenesis. The endocrine status of men with spinal cord injury has been examined in several studies that provided contradictory results (Table 6.1). Some studies in humans [6, 11–14] and animals [15, 16] have reported different hormone abnormalities associated with spinal cord injury, but no consistent correlation with the semen quality was shown. It was also not clear if these abnormalities were primary or secondary. We studied this problem in a group of 66 men with spinal cord injury and found no association between semen quality and serum levels of luteinizing hormone, follicle-stimulating hormone, testosterone, or prolactin [17]. The only exception was in a subgroup of subjects who had elevated levels of follicle-stimulating hormone. In each case, the patient was azoospermic, even patients with only small elevations of follicle-stimulating hormone. Hormonal alterations are unlikely to be a major contributor to poor semen quality in men with spinal cord injury [18–22].

Role of Scrotal Temperature

Elevated scrotal/testicular temperature was one of the first hypotheses to explain the origin of semen abnormalities in men with spinal cord injury. It is common knowledge that spermatogenesis is temperature-sensitive and proceeds optimally at 35°C. Higher scrotal temperatures could have detrimental effects on sperm production [23]. It was assumed that men with spinal cord injury could have scrotal hyperthermia as a result of generalized scrotal thermoregulatory dysfunction or because of sitting in a wheelchair for prolonged periods [24]. Some studies showed

Table 6.1 Principal results of the studies of endocrine status of men with spinal cord injuries

	Luteinizing hormone	Follicle-stimulating hormone	Testosterone	Prolactin
No difference from control	Huang et al. [19]	Naftchi et al. [21]	Huang et al. [19]	Huang et al. [19]
	Tsitouras et al. [20]	Tsitouras et al. [20]	Naftchi et al. [21]	Brackett et al. [17]
		Huang et al. [22]	Brackett et al. [17]	Naderi et al. [14]
Lower than control	Naftchi et al. [21]	Brackett et al. [17]	Tsitouras et al. [20]	
	Brackett et al. [17]	Safarinejad et al. [23]	Safarinejad et al. [23]	
	Safarinejad et al. [23]	Naderi et al. [14]	Naderi et al. [14]	
	Naderi et al. [14]	Kostovski et al. [12]	Kostovski et al. [12]	
	Kostovski et al. [12]			
Higher than control		Huang et al. [19]		
Outside reference range		Huang et al.—high, 18.7% [19]	Tsitouras et al. low, 45% [20]	Huang et al.—high, 25% [19]

Endocrine profiles of spinal cord injury men were not shown to follow any specific pattern and/or to be significantly related to impairments in semen quality

that men with spinal cord injury sitting in wheelchairs had higher scrotal temperatures compared to able-bodied men, sitting in armchairs [7, 25]. Brindley reported an inverse correlation between scrotal temperatures and motile sperm counts in men with spinal cord injury [25]. However, we did not find any difference between control subjects and spinal cord-injured subjects in oral temperature, scrotal temperature, or the difference between these two parameters [26]. Furthermore, men with spinal cord injury who were ambulatory (i.e., not in wheelchairs) still had impaired semen quality [26], indicating that some aspect of spinal cord injury, other than the simple act of sitting in a wheelchair, contributes to abnormal semen quality in these men. Supporting this idea is the fact that no study has found improvement in semen quality by cooling the scrotum of men with spinal cord injury.

Studies of scrotal temperature in noninjured men have suggested that short-term versus long-term exposure to elevated temperature causes reversible versus irreversible changes in the seminiferous tubules [27, 28]. In men with spinal cord injury, however, both cross-sectional [29] and longitudinal [30] studies have shown that semen parameters were not significantly related to the duration of the postinjury period, suggesting a stable (and null) pattern for the measures across time. In light of these facts, it appears that no strong evidence exists to support the role of elevated scrotal temperature as a leading etiologic factor of the semen abnormalities in men with spinal cord injury.

Role of Bladder Management

No bladder management regime has been associated with normal semen quality in men with spinal cord injury. However, some studies have shown that the use of intermittent catheterization is associated with better sperm motility than the use of indwelling urethral catheters, suprapubic catheters, or spontaneous voiding [31, 32]. Although semen quality is improved with intermittent catheterization versus the other methods mentioned, it does not become normalized. Bladder management, then, does not seem to be a significant cause of impaired semen quality in men with spinal cord injury.

Role of Ejaculation Frequency

The majority of men with spinal cord injury cannot ejaculate without medical assistance. It has been hypothesized that long periods between ejaculations may result in reproductive tract stasis which can negatively affect sperm. However, most studies investigating the effect of repeated ejaculation on semen quality in men with spinal cord injury found no improvement in semen parameters [9, 33–37]. Only one group reported a moderate increase in sperm motility and sperm morphology after 3 months of weekly ejaculations with penile vibratory stimulation [38]. These findings indicate that frequency of ejaculation is not the sole factor causing abnormal semen quality in men with spinal cord injury.

Interesting data were presented by Ohl et al., suggesting that spinal cord injury could result in fundamental changes in sperm transport and storage [10]. In eight patients with spinal cord injury, bilateral seminal vesicle aspiration was performed immediately before electroejaculation or penile vibratory stimulation. The seminal vesicle aspirates contained large numbers of poor quality sperm. It should be noted that normal men do not have large numbers of sperm in seminal vesicles. Duration of abstinence did not correlate with the number of seminal vesicle sperm. Furthermore, the semen parameters in samples obtained immediately after seminal vesicle aspiration were significantly better compared to historical ejaculated parameters [10]. The authors concluded that altered transport with stagnation of sperm in the seminal vesicles could be a primary source of semen with poor quality in men with spinal cord injury. It was also shown that factors within the seminal plasma contribute to poor semen abnormalities in men with spinal cord injury [39]. This issue will be discussed in more detail later in this chapter.

Studies of Oxidative Stress in Men with Spinal Cord Injury

In addition to the aforementioned putative causes that have been investigated, there is increasing evidence that oxidative stress is an important mechanism contributing to sperm damage in this group of patients. The generation of reactive oxygen species and their relation to semen quality in men with spinal cord injury has been investigated in several studies.

Electric Current and Reactive Oxygen Species

The first study to demonstrate elevated reactive oxygen activity in the semen of men with spinal cord injury was published by Rajasekaran et al. [40]. At the time of this study, electroejaculation was the most common method of obtaining semen from men with spinal cord injury. Electroejaculation is performed by passing electricity into the pelvic region via a probe inserted into the rectum. The authors hypothesized that this electric current induced sperm damage in men with spinal cord injury. The study consisted of two experiments. During the first experiment, sperm from healthy men was incubated with a normal and an electrolyzed medium. Reactive oxygen species levels and sperm motility were measured in each group of samples. The second experiment included measurements of reactive oxygen species generation in semen from men with spinal cord injury and normal controls. In subjects with spinal cord injury, semen samples were obtained by electroejaculation.

The results of this study showed that when sperm from control subjects were incubated with electrolyzed physiologic medium, a significant and time-dependent decrease occurred in sperm motility and sperm viability, and these decreases were associated with an increased generation of reactive oxygen species. The second experiment demonstrated a significant increase in reactive oxygen species generation in semen from subjects with spinal cord injury compared to semen from control subjects. In the latter group, ejaculates were collected by masturbation. These findings led authors to conclude that, in patients with spinal cord injury, the electric current was a likely cause of poor quality of semen obtained by electroejaculation, and this effect was mediated by increased the production of reactive oxygen species [40].

Reactive Oxygen Species in Whole Semen Versus Washed Sperm

The purpose of a study performed by de Lamirande et al. was to determine whether whole semen samples versus washed spermatozoa obtained from men with spinal cord injury produced excessive amounts of reactive oxygen species [41]. This study included three groups of men: healthy volunteers ($n=20$), infertile able-bodied men ($n=166$), and subjects with spinal cord injury ($n=21$). In the latter group, semen was obtained by masturbation after butylbromide and physostigmine injections in 19 patients and by electroejaculation in the remaining two men. Formation of reactive oxygen species was measured in neat semen and in Percoll-washed spermatozoa of all subjects.

The presence of reactive oxygen species in whole semen was detected in 97% of subjects with spinal cord injury compared to 40% and 15% in infertile able-bodied men and volunteers, respectively. Compared to a threshold value of 10 mV/s/10^9, reactive oxygen species production was elevated in 81% of patients with spinal cord injury, 25% of infertile able-bodied men, and 10% of healthy controls. In healthy controls and in infertile able-bodied subjects, the levels of reactive oxygen species measured in semen were, respectively, 40 and 14 times lower than those detected in semen from subjects with spinal cord injury. No correlation was found between reactive oxygen species production and level or duration of injury.

After centrifugation on Percoll gradients, sperm from men with spinal cord injury continued to generate large amounts of reactive oxygen species. High reactive oxygen species production by Percoll-washed spermatozoa was found in 75% of men with spinal cord injury, 20% of infertile men, and 5% of healthy controls. The mean reactive oxygen species levels in washed spermatozoa from men with spinal cord injury were sixfold higher than that of infertile patients, and 140-fold higher than that of normal volunteers. There was a significant inverse relationship between levels of reactive oxygen species and percentage of motile sperm in Percoll-washed specimens from patients with spinal cord injury.

Results of this study showed that semen samples and Percoll-washed sperm samples from subjects with spinal cord injury produced reactive oxygen species at a higher frequency and at higher levels than equivalent samples from normal men or infertile men. In men with spinal cord injury, levels of reactive oxygen species correlated negatively with sperm motility [41]. These data suggest that the role of reactive oxygen species as a mechanism of sperm damage leading to infertility could be more important in men with spinal cord injury compared to the general population or to the infertile population.

Reactive Oxygen Species and Sperm Characteristics

The generation of reactive oxygen species and its relation to semen characteristics in men with spinal cord injury was investigated by our group [42]. This study included 24 men with spinal cord injury and 19 able-bodied controls. In the spinal cord-injured patients, semen was obtained by penile vibratory stimulation ($n=15$), electroejaculation ($n=8$), and masturbation ($n=1$). Measurements of reactive oxygen species formation were performed before and after stimulation with N-formyl-methionyl-leucyl-phenylalanine and 12-myristate 13-acetate phorbol ester. These two substances trigger the generation of reactive oxygen species by leukocytes and spermatozoa, respectively.

The study showed that mean levels of reactive oxygen species in unstimulated and stimulated specimens were significantly higher in spinal cord-injured men compared to controls. The actual values reflecting the reactive oxygen species activity in the spinal cord-injured group were from 250 to 2,000 times higher than that of the control group. The incidence of samples positive for reactive oxygen species specimens in unstimulated controls and men with spinal cord injury was 47.3% versus 100%, respectively. It was also found that the levels of reactive oxygen species in semen from men with spinal cord injury correlated negatively with sperm motility and positively with white blood cell concentrations. Interestingly, the levels of reactive oxygen species did not differ between antegrade and retrograde samples or between different methods of ejaculation (penile vibratory stimulation and electroejaculation). Therefore, the high levels of reactive oxygen species in semen specimens obtained by electroejaculation and vibratory stimulation may not be due exclusively to the effects of electrical current, as was suggested by Rajasekaran et al. [40].

As can be seen from the above studies, reactive oxygen species production is elevated in semen from patients with spinal cord injury, and increased oxidative stress may be an important mechanism of impaired sperm quality in this group of men. The next section of this chapter will discuss the potential sources of reactive oxygen species in semen from patients with spinal cord injury, the consequences of this oxidative stress elevation, and the possible applications of this information in the treatment of infertility in these patients.

Sources of Reactive Oxygen Radicals in Semen from Men with Spinal Cord Injury

Human ejaculate consists of several types of cells including mature and immature spermatozoa, germ cells from different stages of the spermatogenic process, epithelial cells, and leukocytes. Of these different cell types, leukocytes and spermatozoa have been shown to be the two principal sources of production of free radicals [43].

Effect of Leukocytes

Ejaculates from men with spinal cord injury are known to have increased leukocyte counts (Fig. 6.1) [44, 45]. The main sources of leukocytes in human ejaculate are the prostate gland, seminal vesicles, and epididymis [46]. Our studies showed no evidence of chronic or acute prostate gland inflammation in leukocytospermic patients with spinal cord injury [47], and we did not find any white blood cells in the vasal aspirates from these subjects [48]. These data indicate that the seminal vesicles are the most likely origin of leukocytospermia in men with spinal cord injury.

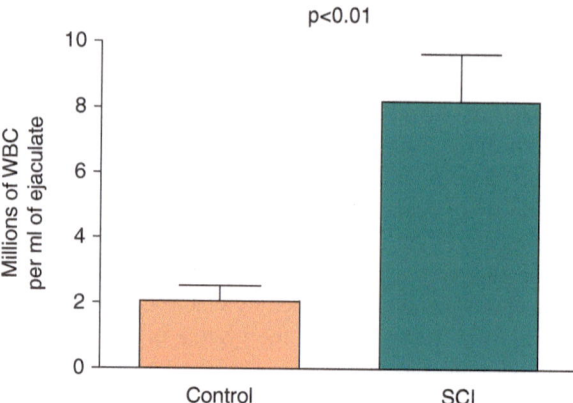

Fig. 6.1 Studies have shown that semen of men with spinal cord injury (SCI) contains higher concentrations of white blood cells (WBC) compared with semen of able-bodied, healthy control subjects

Leukocytes can produce large amounts of reactive oxygen species. A positive correlation has been reported between seminal leukocyte counts and reactive oxygen species production [49, 50]. Of different leukocyte subtypes, peroxidase-positive cells, namely, neutrophils and macrophages, are predominant sources of reactive oxygen species production [51]. In ejaculates obtained by electroejaculation, these two leukocyte subpopulations, as identified by immunohistochemical staining, were the predominant contributors to leukocytospermia in men with spinal cord injury [52]. Lymphocytes were also found to be significant contributors to leukocytospermia in men with spinal cord injury. Immunophenotypic analysis by flow cytometry showed that the greater fraction were T cells, many of which coexpressed the human leukocyte antigen HLA-DR and CD25, suggesting they were in an activated state. No significant B-cell population was evident. [44].

The activation state of leukocytes plays a crucial role in determining reactive oxygen species output because activated white blood cells can produce up to 100-fold increases in reactive oxygen species compared with nonactivated cells [53]. This effect is mediated by an increase in reduced nicotinamide adenine dinucleotide phosphate production via the hexose monophosphate shunt [54]. The myeloperoxidase system of neutrophils and macrophages is also activated, resulting in a respiratory burst and production of large amounts of superoxide and other reactive oxygen species.

Effect of Cytokines

Elevated concentrations of the proinflammatory cytokines interleukin 1 beta, interleukin 6, and tumor necrosis factor α have been detected in the semen of men with spinal cord injury [55], reflecting activation of T-lymphocytes [44] (Fig. 6.2).

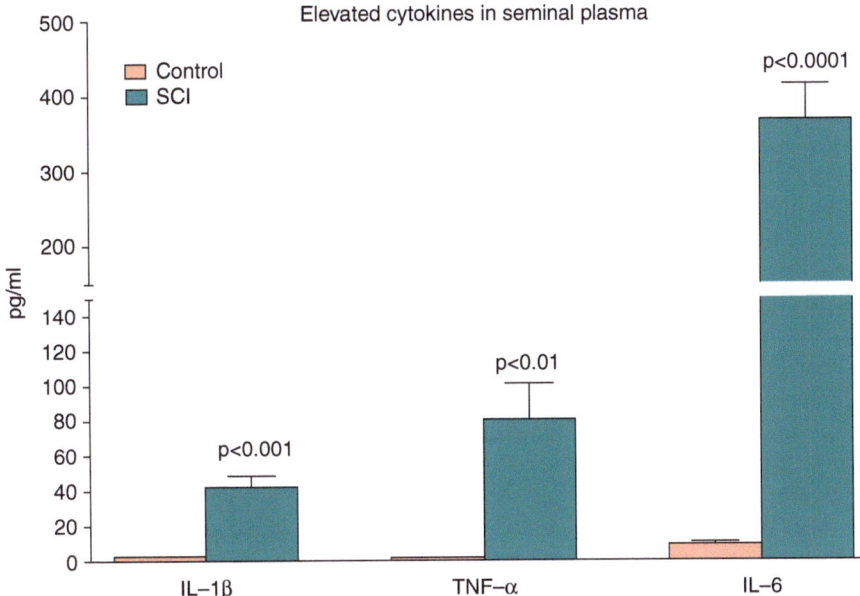

Fig. 6.2 Cytokines can be detrimental to sperm cells. Concentrations of the proinflammatory cytokines, interleukin 1β (1IL-1β), tumor necrosis factor α (TNF-α), and interleukin 6 (IL-6) were significantly elevated in semen of men with spinal cord injury (SCI) compared with semen of control subjects. pg/ml = picograms per milliliter

Inactivation of these cytokines, by adding monoclonal antibodies or receptor blockers to semen from men with spinal cord injury, improves sperm motility [56, 57]. Interleukins are important mediators of free radical generation in many tissues, and the role of cytokines as mediators of oxidative stress is well known. Supporting this notion is the observation of a positive correlation between seminal reactive oxygen species production and seminal plasma concentrations of cytokines such as interleukin 6 [58, 59], interleukin 1, and tumor necrosis factor α [60, 61] in infertile ablebodied men. Interleukin 1 and tumor necrosis factor α were also shown to stimulate reactive oxygen species production in fertile donor semen [62]. Thus, activated seminal leukocytes have the potential to cause oxidative stress elevation in men with spinal cord injury.

Effect of Immature Sperm

Even after complete separation of sperm from leukocytes by density gradient and magnetic beads coated with leukocyte-specific CD45 antibodies, reactive oxygen species production can still be recorded, indicating the ability of spermatozoa to generate reactive oxygen species [63]. This ability inversely correlates with the sperm maturation state. During the process of spermiogenesis, surplus cytoplasm is normally extruded, and the sperm cell takes on a condensed, elongated form. If this process is defective, residual cytoplasm forms a cytoplasmic droplet in the sperm mid-region. These spermatozoa are immature and functionally and morphologically abnormal. The residual cytoplasm contains high concentration of cytosolic enzyme glucose-6-phosphate dehydrogenase, which controls the rate of glucose flux and intracellular production of b-nicotinamide adenine dinucleotide phosphate through the hexose monophosphate shunt [64]. Nicotinamide adenine dinucleotide phosphate contributes to the reactive oxygen species production by nicotinamide adenine dinucleotide phosphate oxidase located within the sperm membrane and nicotinamide adenine dinucleotide phosphate-dependent oxidoreductase in the mitochondria [65, 66]. As a consequence, immature sperm with retained cytoplasm produce increased amounts of reactive oxygen species as compared to mature, morphologically normal sperm.

The maturation stage of sperm development, along with cytoplasmic extrusion, involves other changes, including the sperm plasma membrane remodeling. This remodeling step facilitates the formation of the sites for zona pellucida and hyaluronic acid binding [67]. Immature sperm with cytoplasmic retention are characterized by low densities of zona pellucida binding sites and also of hyaluronic acid receptors [68]. Sperm hyaluronic acid binding capacity can be tested by evaluating the percentage binding of sperm to hyaluronic acid-coated slides. After application of semen to the slide, it can be seen that mature sperm with a high density of hyaluronic acid receptors exhibits permanent binding, while the immature sperm does not bind and swims freely. We have recently investigated hyaluronic acid binding in sperm from men with spinal cord injury and compared it to that of healthy noninjured control subjects [69]. This study included 13 spinal cord-injured subjects and 13 control subjects. Hyaluronic acid binding was significantly lower in spinal cord-injured subjects compared to the control group (55.7 ± 3.8 versus 82.0 ± 2.8, $p < 0.001$) (Fig. 6.3). A hyaluronic acid binding score of 65% is considered a threshold value, as evidenced by clinical outcomes [70]. Only 3 of the 13 spinal cord-injured subjects had a hyaluronic acid binding score higher than 65%, while in the control group, 12 of 13 had a hyaluronic acid binding score higher than 65%.

These results seem to be consistent with an earlier finding showing increased incidences of sperm with cytoplasmic droplets compared to ejaculates of healthy control subjects [42]. It should be noted that the effects of reactive oxygen species produced by immature sperm (intrinsic) and leukocytes (extrinsic) may differ. For example, it has been shown that while both intrinsic and extrinsic reactive oxygen species negatively affect the integrity of deoxyribonucleic acid (DNA) (explained below), the correlation is much stronger for the intrinsic reactive oxygen species production [71]. These data suggest that reactive oxygen species produced by immature sperm cells may have a greater capacity to damage fertility potential.

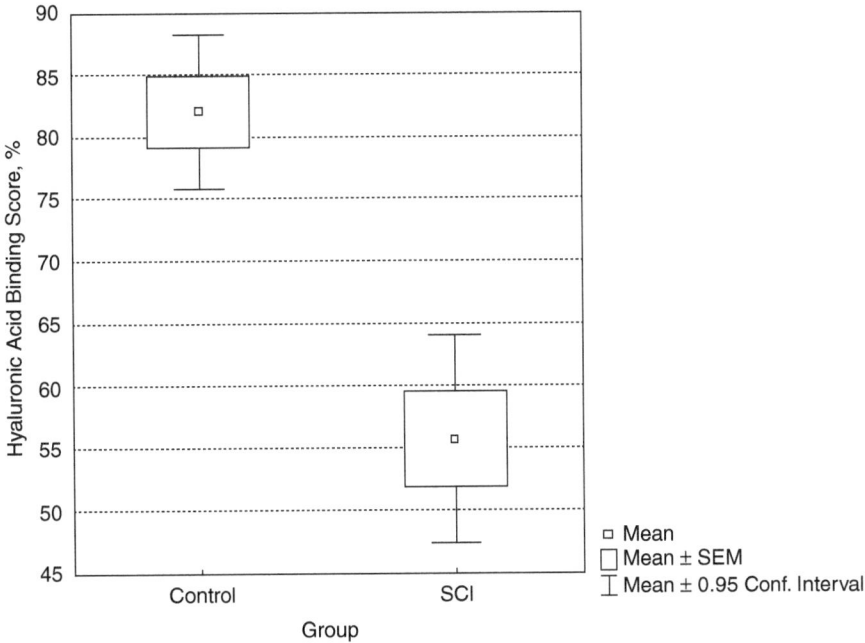

Fig. 6.3 The hyaluronic acid binding score was significantly lower in sperm from men with spinal cord injury (SCI) compared with that of healthy, noninjured control subjects. This deficit may be related to the presence of increased reactive oxygen species and immature sperm in the semen. *SEM* standard error of the mean, *Conf. Interval* confidence interval

Consequences of Oxidative Stress in Semen of Men with Spinal Cord Injury

While leukocytospermia and increased numbers of immature sperm are potential sources of reactive oxygen species in semen of men with spinal cord injury, several other abnormalities, which are characteristic of this group of patients, could be the result of sperm oxidative stress.

Seminal reactive oxygen species, when present in excess, damage different molecules, including lipids, proteins, nucleic acids, and sugars [72]. These toxic effects can result in decreased sperm motility, decreased sperm viability, DNA damage, impaired sperm function, and hyperviscosity of the semen [73]. All of these defects are highly prevalent in semen of men with spinal cord injury [24].

Spermatozoa are vulnerable to the damage induced by excessive reactive oxygen species because their plasma membranes contain large quantities of polyunsaturated fatty acids. Peroxidation of these molecules could decrease membrane flexibility and therefore tail motion. This mechanism of how reactive oxygen species exert their effects on sperm motility was introduced in 1979 [74]. The levels of lipid peroxidation in spermatozoa have been shown to be directly correlated with the loss of motility [75]. Later, several other hypotheses explaining the link between increased reactive oxygen species levels and impaired sperm motility were proposed, including inhibition of enzymes important for intracellular energy production by H_2O_2 and axonemal protein phosphorylation [76, 77]. High levels of seminal reactive oxygen species can also disrupt the inner and outer mitochondrial membranes in spermatozoa [78, 79]. They cause the release of the cytochrome-C protein and activate caspases and apoptosis, resulting in necrospermia [80].

Decreased sperm motility and decreased sperm viability are characteristic features of semen from men with spinal cord injury [24]. In contrast to able-bodied men, most immotile spermatozoa in the semen from men with spinal cord injury are dead. It was shown that the dead-to-live immotile sperm ratio in spinal cord-injured subjects was more than double that in able-bodied subjects (7:3 versus 3:7) [81]. Apoptosis may play an important role in these changes. Experimental data shows that spinal cord injury in rats is associated with decreased sperm mitochondrial transmembrane potential and decreased sperm viability, suggesting excessive apoptosis [16, 82].

Increased levels of reactive oxygen species can also negatively affect the integrity of DNA in the sperm nucleus. Several forms of sperm DNA damage could be caused by reactive oxygen species, including chromatin cross-linking, chromosome deletion, DNA single- and double-stranded breaks, and base oxidation [83, 84]. With the use of flow cytometry, it has been shown that sperm from men with spinal cord injury have a high degree of abnormal chromatin condensation and reduced binding [85].

DNA fragmentation in sperm from men with spinal cord injury was also investigated by our group [86]. The study consisted of three experiments. In experiment 1, we compared the DNA fragmentation index in sperm from men with spinal cord injury to that of able-bodied controls. This experiment showed that the mean DNA fragmentation index was fourfold higher in the spinal cord injury group compared with the control group, and there was no overlap in the DNA fragmentation index between these two groups (Fig. 6.4). As was discussed earlier, chronic anejaculation is considered to be one of the possible explanations of semen abnormalities seen in men with spinal cord injury. To examine this possibility, we performed experiment 2 in which we compared the sperm DNA fragmentation index in two semen specimens obtained 3 days apart from the same spinal cord-injured subjects. No significant difference was found in the sperm DNA fragmentation between the two specimens. The purpose of experiment 3 was to determine if necrospermia, leukocytospermia, or semen processing in men with spinal cord injury contribute to their sperm DNA fragmentation index. In this experiment, the DNA fragmentation index in unprocessed semen samples was compared with that of semen samples processed on a gradient (i.e., free of dead sperm and leukocytes). The results of experiment 3 found no significant difference between mean DNA fragmentation index in aliquots of neat versus processed semen in spinal cord-injured subjects. Although removal of leukocytes did not result in a change in the DNA fragmentation index, it is possible that their negative effects on sperm were exerted prior to

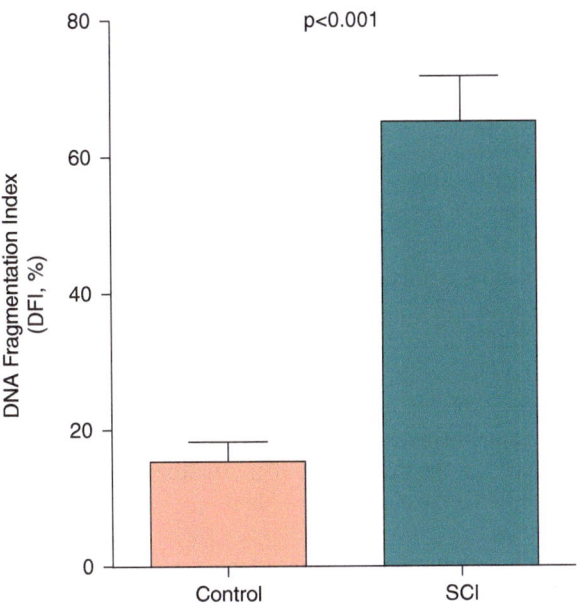

Fig. 6.4 A higher percentage of sperm cells from men with spinal cord injury (SCI) contain DNA damage compared with sperm cells of noninjured control subjects

sperm processing. Thus, it appears that men with spinal cord injury have significantly greater sperm DNA damage, which may be related to high levels of oxidative stress in semen.

Complex relationships exist between apoptosis and DNA damage. Induction of apoptosis by reactive oxygen species results in a high frequency of single- and double-stranded DNA strand breaks in a process referred to karyorrhexis. Severe DNA damage can initiate the apoptosis pathway. Agarwal and Said have suggested that in the context of male infertility, there may be an interaction between seminal reactive oxygen species, sperm DNA damage, and apoptosis, and this interaction may constitute a unified pathogenic molecular mechanism [87].

Semen from men with spinal cord injury is typically highly viscous. Hyperviscous seminal plasma has been reported to be associated with elevated levels of malondialdehyde, an unsaturated carbonyl product of oxidative stress indicating excessive lipid peroxidation [88]. Hyperviscosity has also been shown to be linked to reduced seminal plasma antioxidant capacity [89]. The mechanism of change in seminal viscosity due to oxidative stress could be related to altered interactions between oxidized proteins in the seminal plasma [90].

Increased levels of reactive oxygen species can impair sperm function. This phenomenon could be attributed to changes in membrane fluidity and acrosome integrity, resulting in decreased capacity for sperm-oocyte fusion [91]. Sperm from men with spinal cord injury may have functional impairments that could diminish the capacity of their sperm to bind to the oocyte. A study by Denil et al. [92] showed decreased bovine cervical mucus penetration and decreased hamster egg penetration in sperm from spinal cord-injured subjects versus controls. Sperm from men with spinal cord injury was also reported to have a high degree of acrosomal abnormalities [85].

Acrosin (EC 3.4.21.10) is a sperm acrosomal proteinase with trypsin-like substrate specificity, located in the acrosomal matrix as an enzymatically inactive zymogen. Evidence suggests that its active form, acrosin, is necessary for normal fertilization in humans. If acrosin is reduced, absent, or inhibited, sperm binding to, and penetration of, the zona pellucida is severely impaired [93]. We have recently shown that sperm from men with spinal cord injury is characterized by lower acrosin activity compared to healthy men [69]. These findings indicate that sperm from men with spinal cord injury could have functional defects in sperm-oocyte fusion, resulting from oxidative damage.

Oxidative stress results from an imbalance between the production of reactive oxygen species and their efficient removal by available antioxidant systems. Seminal plasma contains different reactive oxygen species scavengers which take part in the protection of spermatozoa from oxidative stress [94]. Exhaustion of seminal plasma antioxidant capacity facilitates sperm damage by free radicals.

It is known that seminal plasma is a major contributor to semen abnormalities in men with spinal cord injury (Fig. 6.5). For example, seminal plasma of spinal cord-injured men rapidly inhibits motility of sperm from normal men. Similarly, seminal plasma from normal men improves the motility of sperm from spinal cord-injured men [39]. Further evidence that an abnormal seminal plasma environment impairs sperm of men with spinal cord injury comes from a study measuring sperm motility and sperm viability in ejaculates versus vas deferens aspirates of the same group of spinal cord-injured subjects [48]. Because sperm from the vas deferens has not yet been subjected to the effects of the seminal plasma, a direct comparison of these sperm sources provided information about the effects of seminal plasma on sperm function in men with spinal cord injury. The results of this study showed that in patients with spinal cord injury, but not in able-bodied controls, sperm motility and sperm viability were significantly lower in ejaculated specimens (Fig. 6.6). These data provided evidence that, in men with spinal cord injury, seminal plasma is toxic to the sperm.

Interestingly, sperm obtained from men with spinal cord injury not only lose motility more rapidly than sperm from normal men but this deterioration is also exacerbated when semen is stored at body temperature compared to room temperature. In normal men, this correlation was not found [95]. The possible explanation of this discrepancy is higher reactive oxygen species production by activated leukocytes at body temperature in the semen from men with spinal cord injury. Based on the information presented above, it is reasonable to suggest that elevated levels of reactive oxygen species and/or decreased antioxidant capacity of seminal plasma could be, at least in part, responsible for its detrimental effects on sperm motility and viability. Table 6.2 summarizes characteristics of the semen in men with spinal cord injury, suggesting the presence of increased oxidative stress.

Fig. 6.5 Twenty-seven percent of men with spinal cord injury have *brown-colored semen*. The cause of the *brown color* is unknown and may be related the presence of abnormal constituents in the seminal plasma. Evidence suggests that an abnormal seminal plasma environment contributes to sperm impairments in men with spinal cord injury

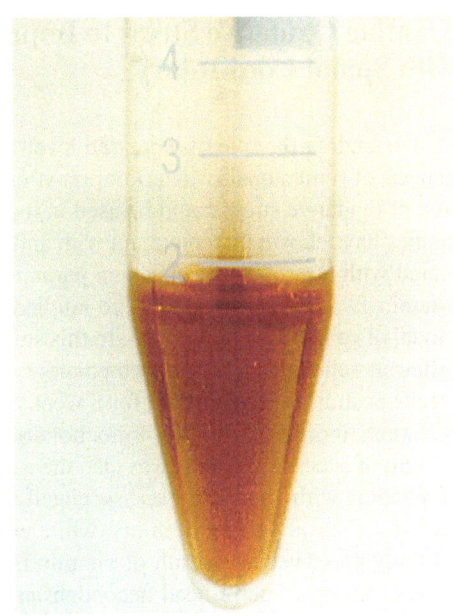

Fig. 6.6 In men with spinal cord injury (SCI), sperm motility was significantly higher when obtained from the vas deferens (VAS) than from the ejaculate (EJAC). In contrast, in control subjects, there was little difference in sperm motility between the two sites. This study provided definitive evidence that seminal plasma was a major contributor to low sperm motility in men with spinal cord injury

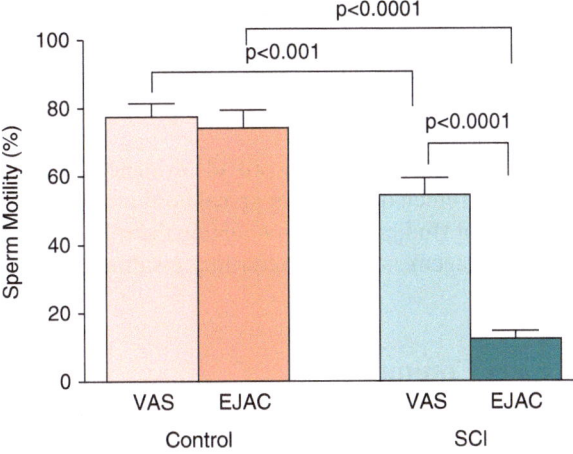

Table 6.2 Characteristics of semen from men with spinal cord injury suggesting increased oxidative stress

Leukocytospermia
Teratozoospermia, increased numbers of immature sperm
Low sperm motility
Necrospermia
Increased DNA fragmentation
Semen hyperviscosity

Treating Oxidative Stress to Improve Semen Quality in Men with Spinal Cord Injury

Understanding the role of increased levels of reactive oxygen species in the pathogenesis of semen quality deterioration after spinal cord injury indicates that correction of oxidative stress could be used in the treatment of these abnormalities. Some studies have shown that treatment with antioxidants, including vitamin E, was associated with improvement of semen parameters in infertile men [96]. The effects of vitamin E on semen quality were studied by Wang et al. in an experimental rat model of spinal cord injury [97]. In this study, rats were given oral vitamin E in two different schedules starting immediately after the injury (maintenance) or 8–10 weeks postinjury (restoration) for 8 weeks. Various sperm parameters were studied including motility, viability, mitochondrial potential, and head decondensation. Weight of accessory glands was also measured.

Feeding with vitamin E was associated with improvement in sperm motility only during the chronic phase of injury, while viability and mitochondrial potential were partially preserved as a result of vitamin E treatment in both restoration and maintenance groups. Sperm head decondensation was significantly less pronounced in rats receiving vitamin E feeding compared to a sham control group. Vitamin E feeding during the chronic phase of injury also resulted in a significant increase in the weight of prostate and seminal vesicles. The results of this study indicate that the antioxidant, vitamin E, attenuated some of the damaging effects of spinal cord injury on sperm motility, viability, and morphology. The partial restoration of prostate and seminal vesicle weight during the chronic phase implies that reactive oxygen species could also be involved in the damaging effects of the spinal cord injury on these glands [97].

Taken together, these data provide evidence that oxidative stress may account for decreased semen quality after spinal cord injury. It is hoped that further laboratory and clinical studies will help to define the role of vitamin E and other antioxidants in the management of male infertility resulting from spinal cord injury.

Expert Commentary

A number of reasons for poor sperm quality in men with spinal cord injury have been postulated; however, we believe that no single factor has been convincingly shown to be the root cause, and it is likely that the etiology of this problem is multifactorial. Among these factors, elevated oxidative stress is clearly an important pathogenic mechanism leading to sperm damage and subsequent infertility resulting from spinal cord injury. Several studies have established a relationship between poor semen quality and the generation of reactive oxygen species in men with spinal cord injury. Semen from these men is characterized by higher concentrations of leukocytes and immature spermatozoa, both of which are important sources of reactive oxygen species production. Furthermore, other seminal abnormalities found in men with spinal cord injury may result from increased oxidative stress.

Five-Year View and Key Issues

While much evidence indicates a role for oxidative stress in the development of infertility in men with spinal cord injury, many unanswered questions still remain. Future research should take several directions:

- Measurements of the changes in antioxidant capacity of seminal plasma in men with spinal cord injury.
- Analysis of the correlation between antioxidant capacity of the seminal plasma and its toxic effects on sperm.
- Studies of the effects of antioxidants as an in vitro and possibly in vivo treatment of semen abnormalities in men with spinal cord injury.
- Investigation of the role of apoptosis in the development of semen abnormalities in men with spinal cord injury and the correlation between apoptosis and seminal plasma antioxidant capacity/seminal reactive oxygen species production.

Results of these studies will enhance our understanding of the underlying pathophysiology of infertility in men with spinal cord injury. These data may also help introduce new methods of treatment of semen abnormalities in this group of patients.

References

1. Spinal cord injury—facts and figures at a glance. 2009. http://www.spinalcord.uab.edu/. Accessed 10 Sept 2009.
2. Elliott S. Sexual dysfunction and infertility in men with spinal cord disorders. In: Lin V, editor. Spinal cord medicine: principles and practice. New York: Demos Medical Publishing; 2003. p. 349–65.
3. Brackett NL, Lynne CM, Ibrahim E, Ohl DA, Sonksen J. Treatment of infertility in men with spinal cord injury. Nat Rev Urol. 2010;7:162–72.
4. Brackett NL, Ibrahim E, Iremashvili V, Aballa TC, Lynne CM. Treatment of ejaculatory dysfunction in men with spinal cord injury: a single-center experience of more than 18 years. J Urol. 2010;183:2304–8.
5. Kafetsoulis A, Brackett NL, Ibrahim E, Attia GR, Lynne CM. Current trends in the treatment of infertility in men with spinal cord injury. Fertil Steril. 2006;86:781–9.
6. Wang YH, Huang TS, Lien IN. Hormone changes in men with spinal cord injuries. Am J Phys Med Rehabil. 1992;71:328–32.
7. Wang YH, Huang TS, Lin MC, Yeh CS, Lien IN. Scrotal temperature in spinal cord injury. Am J Phys Med Rehabil. 1993;72:6–9.
8. Ohl DA, Denil J, Fitzgerald-Shelton K, et al. Fertility of spinal cord injured males: effect of genitourinary infection and bladder management on results of electroejaculation. J Am Paraplegia Soc. 1992;15:53–9.
9. Beretta G, Chelo E, Zanollo A. Reproductive aspects in spinal cord injured males. Paraplegia. 1989;27:113–8.
10. Ohl DA, Menge AC, Jarow JP. Seminal vesicle aspiration in spinal cord injured men: insight into poor sperm quality. J Urol. 1999;162:2048–51.
11. Kostovski E, Iversen PO, Birkeland K, Torjesen PA, Hjeltnes N. Decreased levels of testosterone and gonadotrophins in men with long-standing tetraplegia. Spinal Cord. 2008;46:559–64.
12. Bors E, Engle ET, Rosenquist RC, Holliger VH. Fertility in paraplegic males; a preliminary report of endocrine studies. J Clin Endocrinol Metab. 1950;10:381–98.

13. Shim HB, Kim YD, Jung TY, Lee JK, Ku JH. Prostate-specific antigen and prostate volume in Korean men with spinal cord injury: a case-control study. Spinal Cord. 2008;46:11–5.
14. Naderi AR, Safarinejad MR. Endocrine profiles and semen quality in spinal cord injured men. Clin Endocrinol (Oxf). 2003;58:177–84.
15. Huang HF, Li MT, Giglio W, Anesetti R, Ottenweller JE, Pogach LM. The detrimental effects of spinal cord injury on spermatogenesis in the rat is partially reversed by testosterone, but enhanced by follicle-stimulating hormone. Endocrinology. 1999;140:1349–55.
16. Huang HF, Li MT, Wang S, Barton B, Anesetti R, Jetko JA. Effects of exogenous testosterone on testicular function during the chronic phase of spinal cord injury: dose effects on spermatogenesis and Sertoli cell and sperm function. J Spinal Cord Med. 2004;27:55–62.
17. Brackett NL, Lynne CM, Weizman MS, Bloch WE, Abae M. Endocrine profiles and semen quality of spinal cord injured men. J Urol. 1994;151:114–9.
18. Huang HF, Linsenmeyer TA, Li MT, et al. Acute effects of spinal cord injury on the pituitary-testicular hormone axis and Sertoli cell functions: a time course study. J Androl. 1995;16:148–57.
19. Tsitouras PD, Zhong YG, Spungen AM, Bauman WA. Serum testosterone and growth hormone/insulin-like growth factor-I in adults with spinal cord injury. Horm Metab Res. 1995;27:287–92.
20. Naftchi NE, Viau AT, Sell GH, Lowman EW. Pituitary-testicular axis dysfunction in spinal cord injury. Arch Phys Med Rehabil. 1980;61:402–5.
21. Huang HF, Linsenmeyer TA, Anesetti R, Giglio W, Ottenweller JE, Pogach L. Suppression and recovery of spermatogenesis following spinal cord injury in the rat. J Androl. 1998;19:72–80.
22. Safarinejad MR. Level of injury and hormone profiles in spinal cord-injured men. Urology. 2001;58:671–6.
23. Zorgniotti A, Reiss H, Toth A, Sealfon A. Effect of clothing on scrotal temperature in normal men and patients with poor semen. Urology. 1982;19:176–8.
24. Brackett NL, Nash MS, Lynne CM. Male fertility following spinal cord injury: facts and fiction. Phys Ther. 1996;76:1221–31.
25. Brindley GS. Deep scrotal temperature and the effect on it of clothing, air temperature, activity, posture and paraplegia. Br J Urol. 1982;54:49–55.
26. Brackett NL, Lynne CM, Weizman MS, Bloch WE, Padron OF. Scrotal and oral temperatures are not related to semen quality of serum gonadotropin levels in spinal cord-injured men. J Androl. 1994;15:614–9.
27. Dada R, Gupta NP, Kucheria K. Spermatogenic arrest in men with testicular hyperthermia. Teratog Carcinog Mutagen. 2003;(Suppl 1):235–43.
28. Morgentaler A, Stahl BC, Yin Y. Testis and temperature: an historical, clinical, and research perspective. J Androl. 1999;20:189–95.
29. Brackett NL, Ferrell SM, Aballa TC, Amador MJ, Lynne CM. Semen quality in spinal cord injured men: does it progressively decline postinjury? Arch Phys Med Rehabil. 1998;79:625–8.
30. Iremashvili V, Brackett NL, Ibrahim E, et al. Semen quality remains stable during the chronic phase of spinal cord injury: a longitudinal study. J Urol. 2010;184(5):2073–7.
31. Rutkowski SB, Middleton JW, Truman G, Hagen DL, Ryan JP. The influence of bladder management on fertility in spinal cord injured males. Paraplegia. 1995;33:263–6.
32. Ohl DA, Bennett CJ, McCabe M, Menge AC, McGuire EJ. Predictors of success in electroejaculation of spinal cord injured men. J Urol. 1989;142:1483–6.
33. Momen MN, Fahmy I, Amer M, Arafa M, Zohdy W, Naser TA. Semen parameters in men with spinal cord injury: changes and aetiology. Asian J Androl. 2007;9:684–9.
34. Das S, Dodd S, Soni BM, Sharma SD, Gazvani R, Lewis-Jones DI. Does repeated electroejaculation improve sperm quality in spinal cord injured men? Spinal Cord. 2006;44:753–6.
35. Siosteen A, Forssman L, Steen Y, Sullivan L, Wickstrom I. Quality of semen after repeated ejaculation treatment in spinal cord injury men. Paraplegia. 1990;28:96–104.
36. Heruti RJ, Katz H, Menashe Y, et al. Treatment of male infertility due to spinal cord injury using rectal probe electroejaculation: the Israeli experience. Spinal Cord. 2001;39:168–75.

37. Sonksen J, Ohl DA, Giwercman A, Biering-Sorensen F, Skakkebaek NE, Kristensen JK. Effect of repeated ejaculation on semen quality in spinal cord injured men. J Urol. 1999;161:1163–5.

38. Hamid R, Patki P, Bywater H, Shah PJ, Craggs MD. Effects of repeated ejaculations on semen characteristics following spinal cord injury. Spinal Cord. 2006;44:369–73.

39. Brackett NL, Davi RC, Padron OF, Lynne CM. Seminal plasma of spinal cord injured men inhibits sperm motility of normal men. J Urol. 1996;155:1632–5.

40. Rajasekaran M, Hellstrom WJ, Sparks RL, Sikka SC. Sperm-damaging effects of electric current: possible role of free radicals. Reprod Toxicol. 1994;8:427–32.

41. de Lamirande E, Leduc BE, Iwasaki A, Hassouna M, Gagnon C. Increased reactive oxygen species formation in semen of patients with spinal cord injury. Fertil Steril. 1995;63:637–42.

42. Padron OF, Brackett NL, Sharma RK, Lynne CM, Thomas Jr AJ, Agarwal A. Seminal reactive oxygen species and sperm motility and morphology in men with spinal cord injury. Fertil Steril. 1997;67:1115–20.

43. Aitken RJ, Buckingham DW, Brindle J, Gomez E, Baker HW, Irvine DS. Analysis of sperm movement in relation to the oxidative stress created by leukocytes in washed sperm preparations and seminal plasma. Hum Reprod. 1995;10:2061–71.

44. Basu S, Lynne CM, Ruiz P, Aballa TC, Ferrell SM, Brackett NL. Cytofluorographic identification of activated T-cell subpopulations in the semen of men with spinal cord injuries. J Androl. 2002;23:551–6.

45. Aird IA, Vince GS, Bates MD, Johnson PM, Lewis-Jones ID. Leukocytes in semen from men with spinal cord injuries. Fertil Steril. 1999;72:97–103.

46. Pentyala S, Lee J, Annam S, et al. Current perspectives on pyospermia: a review. Asian J Androl. 2007;9:593–600.

47. Randall JM, Evans DH, Bird VG, Aballa TC, Lynne CM, Brackett NL. Leukocytospermia in spinal cord injured patients is not related to histological inflammatory changes in the prostate. J Urol. 2003;170:897–900.

48. Brackett NL, Lynne CM, Aballa TC, Ferrell SM. Sperm motility from the vas deferens of spinal cord injured men is higher than from the ejaculate. J Urol. 2000;164:712–5.

49. Whittington K, Harrison SC, Williams KM, et al. Reactive oxygen species (ROS) production and the outcome of diagnostic tests of sperm function. Int J Androl. 1999;22:236–42.

50. Sharma RK, Pasqualotto AE, Nelson DR, Thomas Jr AJ, Agarwal A. Relationship between seminal white blood cell counts and oxidative stress in men treated at an infertility clinic. J Androl. 2001;22:575–83.

51. Agarwal A, Makker K, Sharma R. Clinical relevance of oxidative stress in male factor infertility: an update. Am J Reprod Immunol. 2008;59:2–11.

52. Trabulsi EJ, Shupp-Byrne D, Sedor J, Hirsch IH. Leukocyte subtypes in electroejaculates of spinal cord injured men. Arch Phys Med Rehabil. 2002;83:31–4.

53. Plante M, de Lamirande E, Gagnon C. Reactive oxygen species released by activated neutrophils, but not by deficient spermatozoa, are sufficient to affect normal sperm motility. Fertil Steril. 1994;62:387–93.

54. Said TM, Agarwal A, Sharma RK, Thomas Jr AJ, Sikka SC. Impact of sperm morphology on DNA damage caused by oxidative stress induced by beta-nicotinamide adenine dinucleotide phosphate. Fertil Steril. 2005;83:95–103.

55. Basu S, Aballa TC, Ferrell SM, Lynne CM, Brackett NL. Inflammatory cytokine concentrations are elevated in seminal plasma of men with spinal cord injuries. J Androl. 2004;25:250–4.

56. Brackett NL, Cohen DR, Ibrahim E, Aballa TC, Lynne CM. Neutralization of cytokine activity at the receptor level improves sperm motility in men with spinal cord injuries. J Androl. 2007;28:717–21.

57. Cohen DR, Basu S, Randall JM, Aballa TC, Lynne CM, Brackett NL. Sperm motility in men with spinal cord injuries is enhanced by inactivating cytokines in the seminal plasma. J Androl. 2004;25:922–5.

58. Nandipati KC, Pasqualotto FF, Thomas Jr AJ, Agarwal A. Relationship of interleukin-6 with semen characteristics and oxidative stress in vasectomy reversal patients. Andrologia. 2005; 37:131–4.

59. Camejo MI, Segnini A, Proverbio F. Interleukin-6 (IL-6) in seminal plasma of infertile men, and lipid peroxidation of their sperm. Arch Androl. 2001;47:97–101.

60. Martinez P, Proverbio F, Camejo MI. Sperm lipid peroxidation and pro-inflammatory cytokines. Asian J Androl. 2007;9:102–7.

61. Sanocka D, Jedrzejczak P, Szumala-Kaekol A, Fraczek M, Kurpisz M. Male genital tract inflammation: the role of selected interleukins in regulation of pro-oxidant and antioxidant enzymatic substances in seminal plasma. J Androl. 2003;24:448–55.

62. Buch JP, Kolon TF, Maulik N, Kreutzer DL, Das DK. Cytokines stimulate lipid membrane peroxidation of human sperm. Fertil Steril. 1994;62:186–8.

63. Aitken RJ, Buckingham DW, West K, Brindle J. On the use of paramagnetic beads and ferrofluids to assess and eliminate the leukocytic contribution to oxygen radical generation by human sperm suspensions. Am J Reprod Immunol. 1996;35:541–51.

64. Fisher HM, Aitken RJ. Comparative analysis of the ability of precursor germ cells and epididymal spermatozoa to generate reactive oxygen metabolites. J Exp Zool. 1997;277:390–400.

65. Aitken RJ, Buckingham DW, West KM. Reactive oxygen species and human spermatozoa: analysis of the cellular mechanisms involved in luminol- and lucigenin-dependent chemiluminescence. J Cell Physiol. 1992;151:466–77.

66. Gavella M, Lipovac V. NADH-dependent oxidoreductase (diaphorase) activity and isozyme pattern of sperm in infertile men. Arch Androl. 1992;28:135–41.

67. Huszar G, Sbracia M, Vigue L, Miller DJ, Shur BD. Sperm plasma membrane remodeling during spermiogenetic maturation in men: relationship among plasma membrane beta 1,4-galactosyltransferase, cytoplasmic creatine phosphokinase, and creatine phosphokinase isoform ratios. Biol Reprod. 1997;56:1020–4.

68. Huszar G, Ozenci CC, Cayli S, Zavaczki Z, Hansch E, Vigue L. Hyaluronic acid binding by human sperm indicates cellular maturity, viability, and unreacted acrosomal status. Fertil Steril. 2003;79 Suppl 3:1616–24.

69. Iremashvili V, Brackett NL, Ibrahim E, Aballa TC, Bruck D, Lynne CM. Hyaluronic acid binding and acrosin activity are decreased in sperm from men with spinal cord injury. Fertil Steril. 2010;94(5):1925–7.

70. Huszar G, Ozkavukcu S, Jakab A, Celik-Ozenci C, Sati GL, Cayli S. Hyaluronic acid binding ability of human sperm reflects cellular maturity and fertilizing potential: selection of sperm for intracytoplasmic sperm injection. Curr Opin Obstet Gynecol. 2006;18:260–7.

71. Henkel R, Kierspel E, Stalf T, et al. Effect of reactive oxygen species produced by spermatozoa and leukocytes on sperm functions in non-leukocytospermic patients. Fertil Steril. 2005; 83:635–42.

72. Pryor WA, Houk KN, Foote CS, et al. Free radical biology and medicine: it's a gas, man! Am J Physiol Regul Integr Comp Physiol. 2006;291:R491–511.

73. Tremellen K. Oxidative stress and male infertility–a clinical perspective. Hum Reprod Update. 2008;14:243–58.

74. Jones R, Mann T, Sherins R. Peroxidative breakdown of phospholipids in human spermatozoa, spermicidal properties of fatty acid peroxides, and protective action of seminal plasma. Fertil Steril. 1979;31:531–7.

75. Gomez E, Irvine DS, Aitken RJ. Evaluation of a spectrophotometric assay for the measurement of malondialdehyde and 4-hydroxyalkenals in human spermatozoa: relationships with semen quality and sperm function. Int J Androl. 1998;21:81–94.

76. Aitken RJ, Fisher HM, Fulton N, et al. Reactive oxygen species generation by human spermatozoa is induced by exogenous NADPH and inhibited by the flavoprotein inhibitors diphenylene iodonium and quinacrine. Mol Reprod Dev. 1997;47:468–82.

77. de Lamirande E, Gagnon C. Reactive oxygen species and human spermatozoa. I. Effects on the motility of intact spermatozoa and on sperm axonemes. J Androl. 1992;13:368–78.

78. de Lamirande E, Gagnon C. Reactive oxygen species and human spermatozoa. II. Depletion of adenosine triphosphate plays an important role in the inhibition of sperm motility. J Androl. 1992;13:379–86.

79. de Lamirande E, Jiang H, Zini A, Kodama H, Gagnon C. Reactive oxygen species and sperm physiology. Rev Reprod. 1997;2:48–54.
80. Wang X, Sharma RK, Sikka SC, Thomas Jr AJ, Falcone T, Agarwal A. Oxidative stress is associated with increased apoptosis leading to spermatozoa DNA damage in patients with male factor infertility. Fertil Steril. 2003;80:531–5.
81. Brackett NL, Bloch WE, Lynne CM. Predictors of necrospermia in men with spinal cord injury. J Urol. 1998;159:844–7.
82. Nunez R, Murphy TF, Huang HF, Barton BE. Use of SYBR14, 7-amino-actinomycin D, and JC-1 in assessing sperm damage from rats with spinal cord injury. Cytometry A. 2004;61:56–61.
83. Aitken RJ, Krausz C. Oxidative stress, DNA damage and the Y chromosome. Reproduction. 2001;122:497–506.
84. Kemal Duru N, Morshedi M, Oehninger S. Effects of hydrogen peroxide on DNA and plasma membrane integrity of human spermatozoa. Fertil Steril. 2000;74:1200–7.
85. Engh E, Clausen OP, Purvis K, Stien R. Sperm quality assessed by flow cytometry and accessory sex gland function in spinal cord injured men after repeated vibration- induced ejaculation. Paraplegia. 1993;31:3–12.
86. Brackett NL, Ibrahim E, Grotas JA, Aballa TC, Lynne CM. Higher sperm DNA damage in semen from men with spinal cord injuries compared with controls. J Androl. 2008;29:93–9. discussion 100–101.
87. Agarwal A, Said TM. Oxidative stress, DNA damage and apoptosis in male infertility: a clinical approach. BJU Int. 2005;95:503–7.
88. Aydemir B, Onaran I, Kiziler AR, Alici B, Akyolcu MC. The influence of oxidative damage on viscosity of seminal fluid in infertile men. J Androl. 2008;29:41–6.
89. Siciliano L, Tarantino P, Longobardi F, Rago V, De Stefano C, Carpino A. Impaired seminal antioxidant capacity in human semen with hyperviscosity or oligoasthenozoospermia. J Androl. 2001;22:798–803.
90. Traverso N, Menini S, Maineri EP, et al. Malondialdehyde, a lipoperoxidation-derived aldehyde, can bring about secondary oxidative damage to proteins. J Gerontol A Biol Sci Med Sci. 2004;59:B890–5.
91. Agarwal A, Saleh RA. Role of oxidants in male infertility: rationale, significance, and treatment. Urol Clin North Am. 2002;29:817–27.
92. Denil J, Ohl DA, Menge AC, Keller LM, McCabe M. Functional characteristics of sperm obtained by electroejaculation. J Urol. 1992;147:69–72.
93. Liu DY, Baker HW. Inhibition of acrosin activity with a trypsin inhibitor blocks human sperm penetration of the zona pellucida. Biol Reprod. 1993;48:340–8.
94. Balercia G, Armeni T, Mantero F, Principato G, Regoli F. Total oxyradical scavenging capacity toward different reactive oxygen species in seminal plasma and sperm cells. Clin Chem Lab Med. 2003;41:13–9.
95. Brackett NL, Santa-Cruz C, Lynne CM. Sperm from spinal cord injured men lose motility faster than sperm from normal men: the effect is exacerbated at body compared to room temperature. J Urol. 1997;157:2150–3.
96. Kessopoulou E, Powers HJ, Sharma KK, et al. A double-blind randomized placebo cross-over controlled trial using the antioxidant vitamin E to treat reactive oxygen species associated male infertility. Fertil Steril. 1995;64:825–31.
97. Wang S, Wang G, Barton BE, Murphy TF, Huang HF. Beneficial effects of vitamin E in sperm functions in the rat after spinal cord injury. J Androl. 2007;28:334–41.

Part II
Clinical Management of Male Infertility

Chapter 7
Endocrinopathies

Sam Haywood, Eric L. Laborde, and Robert E. Brannigan

Spermatogenesis depends on an intricate interplay of hormonal factors both centrally and in the testis. Centrally, the hypothalamus releases gonadotropin-releasing hormone (GnRH), which acts on the anterior pituitary to cause secretion of luteinizing hormone (LH) and follicle-stimulating hormone (FSH). At the level of the testis, FSH acts on Sertoli cells to induce the maturation process in spermatogonia. LH exerts its effect on Leydig cells, stimulating production of testosterone [1]. Effective spermatogenesis requires local testosterone concentrations to be much higher than serum concentrations [2]. This intratesticular testosterone then acts indirectly to stimulate germ cell maturation through actions on Sertoli cells [1, 2].

Although endocrinopathies only account for a small minority of cases of male infertility, about 1–2% [3], the treatment of these conditions offers patients a strategy of directed therapy. Broad classification of endocrinopathies involves two main categories: hormonal deficiency and hormonal excess, with specific hormonal abnormalities falling under each of the previously mentioned categorizations.

Hormonal Deficiency

Hypogonadotropic Hypogonadism

As the name suggests, hypogonadotropic hypogonadism is a state of testosterone deficiency associated with subnormal levels of gonadotropins (FSH and LH). Etiologies of hypogonadotropic hypogonadism can be numerous and are divided into congenital and acquired causes.

S. Haywood, BA (✉) • E.L. Laborde, MD • R.E. Brannigan, MD
Department of Urology, Northwestern University Feinberg School of Medicine,
Galter Pavilion, Suite 20-150 675 N. Saint Clair Street, Chicago, IL 60611, USA
e-mail: r-brannigan@northwestern.edu

S.J. Parekattil, A. Agarwal (eds.), *Male Infertility for the Clinician*,
© Springer Science+Business Media New York 2013

Kallmann syndrome is one identified congenital etiology of hypogonadotropic hypogonadism. Inherited in an X-linked recessive fashion, Kallmann syndrome can arise due to a variety of mutations, the most prevalent of which involves the KAL1 gene. Features include hypogonadism as well as anosmia, facial defects, renal agenesis, and neurologic abnormalities [4]. The hypogonadism and associated clinical sequelae (delayed puberty, infertility) result from a failure of migration of GnRH-secreting neurons. This failure of migration leads to absence of GnRH secretion which in turn leads to absent LH and FSH secretion [3].

Hypogonadotropic hypogonadism can also be acquired, as in the case of pituitary insufficiency resulting from pituitary tumors, surgery, infarct, or infiltrative disease. Regardless of the myriad etiologies of hypogonadotropic hypogonadism, the underlying disturbance is low gonadotropin levels, and treatment can be affected through pharmacologic replacement.

Treating hypogonadotropic hypogonadism involves replacement of the deficient hormones through gonadotropin therapy. Agents used in this therapy include human chorionic gonadotropin (hCG), human menopausal gonadotropin (hMG), and recombinant follicle-stimulating hormone (rFSH). Human chorionic gonadotropin use stems from its properties as an LH analogue, acting at the Leydig cell to stimulate androgen secretion. Human menopausal gonadotropin is a product purified from the urine of postmenopausal women that contains both LH and FSH. Regimens of gonadotropin therapy for men with hypogonadotropic hypogonadism typically begin with hCG administration alone for 3–6 months. Dosages range from 1,000 to 1,500 USP units either IM or SC three times per week. Adequacy of therapy can be assessed by measuring serum testosterone levels, with the goal of achieving sustained normal levels. Although the pertinent goal for spermatogenesis is adequate intratesticular testosterone concentrations, this value is not normally assessed in gonadotropin replacement therapy. However, intratesticular testosterone levels show linear correlation with administered hCG dosage [5]. After titration to sustained normal testosterone levels, usually after 3–6 months of hCG monotherapy, therapy is initiated to replace FSH levels. One method of FSH replacement involves hMG given at doses of 75–150 IU IM/SC three times a week at a separate injection site. Alternatively, rFSH can be used at dosages of 150 IU SC three times a week [6]. Relative efficacy of hMG versus rFSH has been studied to some extent in women undergoing IVF, but comparisons in male patients are lacking. Replacing gonadotropins in this manner has shown promising results as more than 90% of treated males experience spermatogenesis [3]. The time to spermatogenesis can be quite variable, with the average response occurring in about 6–9 months. However, therapy may be required for up to 1–2 years before a response may occur, and some individuals unfortunately never respond to this modality [7]. An Australian study of 38 men with hypogonadotropic hypogonadism found that median time to first sperm in the ejaculate was 7.1 months, while median time to conception was 28.2 months [8].

While spermatogenesis occurs in a strong majority of patients, sperm concentrations achieved through gonadotropin therapy still sometimes fall below goal ranges (<20 million sperm/mL). Despite this, fertility outcomes with gonadotropin therapy are very good. In a study of 24 men with hypogonadotropic hypogonadism treated with gonadotropin therapy, 22 men achieved pregnancy, even though mean sperm concentration was 16.7 million sperm/mL [9]. A retrospective study of Japanese men found sperm production in 71% of men treated with hCG (3,000 IU) and hMG (75 IU), provided testicular size was greater than prepubertal sizes (>4 mL) [10]. A recently published Saudi Arabian paper studied 87 infertile men with hypogonadotropic hypogonadism treated with IM gonadotropins for a median of 26 months, with the primary outcome of fertility. Overall, 35 of the 87 patients (40%) were able to achieve pregnancy [11].

An important area of newer research focuses on determining predictors of response to gonadotropin therapy. The aforementioned long-term study in Japanese men found a correlation between testicular size pretreatment and response to gonadotropin therapy. Men with testicular size >4 mL had a 71% chance of responding to treatment, whereas men with testicular size <4 mL had only a 36% chance of responding to treatment [10]. In addition, the above Saudi Arabian study found that only pretreatment testicular size was predictive of conception. In particular, responders to treatment had a mean testicular pretreatment volume of 9.0 ± 3.6 mL, while the pretreatment testicular volume of nonresponders was only 5.7 ± 2.0 mL. Interestingly, there was no significant difference in conception rates between men with hypogonadotropic hypogonadism due to congenital or acquired etiologies [11]. Larger baseline testicular size has also been shown as an independent predictor of response time to gonadotropin therapy, and achieving summed testis volume >20 mL after treatment increased the odds of achieving both goal sperm parameters and pregnancy by at least twofold [8]. It is worth noting that the lower sperm concentrations found in these studies, while below traditional goals of infertility management, may allow for pregnancy with adjunctive use of assisted reproductive therapies such as intrauterine insemination or in vitro fertilization. Additionally, such medical treatment may allow increased efficacy of surgical sperm extraction.

Another method of treatment for men with hypogonadotropic hypogonadism involves the use of antiestrogen agents. These agents competitively bind to estrogen receptor sites in the hypothalamus. Normally, estradiol acts via negative feedback at this endocrine center to inhibit gonadotropin secretion. By binding at these sites, antiestrogen agents block estradiol's feedback inhibition of the hypothalamus and thus increase the hypothalamic secretion of GnRH. The increased secretion of GnRH leads to increased pituitary secretion of gonadotropins, which thereby stimulates an increase in intratesticular testosterone production. The most commonly used agent in this class is clomiphene citrate, but similar agents include tamoxifen, raloxifene, and toremifene. These drugs have been previously studied in the setting of empiric therapy for idiopathic infertility with mixed results [7]. However, the directed use of clomiphene in patients with proven hypogonadotropic hypogonadism has shown to be useful in limited settings. An American study treated four men with hypogonadotropic hypogonadism with clomiphene citrate 50 mg three times a week and found improved testosterone levels and semen parameters in three of these patients. Subsequently, two of these three men achieved documented pregnancy [12]. Similar success at the biochemical level has also been described in case reports, although fertility was not a goal of these treatments [13, 14]. Clomiphene treatment of male infertility can be associated with such side effects as visual disturbances, GI upset, weight gain, hypertension, and insomnia [7].

It is worth noting that exogenous GnRH treatment represents another avenue of medical therapy for hypogonadotropic hypogonadism. Synthetic analogues of GnRH can be administered to stimulate secretion of gonadotropins. However, the short half-life of these agents combined with the necessary pulsatile release to recreate normal physiology requires a method of frequent administration, such as frequent injections, nasal sprays, or an implantable pump. These methods are obviously less convenient, and further, studies have not shown this treatment has a strong benefit for hypogonadotropic hypogonadism [15].

Hypergonadotropic Hypogonadism

In hypergonadotropic hypogonadism, the main perturbation is an inadequate or absent function of the testes. Gonadotropins are appropriately elevated secondary to lack of negative feedback from estradiol, testosterone, and inhibin B from the testis. Without appropriate androgen secretion, spermatogenesis is impaired. These men also typically have significant testicular atrophy with fibrosis and markedly reduced germ cell number, also leading to abnormally low levels of spermatogenesis. Hypergonadotropic hypogonadism can occur as a result of genetic etiologies (e.g., Klinefelter syndrome) or from acquired conditions. Acquired etiologies of hypergonadotropic hypogonadism include destruction of normal gonadal tissue from chemotherapy or radiation, trauma, mumps orchitis, or androgen decline in the aging male. Men with hypergonadotropic hypogonadism not desiring fertility can be treated with exogenous testosterone therapy, but men trying to conceive should generally not be given exogenous testosterone. The treatment for men trying to conceive is less well characterized. Aromatase inhibitors have been suggested as treatment for men with Klinefelter syndrome [4]. A small cohort of patients with Klinefelter syndrome treated with aromatase inhibitors showed hormonal improvements with treatment, although the study did not comment on semen parameters in the Klinefelter subset. In particular, for this subset of patients, testolactone therapy was more efficacious with respect to hormonal levels than anastrazole [16].

It is important to mention the additional potential advantage in the setting of surgical sperm extraction after adjuvant medical therapy in men with Klinefelter syndrome. Surgical sperm extraction alone has resulted in successful retrieval in up to 50% of attempts [17]. Ramasamy et al. retrospectively studied 68 azoospermic men with Klinefelter syndrome. Of these 68, 56 men were treated for low testosterone levels (<300 ng/dL) with a combination of medical therapies (aromatase inhibitors, hCG, clomiphene) before microdissection TESE. Of the 56 men receiving medical therapy before TESE, 28 received testolactone alone, 12 received testolactone and weekly hCG, 9 received anastrozole alone, 1 received anastrozole and hCG, and 4 received hCG alone. Three patients total received clomiphene citrate. While there was no difference among specific agents in terms of successful sperm extraction, these medical regimens collectively resulted in improved sperm retrieval when patients responded to medical therapies with posttreatment testosterone >250 ng/dL. More specifically, successful sperm extraction was seen in 77% of men with posttreatment testosterone >250 ng/dL versus 55% of men with posttreatment testosterone <250 ng/dL [17].

Hypothyroidism

Thyroid hormones are essential in organ development and routine metabolism. However, there have been few studies evaluating hypothyroidism and male reproduction. Hypothyroidism has long been associated with diminished libido and erectile dysfunction [18]. Additionally, a recent study by Meeker et al. revealed a correlation between thyroxine (T4) level and sperm concentration, with higher T4 being correlated with better sperm concentrations [19]. Sperm concentration may not be the only parameter affected, as a study by Krassas et al. showed that men with hypothyroidism have a lower than normal percentage of sperm with normal morphology. Correcting the hypothyroidism resulted in 76% of the patients having a normal morphology [20]. Overall, there is a relative scarcity of data regarding hypothyroidism and semen parameters. Nonetheless, these studies do suggest a link between thyroid function and spermatogenesis.

Hormonal Excess

Androgen Excess

Within the hypothalamic–pituitary–testis axis, testosterone exerts negative feedback inhibition on the hypothalamic secretion of GnRH. This effect is indirect and thought to occur via aromatization of testosterone to estradiol. Acting in this manner, excess circulating testosterone can suppress this axis and cause inhibition of spermatogenesis. Testosterone excess can result from exogenous testosterone administration or from endogenous production. Therapeutic administration can inadvertently result in testosterone excess, but testosterone excess can also result from the illicit use of anabolic steroids. Regardless of the cause, exogenous androgens typically suppress gonadotropin secretion with resultant decreased levels of intratesticular testosterone and decreased spermatogenesis. Diagnosis is suggested by normal to high serum testosterone levels with suppressed gonadotropins. The first step in treating a male with suspected androgen excess is to remove the exogenous source. Return of spermatogenesis usually occurs within 4 months but in some instances can take up to 3 years [21, 22]. If sperm parameters do not improve adequately or are slow to improve, some evidence suggests beneficial effects of gonadotropin therapy in improving intratesticular testosterone levels [22, 23]. If response to treatment remains suboptimal after a trial of gonadotropin therapy, limited evidence suggests a possible use of clomiphene in reestablishing the hypothalamic–pituitary–testis axis [24].

Androgen excess can also result from endogenous androgen production. The most common endogenous source is congenital adrenal hyperplasia, although functional tumors (adrenal or testicular) and androgen insensitivity syndromes could also be responsible [3]. These etiologies have their own treatment strategies that will not be discussed here, but consideration should be given to their presence for complete patient care.

Estrogen Excess

As mentioned earlier, testosterone's ability to inhibit GnRH secretion at the hypothalamus is mediated through conversion to estrogens. A primary excess of estrogens can act similarly to inhibit the hypothalamic–pituitary–testis axis and thus contribute to decreased fertility. While estrogens are produced in the testis along with testosterone, the main source of estrogens in males is peripheral aromatization of testosterone by the enzyme aromatase, found in adipose tissue. The rising prevalence of obesity in our society puts more men at risk for estrogen excess. In particular, the ratio of testosterone to estradiol (T:E2) appears to be an important measure of estrogen excess, with a goal ratio >10:1 sought by many clinicians. Pavlovich et al. examined a cohort of infertile men and found significantly reduced T:E2 ratios in the infertile men compared to a fertile control group (6.9 vs. 14.5) [25].

Treatment of relative estrogen excess involves inhibitors of the aromatase enzyme. There are two main classes of aromatase inhibitors: steroidal agents (e.g., testolactone) and nonsteroidal agents (e.g., anastrozole). Both have shown utility in treatment of infertile men with low T:E2 ratios. The above Pavlovich study treated 63 men with male factor infertility and low T:E2 ratios with testolactone, 50–100 mg twice daily. Treatment was effective in improving both T:E2 ratio and sperm quality, as defined by concentrations and motility [25]. A more recent study by Raman and Schlegel treated 140 infertile men with abnormal T:E2 ratios with either testolactone (100–200 mg daily) or anastrozole (1 mg daily). Both treatment arms showed improvement in T:E2 ratio as well as improved sperm concentration and motility. Further, the study did not show any significant difference between the two classes of aromatase inhibitors in terms of hormonal profile or semen analysis, except in the setting of Klinefelter syndrome, where testolactone was superior in treating the abnormal T:E2 ratios [16]. These studies combined show a clear role for aromatase inhibitors in infertile men with abnormal T:E2 ratios. This treatment strategy may be of particular importance in obese patients [26].

Thyroid Excess

As was touched upon earlier, the role of thyroid hormones in spermatogenesis is not entirely clear. However, hyperthyroidism appears to adversely affect semen parameters. Abalovich et al. found that patients with hyperthyroidism have lower bioavailable testosterone, higher sex-hormone-binding globulin, and higher LH levels compared to controls [27]. Hyperthyroid patients were reported to have markedly impaired semen parameters, including low motility, low ejaculate volume, low sperm concentration, and abnormal morphology. The authors noted that 85% of the seminal abnormalities normalized on semen testing conducted 7–19 months after achievement of euthyroid status. A more recent study also found that hyperthyroidism can impair semen parameters [28]. The authors of this study reported that hyperthyroid patients had significantly lower sperm motility than controls. Motility was improved after euthyroid status was achieved with medical thyroid ablation. Just as with hypothyroidism, there is a scarcity of data regarding hyperthyroidism and spermatogenesis. However, the available studies seem to suggest that hyperthyroidism can adversely affect semen parameters.

Prolactin Excess

Hyperprolactinemia, an excess of the hormone prolactin, is another hormonal etiology of male infertility. The diagnosis is relatively straightforward, as hyperprolactinemia can be detected on routine serum testing, but determination of a particular etiology can be more challenging. Hyperprolactinemia can occur in the case of hypothyroidism, liver disease, stress, use of certain medications (i.e., phenothiazines, tricyclic antidepressants), and with functional pituitary adenomas (prolactinomas). Clinical suspicion must be high for excess prolactin, as the manifestations can range from asymptomatic in many patients to galactorrhea or hypoandrogenic states (i.e., low libido, erectile dysfunction) in affected patients. Patients with pituitary adenomas may also present with bilateral temporal visual field defects. This state, known as bitemporal hemianopsia, is the result of the close anatomic proximity of the pituitary gland to the optic chiasm. Growth of the pituitary tumor compresses the optic nerve, leading to visual field deficits.

Hyperprolactinemia can cause male infertility through its inhibitory effects on the hypothalamus. The high levels of prolactin suppress secretion of GnRH from the hypothalamus, which subsequently impairs the release of gonadotropins, the production of testosterone, and spermatogenesis. The multiple effects on the hypothalamic–pituitary–testicular axis can result in a patient presenting with multiple problems such as decreased libido, inability to achieve erection, and abnormal semen parameters.

Once the diagnosis of hyperprolactinemia is made, the practitioner should obtain an MRI study focusing on the pituitary gland. If a prolactinoma is found, it can be characterized based on its size and appearance. The main differentiation is between microadenomas, lesions <10 mm, and macroadenomas, which are lesions >10 mm. If a prolactinoma is discovered, medical therapy focuses on blocking the secretion of prolactin through the use of dopamine agonists. Examples of these agents include bromocriptine, cabergoline, pergolide, and quinagolide, with the most well-characterized agents being bromocriptine and cabergoline. These agonists make use of the natural inhibition of prolactin secretion by dopamine. This can actually cause regression of the tumor, although the process generally occurs over months. Possible side effects of dopamine agonists include nausea, vomiting, and postural hypotension. While inhibition of excess prolactin secretion prevents the disruption of the hypothalamic–pituitary axis, there have been few studies specifically elucidating the effects of these dopamine agonists on spermatogenesis and fertility. A 1974 study treated men with functional prolactinomas and hypogonadism with bromocriptine and found no increase in sperm motility [29]. However, more recently, DeRosa and colleagues compared bromocriptine and cabergoline in such patients.

Both treatments showed overall improvements in sperm number, motility, rapid progression, and morphology within 6 months of therapy [30]. A subsequent study from the same institution compared seminal fluid parameters between men with prolactinomas and control men. After 24 months of treatment with cabergoline (initial dose 0.5 mg weekly, subsequently titrated to PRL levels), two-thirds of men showed restored gonadal function as compared against healthy control men [31].

Comparing cabergoline and bromocriptine, it appears that cabergoline is more efficacious at normalization of prolactin levels and regressing tumor burden [32]. Further, a higher percentage of patients show a clinical response to cabergoline when compared with bromocriptine. Finally, there is a higher overall rate of permanent remission and fewer side effects with cabergoline compared to bromocriptine [32]. Considering all of these findings, cabergoline is often the first therapy utilized in treating men with prolactinomas.

While treatment of prolactinomas with dopamine agonists can be effective in many cases, a significant percentage of men may still remain persistently hypogonadotropic. Recent research suggests that clomiphene citrate may be an effective treatment for these men. Ribiero and Abucham treated 14 persistently hypogonadal men with clomiphene (50 mg/day for 12 weeks) and noted both improved testosterone levels and sperm motility [33].

Ablative therapy for prolactinomas—in the form of radiation therapy or transsphenoidal resection—is also available. Ablative therapy is typically reserved for those who fail medical management. Ablative treatments remove the source of prolactin and thus the inhibition of GnRH secretion. Measurement of the patient's gonadotropin levels posttreatment remains important, as further intervention with exogenous gonadotropins may be necessary to optimize therapeutic benefit.

Expert Commentary

Medical treatments for male infertility have traditionally centered on empiric approaches to enhance spermatogenesis. Over the past two decades, improved insight has been gained into the pathophysiology of male infertility and the outcomes associated with empiric therapy. With this insight, more targeted and directed use of medical agents has been described. As such, "empiric therapy" is used with less frequency now than was the case 20 years ago. Many available medical therapies for infertile men are used to optimize the hormonal milieu and thus optimize spermatogenesis. This has indeed been the focus of this chapter. However, numerous other medical agents are used routinely to address other specific pathophysiologic conditions leading to male factor infertility. These agents include antimicrobial drugs, anti-inflammatory medications, and sympathetic agonists. Each of these classes of drugs has clear indications for use in specifically targeted subgroups of infertile men, and they are each described in other specific chapters of this text.

One important point clearly delineated in the literature over recent years is this: empiric medical therapy generally has limited utility and benefit in the treatment of infertile men. While randomized, double-blinded, placebo-controlled studies are costly in terms of time and money, they remain the proving ground for effective medical therapies. More than one agent has failed to pass this test in recent years, but this is a good thing. While the armamentarium of available medical agents for the treatment of male infertility is somewhat limited, this fact should push us to strive harder to gain enhanced insight into the pathophysiological mechanisms leading to decreased male reproductive potential. It is with this enhanced insight into the fundamental problems leading to male infertility that we will develop additional, effective medical therapies.

Five-Year View

The future for medical therapies for male infertility truly hinges on enhanced understanding of the root causes of impaired male reproduction. Much effort is now being expended by leading investigators throughout the world to gain insight into the following:

- The genetic basis of male infertility
- Environmental factors that interfere with male reproductive potential
- Reactive oxygen species and their detrimental effects on sperm DNA/sperm function
- Unexplained infertility (clarifying the pathophysiology)

Each of these broad categories certainly has potential to provide additional targets for directed medical therapies, but this will not come until we gain enhanced understanding of each of these enumerated categories.

An emerging health issue here in the United States and throughout much of the world is metabolic syndrome. As has been clearly shown in numerous studies, metabolic syndrome can negatively affect male reproductive health in a myriad of ways [34]. In addition to promoting lifestyle changes in affected patients, physicians will likely be increasingly called upon to medically address certain problems associated with this syndrome that can hinder male reproduction, such as hypogonadism, diminished libido, erectile dysfunction, and a "proinflammatory" state that may set the stage for abnormally high sperm DNA damage.

Key Issues

Targeted medical therapies for male infertility generally address endocrinopathies, infection, inflammation, and disorders of erection and ejaculation. Empiric medical therapy has gradually been replaced by medical treatments aimed at addressing specific underlying medical problems causing decreased male reproductive potential.

The armamentarium of available medical therapies for male infertility is somewhat limited in terms of numbers of patients suitable for treatment. However, enhanced understanding of the pathophysiological mechanisms causing male factor infertility should broaden opportunities for the development of specifically targeted, effective agents.

References

1. Alukal J, Lamb D, Niederberger C, Makhlouf A. Spermatogenesis in the adult. In: Lipshultz L, Howards S, Niederberger C, editors. Infertility in the male. New York: Cambridge University; 2009. p. 74–89.
2. Caroppo E. Male hypothalamic-pituitary-gonadal axis. In: Lipshultz L, Howards S, Niederberger C, editors. Infertility in the male. New York: Cambridge University; 2009. p. 14–28.
3. Kim HH, Schlegel PN. Endocrine manipulation in male infertility. Urol Clin North Am. 2008;35:303–18.
4. Sussman EM, Chudnovsky A, Niederberger CS. Hormonal evaluation of the infertile male: has it evolved? Urol Clin North Am. 2008;35:147–55.
5. Coviello AD, Matsumoto AM, Bremner WJ, et al. Low-dose human chorionic gonadotropin maintains intratesticular testosterone in normal men with testosterone-induced gonadotropin suppression. J Clin Endocrinol Metab. 2005;90:2595–602.
6. Bouloux PM, Nieschlag E, Burger HG, et al. Induction of spermatogenesis by recombinant follicle-stimulating hormone (puregon) in hypogonadotropic azoospermic men who failed to respond to human chorionic gonadotropin alone. J Androl. 2003;24: 604–11.
7. Schiff JD, Ramirez ML, Bar-Chama N. Medical and surgical management male infertility. Endocrinol Metab Clin North Am. 2007;36:313–31.
8. Liu PY, Baker HW, Jayadev V, Zacharin M, Conway AJ, Handelsman DJ. Induction of spermatogenesis and fertility during gonadotropin treatment of gonadotropin-deficient infertile men: predictors of fertility outcome. J Clin Endocrinol Metab. 2009;94:801–8.
9. Clark ABR, Vantman D, Sherins R. A low sperm concentration does not preclude fertility in men with isolated hypogonadotropic hypogonadism after gonadotropin therapy. Fertil Steril. 1988;50: 343–7.
10. Miyagawa Y, Tsujimura A, Matsumiya K, et al. Outcome of gonadotropin therapy for male hypogonadotropic hypogonadism at university affiliated male infertility centers: a 30-year retrospective study. J Urol. 2005;173:2072–5.
11. Farhat R, Al-Zidjali F, Alzahrani AS. Outcome of gonadotropin therapy for male infertility due to hypogonadotrophic hypogonadism. Pituitary. 2010;13(2):05–10.
12. Whitten SJ, Nangia AK, Kolettis PN. Select patients with hypogonadotropic hypogonadism may respond to treatment with clomiphene citrate. Fertil Steril. 2006;86:1664–8.
13. Ioannidou-Kadis S, Wright PJ, Neely RD, Quinton R. Complete reversal of adult-onset isolated hypogonadotropic hypogonadism with clomiphene citrate. Fertil Steril. 2006;86:1513e5–9.
14. Burge MR, Lanzi RA, Skarda ST, Eaton RP. Idiopathic hypogonadotropic hypogonadism in a male runner is reversed by clomiphene citrate. Fertil Steril. 1997;67:783–5.
15. Boyle K. Nonsurgical treatment: empiric therapy. In: Lipshultz L, Howards S, Niederberger C, editors. Infertility in the male. New York: Cambridge University; 2009. p. 438–53.
16. Raman JD, Schlegel PN. Aromatase inhibitors for male infertility. J Urol. 2002;167:624–9.
17. Ramasamy R, Ricci JA, Palermo GD, Gosden LV, Rosenwaks Z, Schlegel PN. Successful fertility treatment for Klinefelter's syndrome. J Urol. 2009;182:1108–13.
18. Griboff SI. Semen analysis in myxedema. Fertil Steril. 1962;13: 436–43.
19. Meeker JD, Godfrey-Bailey L, Hauser R. Relationships between serum hormone levels and semen quality among men from an infertility clinic. J Androl. 2007;28:397–406.
20. Krassas GE, Papadopoulou F, Tziomalos K, Zeginiadou T, Pontikides N. Hypothyroidism has an adverse effect on human spermatogenesis: a prospective, controlled study. Thyroid. 2008; 18:1255–9.
21. Dohle GR, Smit M, Weber RF. Androgens and male fertility. World J Urol. 2003;21:341–5.
22. Turek PJ, Williams RH, Gilbaugh 3rd JH, Lipshultz LI. The reversibility of anabolic steroid-induced azoospermia. J Urol. 1995;153:1628–30.
23. Menon DK. Successful treatment of anabolic steroid-induced azoospermia with human chorionic gonadotropin and human menopausal gonadotropin. Fertil Steril. 2003;79 Suppl 3: 1659–61.

24. Tan RS, Vasudevan D. Use of clomiphene citrate to reverse premature andropause secondary to steroid abuse. Fertil Steril. 2003;79:203–5.
25. Pavlovich CP, King P, Goldstein M, Schlegel PN. Evidence of a treatable endocrinopathy in infertile men. J Urol. 2001;165:837–41.
26. Roth MY, Amory JK, Page ST. Treatment of male infertility secondary to morbid obesity. Nat Clin Pract Endocrinol Metab. 2008;4:415–9.
27. Abalovich M, Levalle O, Hermes R, et al. Hypothalamic-pituitary-testicular axis and seminal parameters in hyperthyroid males. Thyroid. 1999;9:857–63.
28. Krassas GE, Pontikides N, Deligianni V, Miras K. A prospective controlled study of the impact of hyperthyroidism on reproductive function in males. J Clin Endocrinol Metab. 2002;87: 3667–71.
29. Thorner MO, McNeilly AS, Hagan C, Besser GM. Long-term treatment of galactorrhoea and hypogonadism with bromocriptine. Br Med J. 1974;2:419–22.
30. De Rosa M, Colao A, Di Sarno A, et al. Cabergoline treatment rapidly improves gonadal function in hyperprolactinemic males: a comparison with bromocriptine. Eur J Endocrinol. 1998;138: 286–93.
31. De Rosa M, Ciccarelli A, Zarrilli S, et al. The treatment with cabergoline for 24 month normalizes the quality of seminal fluid in hyperprolactinaemic males. Clin Endocrinol (Oxf). 2006;64:307–13.
32. Gillam MP, Molitch ME, Lombardi G, Colao A. Advances in the treatment of prolactinomas. Endocr Rev. 2006;27:485–534.
33. Ribeiro RS, Abucham J. Recovery of persistent hypogonadism by clomiphene in males with prolactinomas under dopamine agonist treatment. Eur J Endocrinol. 2009;161:163–9.
34. Kasturi SS, Tannir J, Brannigan RE. The metabolic syndrome and male infertility. J Androl. 2008;29:251–9.

Chapter 8
Surgical Treatment for Male Infertility

Sandro C. Esteves and Ricardo Miyaoka

Infertility complaint is common in the urologic office. Approximately 8% of men in reproductive age seek for medical assistance for fertility-related problems. Of these, 1–10% carries conditions that compromise the reproductive potential [1]. The role of the urologist in this context cannot be underestimated, since he/she is trained to diagnose, to counsel, to provide medical or surgical treatment whenever possible, or to correctly refer the male patient for assisted conception. The urologist can also be part of the multi-professional reproductive team in the assisted reproduction unit, being responsible for the previously cited tasks as well as for the sperm surgical retrieval from the epididymis or testicle.

In a group of 2,875 infertile couples attending our tertiary center for male reproduction, potentially surgical correctable conditions were identified in 34.4% of the male partners. About 1/3 of these individuals were azoospermic. Although reconstructive surgery would be possible in only 30% of this subgroup, most of the remaining would be candidates for sperm retrieval techniques if enrolled in assisted reproduction programs. Therefore, surgical management can be offered to more than 50% of our patient population in daily practice (Table 8.1).

Two major breakthroughs occurred in the area of male infertility with regard to treatment. The first was the development of microsurgery, which increased success rates for reconstruction of the reproductive tract. The second was the

S.C. Esteves, MD, PhD (✉) • R. Miyaoka, MD
ANDROFERT, Andrology and Human Reproduction Clinic,
Center for Male Reproduction, Av. Dr. Heitor Penteado, 1464,
Campinas, SP 13075-460, Brazil
e-mail: s.esteves@androfert.com.br; rmiyaoka@androfert.com.br

S.J. Parekattil, A. Agarwal (eds.), *Male Infertility for the Clinician*,
© Springer Science+Business Media New York 2013

Table 8.1 Distribution of diagnostic categories of couples seeking infertility evaluation in a male infertility clinic

Category	N	%
Varicocele	629	21.9
Infectious	72	2.5
Hormonal	54	1.9
Ejaculatory dysfunction	28	1.0
Systemic diseases	11	0.4
Idiopathic	289	10.0
Normal/female factor	492	17.1
Immunologic	54	1.9
Obstruction	359	12.5
Cancer	11	0.4
Cryptorchidism	342	11.9
Genetic	189	6.6
Testicular failure	345	11.9
Total	2,875	

development of intracytoplasmic sperm injection (ICSI) and the demonstration that spermatozoa retrieved from either the epididymis or the testis were capable of fertilization and pregnancy [2, 3]. Thereafter, several sperm retrieval methods have been developed to collect epididymal and testicular sperm for ICSI in azoospermic men. Microsurgery was incorporated to this armamentarium, either for collection of sperm from the epididymis in men with obstructive azoospermia or from the testicle in those with nonobstructive azoospermia (NOA) [2, 4].

This chapter describes the most common surgical treatments for male infertility. It includes not only the reconstructive interventions for the male reproductive system but also the sperm retrieval techniques to be used in cases of obstructive (OA) and NOA. A critical commentary, based on the authors' experience in the surgical management for the infertile male, and a review of important publications from the last 5 years are included. Finally, a list of key issues is provided to summarize the current knowledge in this area.

Surgical Treatments

Varicocele Repair

Varicoceles can be identified in up to 35% of the male population with infertility complaints [1]. The etiology of varicocele formation is likely to be multifactorial, and several theories aim to explain the impact of varicoceles on testicular function, none of them fully elucidating the variable effect of varicocele on human spermatogenesis and male fertility [5–8]. The association between varicocele and infertility is still a matter of debate. However, there is an increased incidence of this condition among infertile men [9]. Moreover, varicocele is associated with reduced semen parameters and testicular size [10]. Lastly, it has been shown that surgical treatment of clinical varicoceles improves semen quality and increases the likelihood of pregnancy [11, 12]. Despite these facts, it is still unclear why most men with varicocele retain fertility and why fertility status is not always improved after treatment [13].

Preoperative Planning and Patient Evaluation

Treatment of varicocele in infertile men aims to restore or improve testicular function. Current recommendations suggest that treatment should be offered for couples with documented infertility whose male partner has a clinically palpable varicocele and abnormal semen analysis. A detailed medical history must be taken and prognostic factors identified. Physical examination with the patient standing in a warm room is the preferred diagnostic method. Varicoceles diagnosed by this method are termed "clinical" and may be graded according to the size. Large varicoceles (grade III) are varicose veins seen through the scrotal skin. Moderate (grade II) and small-sized varicoceles (grade I) are dilated veins palpable without and with the aid of the Valsalva maneuver, respectively [14]. In the presence of bilateral palpable varicocele, it is recommended to perform surgery on both sides at the same operative time [15].

Physical examination may be inconclusive or equivocal in cases of low-grade varicocele and in men with a history of previous scrotal surgery, concomitant hydroceles, or obesity. Imaging studies may be recommended during the evaluation of infertile men for varicocele if physical examination is inconclusive. When a varicocele is not palpable but a retrograde blood flow is detected by other diagnostic methods such as venography, Doppler examination, ultrasonography, scintigraphy, or thermography, the varicocele is termed subclinical [16, 17]. However, the role of subclinical varicocele as a cause of male infertility remains debatable, and current evidence does not support the recommendation for treating infertile men with subclinical varicocele [18, 19].

Preoperative hormone profile including follicle-stimulating hormone (FSH) and testosterone is recommended. Testicular volume should be assessed using a measurement instrument such as the Prader orchidometer or a pachimeter. At least two semen analyses must be obtained and evaluated according to the World Health Organization guidelines [20]. It seems that infertile men either with higher preoperative semen parameters or undergoing varicocele repair for large varicoceles are more likely to show postoperative semen parameters improvement [21]. On the other hand, reduced preoperative testicular volume, elevated serum FSH levels, diminished testosterone concentrations, and subclinical varicocele are negative predictors for fertility improvement after surgery [18, 22–27].

Men with clinical varicoceles presenting with azoospermia may be candidates for surgical repair. In such cases, genetic evaluation including Giemsa karyotyping and polymerase chain Yq microdeletion screening for AZFa, AZFb, and AZFc regions is recommended. A testis biopsy (open or percutaneous) may be obtained to assess testicular histology, which has been shown to be the only valid prognostic factor for restoration of spermatogenesis [20, 28]. The benefit of varicocelectomy in azoospermic men with genetic abnormalities is doubtful and should be carefully balanced. The same caution is valid for patients with atrophic testes and/or history of cryptorchidism, testicular trauma, orchitis, and systemic or hormonal dysfunction due to the fact that varicocele in such cases may not be the cause of infertility but merely coincidental [29].

As for all surgical reconstructive procedures, the evaluation of the female partner's reproductive potential is recommended before an intervention is indicated, and the alternatives to varicocele repair discussed.

Anesthesia and Techniques

Varicocele repair may be carried out using local, regional, or general anesthesia, according solely with the surgeon and patient's preferences. In the authors' practice, we routinely perform microsurgical subinguinal varicocele repair using short-acting propofol intravenous anesthesia associated with the blockage of the spermatic cord using 10 mL of a 2% lidocaine hydrochloride on an outpatient basis [20].

Varicoceles are surgically treated either by open (with or without magnification) or laparoscopic approaches. The main concept is the occlusion of the dilated veins of the pampiniform plexus. The high retroperitoneal and laparoscopic approaches are performed for internal spermatic vein ligation, while the inguinal and subinguinal approaches allow the ligation of the internal and external spermatic and cremasteric veins that may contribute to the varicocele.

Retroperitoneal Techniques

High retroperitoneal open varicocele repair involves incision medial to the anterior superior iliac spine at the level of the internal inguinal ring (Fig. 8.1a). The external oblique muscle is split, the internal oblique muscle is retracted and the peritoneum is teased away. Exposure of the internal spermatic artery and vein is carried out retroperitoneally near the ureter. At this level, only one or two internal spermatic veins are present, but the internal spermatic artery may not be easy to identify. The veins are ligated near to the point of drainage into the left renal vein. Neither the parallel inguinal and retroperitoneal collateral veins that exit the testis and bypass the retroperitoneal area of ligation nor the cremasteric veins can be identified in the retroperitoneal approach. It is believed that these collaterals are the primary cause of recurrence seen in retroperitoneal varicocelectomy. The surgical approach on the right side may be more difficult because the right gonadic vein drains in the inferior vena cava. Laparoscopic varicocelectomy is a retroperitoneal approach using high magnification. The spermatic artery and the lymphatics are easily identified and spared; collateral veins can also be clipped or coagulated. However, external

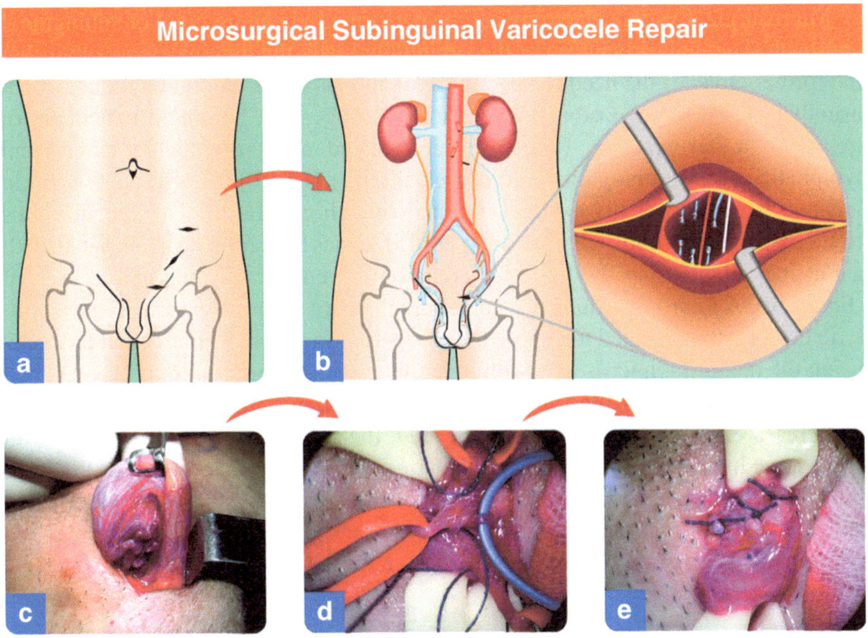

Fig. 8.1 Microsurgical subinguinal varicocele repair. (**a**) Incision sites commonly used for subinguinal, inguinal, and retroperitoneal varicocele repair. (**b**) In the subinguinal approach, a transverse incision is made just below the level of the external inguinal ring. (**c–e**) Intraoperative photographs of the spermatic cord. (**c**) Dilated cremasteric veins are identified by elevating the spermatic cord with a Babcock clamp. (**d**) Testicular artery (*blue vessel loop*), lymphatics (*blue cotton suture*), and dilated varicose veins (*red vessel loops*) are demonstrated. (**e**) Final surgical aspect of varicose veins transected and ligated with nonabsorbable sutures

spermatic veins cannot be treated, thus leading to a recurrence rate of approximately 5 % [30]. Laparoscopy varicocele repair is more invasive and costly, and it is associated with higher complication rates than open procedures [30–32].

Inguinal and Subinguinal Techniques

The classic approach to the inguinal varicocelectomy involves a 5–10-cm incision over the inguinal canal, opening of the external oblique aponeurosis and isolation of the spermatic cord (Fig. 8.1a). The internal spermatic veins are dissected and ligated. An attempt is made to positively identify and spare the testicular artery and the lymphatics. External spermatic veins running parallel to the spermatic cord or perforating the floor of the inguinal canal can be identified and ligated. Although internal and external spermatic veins can be identified macroscopically, the use of magnification facilitates identification and preservation of internal spermatic artery and lymphatics, which may prevent testicular atrophy and hydrocele formation, respectively [33].

Microsurgical varicocelectomy can be performed via an inguinal or subinguinal approach. The main advantage of the subinguinal over the inguinal approach is that the former obviates the need to open the aponeurosis of the external oblique, which usually results in more postoperative pain and a longer time before the patient return to work. In our practice, varicoceles are treated using a testicular artery and lymphatic-sparing subinguinal microsurgical repair [12, 20]. Briefly, a 2.5-cm skin incision is made over the external inguinal ring (Fig. 8.1a, b). The subcutaneous tissue is separated until the spermatic cord is exposed. The cord is elevated with a Babcock clamp, and the posterior cremasteric veins are ligated and transected (Fig. 8.1c). A Penrose drain is placed behind the cord without tension. The cremasteric fascia is then opened to expose the cord structures, and the dissection proceeds using the operating microscope with magnification ranging from 6 to 16x. Dilated cremasteric veins are ligated and transected. Lymphatics and arteries are identified and preserved (Fig. 8.1d). Whenever needed, the cord structures are sprayed with papaverine hydrochloride to increase the arterial beat. All dilated veins of the spermatic cord are identified, tagged with vessel loops, then ligated using nonabsorbable sutures and transected (Fig. 8.1e). Vasal veins are ligated only if they exceed 2 mm in diameter. Sclerosis of small veins is not used.

Postoperative Care

Local dressing and scrotal supporter are kept for 48–72 h and 1 week, respectively. Scrotal ice packing is always recommended to control local edema for the first 48 postoperative hours. Patients are counseled to restrain from physical activity and sexual intercourse for 2–3 weeks. Oral analgesics usually suffice to control postoperative pain. Postoperative follow-up aims to evaluate improvement in semen parameters, complications, and spontaneous or assisted conception. Semen analysis should be performed every 3 months until the semen parameters stabilize or pregnancy occurs.

Reconstructive Surgery of the Vas Deferens and Epididymis

Vasovasostomy and vasoepididymostomy are surgical procedures designed to bypass an obstruction in the male genital tract. Approximately 13% of married men aged 15–44 years reported having had a vasectomy in the United States [34]. As expected, vasectomy frequency increases with older age and greater number of biological children. The number of men seeking for vasectomy reversal due to changes in marital status or reproductive goals has increased and vary from 2% to 6% [35]. In Brazil, it is estimated that 200,000 and 7,000 vasectomies and reversals are annually performed, respectively [36]. While the vast majority of vasovasostomy and vasoepididymostomy procedures are to reverse intentional obstructions, other indications include correction of epididymal or vasal obstructions due to genital infections, iatrogenic injuries related to inguinal or scrotal surgery, especially during the early childhood and postvasectomy pain syndrome [37].

Preoperative Planning and Patient Evaluation

A detailed medical history must be taken and prognostic factors identified. Obstruction intervals from vasectomy to reversal are believed to play a major role in determining surgery outcomes. Patency and pregnancy rates for obstruction intervals up to 15 years are approximately 74% and 40%, respectively [38]. Obstruction intervals longer than 15 years are associated with lower patency and pregnancy rates. Long obstruction intervals are associated with higher incidence of epididymal obstruction, and as a result, vasoepididymostomy (VE) is likely to be required. A computer model based on obstructive interval and patient age was created to determine the need for VE. The model was designed to be 100% sensitive in detecting patients requiring VE. In the test group, the model was 100% sensitive in predicting VE with a specificity of 58.8% [39].

A history of a previous vasectomy reversal attempt does not preclude a new one. Patency and pregnancy rates of 79% and 31%, respectively, are reported for repeated reversals [40]. These authors found that the history of conception with the current partner had been the only significant predictor for a successful pregnancy. History of genital/inguinal surgery should raise concern about the possibility of iatrogenic surgical obstruction. Repair of obstruction in the inguinal canal or retroperitoneum can be technically challenging.

A detailed physical examination should be carried out. Small and soft testes may indicate impaired spermatogenesis. Indurate, irregular epididymis and the presence of hydrocele are often associated with epididymal obstruction and may suggest the need for vasoepididymostomy. Palpation of a granuloma in the vas deferens should be interpreted as a favorable prognostic sign. Its presence means that sperm has leaked at the vasectomy site preventing overpressure within the epididymis tubules and rupture [35, 38, 41]. If a vasal gap is detected, the patient should be advised that a larger incision into the inguinal region may be needed in order to allow a tension-free anastomosis to be performed. Specific laboratory tests are not necessary before reconstructive surgeries. Serum FSH testing is recommended as a marker of testicular reserve only if testicular damage is suspected on physical examination. The usefulness of antibody testing remains controversial, and evidence suggests that late failures following reversals are likely to be technical rather than immunological [42, 43]. Besides, overall conception rates are acceptably high, and the presence of antisperm antibodies does not correlate closely with postsurgical fecundability [44].

The female partner fertility has to be carefully assessed before indicating reconstruction procedures, and alternatives to vasectomy reversal should be discussed. It has been shown that reversal outcomes in men with the same partners are significantly better than those with new partners. The proven fecundity as a couple, shorter obstructive interval, and stronger emotional dedication to achieving conception may act as possible factors for the higher success rate [35, 45]. Female age greater than 40 years is a negative predictor for success [46, 47].

Anesthesia and Techniques

Vasovasostomy and vasoepididymostomy may be safely performed using local, regional, or general anesthesia. In the authors' practice, procedures are carried out on an outpatient basis. Continuous propofol intravenous anesthesia coupled with the blockage of the spermatic cord using 10–20 mL of a 1% lidocaine hydrochloride solution is our preferred anesthetic method.

Incision

2-centimeter longitudinal scrotal incisions are placed in the anterior aspect of the scrotum on each side. The incision is made onto the palpable granuloma or onto the identified vasal gap. Only the vas ends are delivered through the skin incision. The incision may be extended to the inguinal region in case the vasectomy has been performed high in the scrotum, or a large segment has been removed, and also in repeat reconstructions with difficult vasal mobilization. The testis is delivered only if a vasoepididymostomy or a robotic-assisted anastomosis is to be performed.

Approaching the Vas

Microsurgical dissection is carried out onto the region of the prior vasectomy site to free the vas and its vascular pedicle from surrounding scar tissue. Hemostasis is obtained with great care using either bipolar or handheld thermal cautery units. After the vas has been mobilized and its scarred ends excised, patency of the abdominal vas end is confirmed by the introduction of a 24-gauge blunt-tipped angiocatheter into its lumen and injection of 20-mL sterile saline through the catheter. The vas ends must be adequately mobilized in order to allow a complete tension-free anastomosis. Either a microsurgical clamp or holding sutures can be used to accomplish this step according to the surgeon's preference.

Vasal Fluid Examination

Fluid from the testicular vas end is examined both macroscopically and under the optical microscope for the presence of sperm. The presence of copious, clear, watery, or cloudy fluid and motile sperm is associated with excellent patency rates of 94% as opposed to only 60% when no sperm is found in the vasal fluid [35]. Thick toothpaste-like vasal fluid is suggestive of epididymal obstruction [35, 48]. The quality of sperm found in the intravasal fluid and the surgeon's microsurgical skills are the most important factors to determine the type of reconstructive technique. Typically, the presence of sperm or sperm parts, and even a "dry" vas, is associated with adequate patency rates of about 70–80% following vasovasostomies [49, 50]. The vasoepididymostomy is a challenging surgical procedure that should only be attempted by experienced microsurgeons. Meticulous microsurgical technique and high magnification are required for a precise anastomosis of the vas (luminal diameter of 300–400 µm) to the epididymal tubule (luminal diameter of 150–250 µm). Intraoperative sperm harvesting and cryopreservation can be offered during vasoepididymostomy [51].

Vasovasostomy Techniques

Attention to surgical details directly affects the success of reconstructive microsurgeries. These include the accurate mucosa-to-mucosa approximation, a watertight tension-free anastomosis, preservation of the vasal blood supply and healthy tissue (mucosa and muscularis), and an adequate microscopic atraumatic technique.

Modified One-Layer Technique

The modified one-layer technique described by Sharlip is the authors' choice for vasectomy reversal [52]. Our preference is to perform the anastomosis using a 9-0 nylon suture mounted on a taper-pointed needle and with the aid of a vas clamp (ASSI, catalog# MSPK-3678). The operation is performed entirely with the surgeon located on the patient's right side. The first suture is placed in the medial surface of the right vas (zero degree position) (Fig. 8.2a). This suture is placed through the full thickness of the vas wall on the testicular side first taking a generous bite of adventitia and muscularis and a tiny portion of the mucosa. The suture is then passed into the corresponding zero-degree position of the abdominal side taking a bite at the edge of the mucosa and a large portion of the muscularis/adventitia layer. This suture is tied and cut long, so it is easily identified as the procedure continues. The second suture is placed 180° opposite to the first, and again it takes the full aspect of the vas wall, firstly on the testicular side and then on the abdominal one. This suture is also tied and cut long. A third full thickness suture is placed at the 60° position, one third of the distance from the first to the second sutures. Before it is tied, a fourth suture is placed at the 120° position, two thirds of the distance from the first and second sutures. The fourth suture is then tied after careful inspection of their proper placement (Fig. 8.2a). A fifth suture is placed between these two at the 90° position, but only superficially through the muscularis. This completes the anastomosis of the anterior portion of the vas. At this point, four full thickness stitches and one muscular suture have been placed, and half of the total circumference of the vas wall is closed. The vas clamp is then rotated 180°, and verification of accidental back-walling and proper position of full thickness sutures is carried out. After rotation of the vas, two full thickness sutures are then placed at the 240 and 300° positions. These sutures are

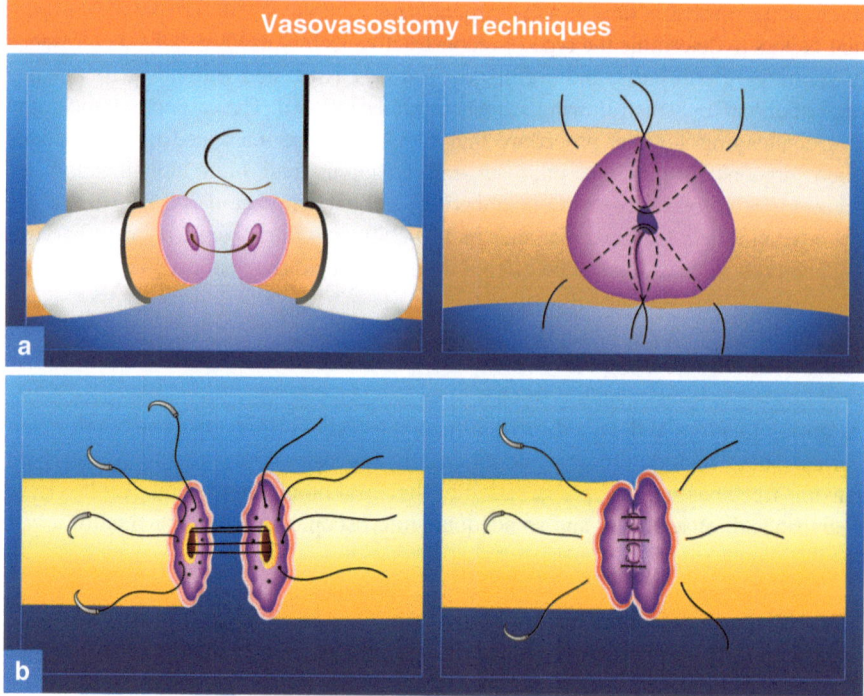

Fig. 8.2 Microsurgical vasovasostomy techniques. Illustration of the modified one-layer (**a**) and the multilayer microdot technique (**b**) (see text for detailed description)

inserted and inspected before being tied. A final suture is placed in the muscularis at the 270° position. This complete the anastomosis, summing up 8 sutures in total instead of 12 as first described by Sharlip. Upon anastomosis completion, the surrounding loose fibrous tissue is sutured over the anastomotic site alleviating tension. Scrotal incision is closed in the routine usual manner.

Two-Layer Technique

This technique, described by Belker, involves the placement of five to eight interrupted 10-0 nylon sutures in the inner mucosal layer and eight to ten 9-0 nylon sutures in the outer muscular and adventitial layer [53]. The use of an approximating clamp and a holding suture is recommended to stabilize the vas ends for the anastomosis. Before suturing begins, the vas ends are placed parallel to each other in such a way that allows the surgeon to look straight down into their lumens. As suturing proceeds, the transected ends of the vas bend toward each other, bringing the suture together without tension. First, three posterior muscular layer sutures are placed in a row so that the knots are outside. At this point, 90° of the circumference is approximated, leaving full access to the mucosa. Then, three posterior mucosal sutures are placed and tied. Subsequently, the far-corner and near-corner sutures are placed and tied alternately until space remains for only two or three sutures in the anterior aspect of the anastomosis. These remaining stitches are then placed and left long and untied until back-walling can be safely ruled out. The sutures are then tied, and the muscular layer is sutured with caution to avoid penetration of the lumen by the outer-layer sutures. Placement of these sutures is easier to perform from the assistant side toward the surgeon's side. Closure of scrotal incision is performed in the usual manner.

Multilayer Microdot Technique

This method, originally described by Goldstein, is adequate to treat markedly discrepant vas diameters in straight or convoluted vas [54]. Vasal ends are prepared with a 90° right angle cut, and methylene blue stain can be used to better visualize the mucosal rings. Planned needle exit points can be marked with microtip marking (Fig. 8.2b). Polypropylene monofilament 10-0 double-armed sutures (70-μm-diameter) with taper-pointed needles are used for the anastomosis. Sutures are placed in an inside-out fashion eliminating the possibility for accidental backwalling. The mucosa and about one-third thickness of the muscularis should be included in each bite, symmetrically on each side of vas ends. Four initial sutures are placed in the anterior aspect of the vas and tied up (Fig. 8.2b). Three 9-0 sutures are then placed exactly in between the previously placed mucosal sutures, just above but not through the mucosa, sealing the gap between the mucosal sutures. The vas is then rotated 180°, and four additional 10-0 sutures are placed completing the mucosal part of the anastomosis. Just prior to tying the last mucosal knot, vas lumen is irrigated with heparinized saline solution to prevent formation of clots. After completion of mucosal layer, 9-0 sutures are placed in between each mucosal suture, again avoiding penetrating the mucosa itself (Fig. 8.2b). Superficial additional adventitia 9-0 sutures should be placed only if necessary. Procedure is completed by approximating the vas sheath with four to six 6-0 sutures.

Robotic-Assisted Technique

Recent reports have shown the feasibility of performing the classic above described techniques using robotic assistance. The robot can offer additional benefits of enhanced imaging (up to ×100 magnification) and control of physiologic tremor [55, 56].

Vasoepididymostomy Techniques

The procedure starts with the placement of a longitudinal incision in the upper scrotum. The testis is delivered through the incision, and the testis and epididymis are thoroughly inspected. The site of obstruction can be often seen as an area where the epididymis changes from a firm, wide caliber to a smaller, softer structure. The distal end of the vas deferens is mobilized in a similar fashion as that described for the vasovasostomy, but usually a longer length is required to perform an epididymal anastomosis. At this point, the microscope is brought into the operating field to aid the surgeon perform the anastomosis. Currently, three variations of the technique have been used for precise approximation of the vas deferens lumen to a single epididymal tubule: end-to-end, end-to-side, and end-to-side intussusception techniques. Prior to the anastomosis, a dilated epididymal tubule must be identified immediately above the level of obstruction. The tubule must be opened and the fluid inspected for the presence of motile sperm. If no sperm are identified, a more proximal site of the epididymis will be required for the anastomosis.

End-to-End Technique

First described by Silber, the end-to-end VE is the most difficult anastomosis to perform [57]. It involves the dissection of a single epididymal tubule, its complete transection, and then its anastomosis to the vas lumen. The epididymis is dissected off the testis for 3–5 cm to provide an adequate length to achieve a tension-free anastomosis. Initially, two 9-0 nylon sutures are placed at the 5 and 7 o'clock positions of the seromuscular surface of the vas, to secure the cut end of the distal vas to the epididymal tunica. Next, four 10-0 nylon sutures mounted in double-armed 70-μm fishhook-shaped taper-pointed needles are placed in a quadrant fashion between the vas mucosa and the epididymal tubule (Fig. 8.3a). These sutures are not tied until all of them have been positioned. The anastomosis is completed by placing several interrupted 9-0 nylon sutures to approximate the seromuscular layer of the vas to the epididymal tunic layer.

End-to-Side Technique

The end-to-side VE, popularized by Thomas, is performed by creating a small window in a loop of the epididymal tubule proximal to the obstruction and by suturing the end of the vas lumen to the open window [58]. The advantages over the end-to-end anastomosis include less dissection and bleeding during the anastomosis because hemostasis can be secured before opening the tubule. Moreover, only one tubule is opened making the identification of the patent tubule more precise and easy. With the tubule opened and sperm presence confirmed, three or four double-armed 10-0 nylon sutures are placed in a quadrant fashion through the edge of the epididymal tubule (Fig. 8.3b). The sutures are placed in the corresponding quadrant of the vasal mucosa and tied. The anastomosis is completed with additional 9-0 nylon sutures between the epididymal tunic and the seromuscular layer of the vas deferens. Lastly, several 9-0 nylon sutures are used to anchor the vas deferens to the parietal layer of the tunica vaginalis. These final sutures are designed to prevent tension on the anastomosis and are placed well away from the vasoepididymostomy site.

Vasoepididymostomy Techniques

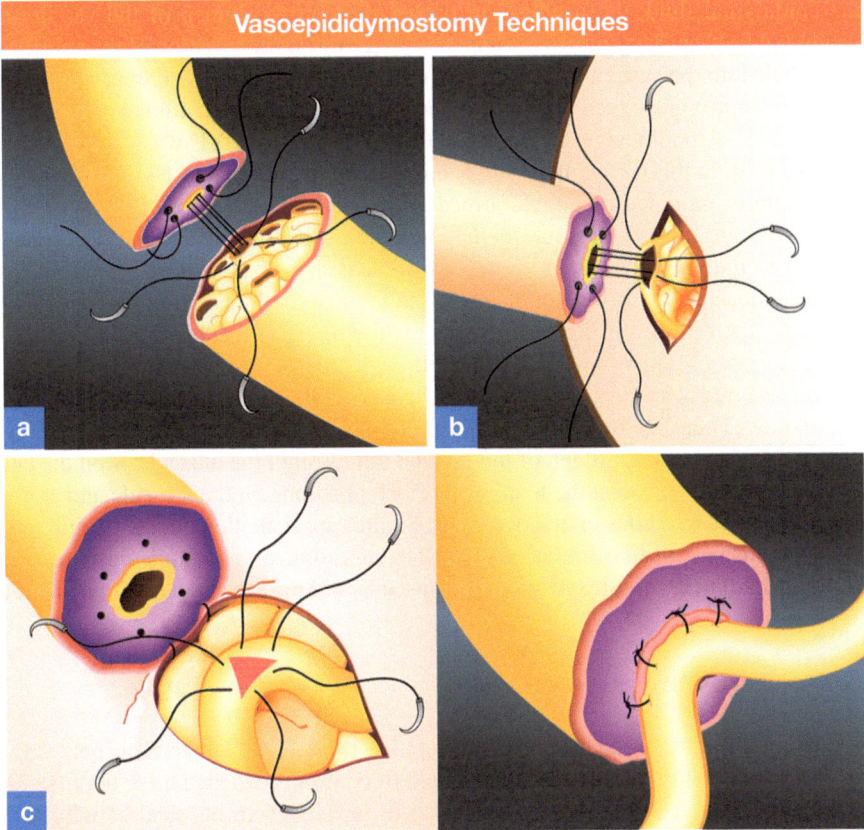

Fig. 8.3 Microsurgical vasoepididymostomy techniques. Illustration of the end-to-end (**a**), end-to-side (**b**), and triangulation end-to-side (**c**) anastomoses (see text for detailed description)

Triangulation End-to-Side Vasoepididymostomy

This technique was introduced by Berger [59] with subsequent modifications by others [60, 61]. It is the simplest and fastest among the three techniques described in this chapter and the authors' choice for vasoepididymostomy. The intention is to combine the precision of the conventional end-to-side anastomosis with a simplified microsuture placement. Rather than a direct approximation of the epididymal tubule to the vas, this method involves pulling the epididymal tubule into the vas lumen. An opening window is made in the epididymal tunic corresponding to the vas diameter. Two 9-0 sutures are used to secure the muscular layer of the vas to the epididymal tunic to avoid tension on the anastomosis site. Three double-armed 10-0 nylon sutures are placed equidistantly in a triangular configuration in the desired epididymal tubule (Fig. 8.3c). Then, the epididymal tubule is carefully opened with microscissors or microknife between the positioned sutures. Once sperm is confirmed in the epididymal fluid, the needles are passed through the lumen of the vas in an inside-out fashion. The sutures are then tied, creating an invagination of the epididymal tubule into the vasal lumen (Fig. 8.3c). Finally, additional 9-0 nylon sutures are placed to approximate the seromuscular layer of the vas to the epididymal tunic.

Recently, a modification of the triangulation end-to-side VE was described by Marmar [60]. In this technique, a single epididymal tubule is exposed, and two 10-0 nylon sutures mounted on double-armed 70-μm bicurve needles are placed on the field. A needle from each suture is mounted on a styrofoam block and positioned parallel to the other with sufficient room for passage of the tip of a microblade between them. A microneedle holder is used to grasp both needles simultaneously and move them from the block to the field while maintaining the parallel arrangement. The tips of both needles are passed through a selected tubule at once. The two sutures are retracted laterally, and a tubulotomy is cut between them with a microknife. Then, all four needles from the epididymal sutures are individually placed into the mucosal lumen of the vas and out through the muscularis on the cut end. Needles are placed at the 8 and 10 o'clock positions on the left side and at the 2 and 4 o'clock positions on the right side. Sutures are tied allowing the epididymal tubule to invaginate into the vas lumen. The anastomosis is completed with 3–4 additional 9-0 nylon sutures through the muscularis of the vas and epididymal tunic.

Postoperative Care

Local dressing and scrotal supporter are kept for 48–72 h and 2 weeks, respectively. Scrotal ice packing is always recommended to control local edema for the first 72 postoperative hours. Patients are counseled to restrain from physical activity and sexual intercourse for 1 or 2 months in cases of vasovasostomy and vasoepididymostomy, respectively. Oral analgesics usually suffice to control postoperative pain. Postoperative follow-up is aimed at evaluating improvement in semen parameters, complications, and spontaneous or assisted conception. Semen analysis should be performed every 2 months after surgery until the semen parameters stabilize or pregnancy occurs.

Transurethral Resection of the Ejaculatory Duct

Ejaculatory duct obstruction (EDO) is a potential surgically correctable cause of male infertility. Congenital obstructions are caused by atresia or stenosis of the ejaculatory ducts, or utricular, mullerian, and wolffian duct cysts. Acquired obstructions may be secondary to trauma or infectious/inflammatory etiologies. Traumatic damage to the ejaculatory ducts may occur after removal of seminal vesicle cysts, pull-through operations for imperforate anus, and even prolonged catheterization or instrumentation. Genital or urinary infection and prostatic abscess may cause stenosis or complete obstruction of the ducts [62]. Prostatic infection may also result in calculus formation and secondary obstruction, while tuberculosis produces genital devastation.

Preoperative Planning and Patient Evaluation

Diagnostic criteria typically include history, physical examination, semen analyses, and transrectal ultrasound evaluation (TRUS). The clinical presentation may be highly variable, and in addition to a history of infertility, complaints may include painful ejaculation, hemospermia, and perineal and/or testicular pain, although patients can be completely asymptomatic. Physical examination is usually normal. Occasionally, the seminal vesicles or a mass is palpable on rectal examination. Prostatic tenderness and/or epididymal enlargement may exist. Hormone profiles are usually normal.

Semen analyses may reveal oligozoospermia or azoospermia, decreased motility, and decreased ejaculate volume. The presence of a low-volume (<1.5 mL) acidic (pH < 7.0) azoospermic ejaculate with absent fructose, palpable vasa, and epididymal thickening is virtually pathognomonic. However, the typical clinical picture may be complicated in cases obstruction is unilateral, partial, or functional [62]. Postejaculate urinalyses are often performed to exclude retrograde ejaculation in patients with low-volume ejaculates.

High-resolution TRUS using with a 5–7 MHz biplanar transducer is recommended in all cases of suspected EDO. The exact definition of obstruction on TRUS, however, is still a matter of debate due to marked variability in the size and shape of the vas deferens, seminal vesicles, and ejaculatory ducts in fertile and infertile men. Common ultrasound findings include dilation of the seminal vesicles (defined as a cross-sectional width of greater than 1.5 cm) or ejaculatory ducts (defined as an internal duct diameter of greater than 2.0 mm), calcifications or calculi in the region of the ejaculatory duct or verumontanum, and midline or eccentrically located prostatic cysts [63–65]. Ultrasound-guided transrectal seminal vesiculography has been shown to provide excellent radiographic visualization of the ejaculatory ducts [66]. Also, TRUS-guided seminal vesicle aspiration and the presence of motile sperm in the aspirates seem to be a useful diagnostic tool since the seminal vesicles are not sperm reservoirs [67]. A testicular biopsy can be done to document the presence of normal spermatogenesis. The authors' preference is to perform a "wet prep" using the percutaneous testicular sperm aspiration (TESA) technique either before or at the time of surgery. In such cases, the presence of motile sperm is highly indicative of obstruction.

Anesthesia and Technique

Transurethral resection of the ejaculatory duct (TURED) is performed using regional or general anesthesia. Our choice is to perform the procedure, as originally described by Farley and Barnes [68], with minor modifications [62]. First, the obstruction is documented using intraoperative vasotomy and vasography. The vas is delivered using a small scrotal incision and dissected free of the associated perivasal vessels. A mixture of injectable saline and radiographic contrast material in a 1:1 ratio is injected into the abdominal end of the vas, together with methylene blue dye, by direct vas puncture with a 30-gauge lymphangiogram needle [62]. Vasography

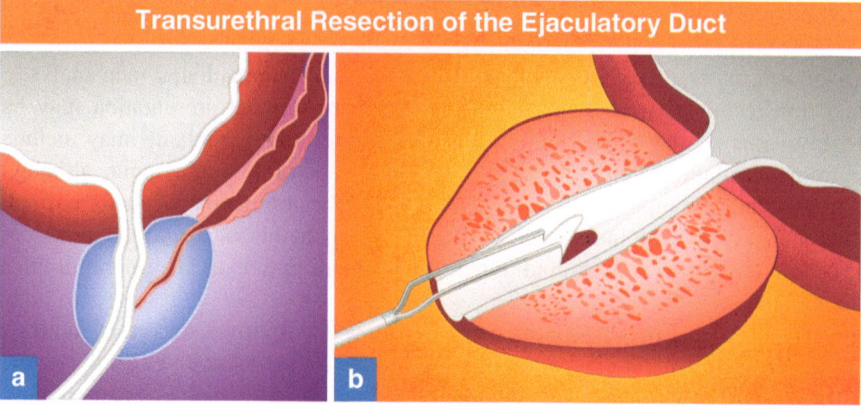

Fig. 8.4 Transurethral resection of the ejaculatory duct. Schematic representation of the ejaculatory duct entering into the prostatic urethra (**a**). A resectoscope loop is used to remove a strip of tissue on the floor of the prostate just proximal to and including a portion of the verumontanum (**b**)

confirms obstruction, whereas dye injection confirms patency by visualization of the effluxing dye mixture during TURED. A 9-0 nylon suture is placed at the muscular layer of the vas to close the vasotomy site. TURED is performed with the patient in the dorsal lithotomy position. A resectoscope with 24-French loop is used to remove a strip of tissue on the floor of the prostate just proximal to and including a portion of the verumontanum (Fig. 8.4a, b). The ducts are considered adequately opened by visualizing its dilated portion and the dye efflux. An 18-French Foley catheter is left in place for 24 h, and the patient is discharged the next day.

Postoperative Care

An indwelling catheter is kept in place for 24–48 h, and patients are discharged the following day. Oral quinolone antibiotics and anti-inflammatory medication are prescribed for 5 days. Scrotal supporter is recommended for 1 week to avoid scrotal edema due to vasotomy. Frequent ejaculation is recommended 3–4 weeks postoperatively, and patients are monitored with monthly semen analyses.

Sperm Retrieval Techniques

Azoospermia, defined as the absence of spermatozoa in the ejaculate after centrifugation, is found in 1–3% of the male population and approximately 10% of infertile males [67]. In this scenario, two different clinical situations exist, i.e., obstructive and nonobstructive azoospermia (NOA). In obstructive azoospermia (OA), spermatogenesis is normal, but a mechanical blockage exists in the genital tract, somewhere between the epididymis and the ejaculatory duct, or the epididymis and vas deferens are totally or partially absent. Acquired OA may be due to vasectomy, failure of vasectomy reversal, postinfectious diseases, surgical procedures in the scrotal, inguinal, pelvic, or abdominal regions, and trauma. Congenital causes of OA include cystic fibrosis, congenital absence of the vas deferens (CAVD), ejaculatory duct or prostatic cysts, and Young's syndrome [67]. NOA comprises a spectrum of testicular histopathology resulting from various causes that include environmental toxins, medications, cryptorchidism, genetic and congenital abnormalities, varicocele, trauma, viral orchitis, endocrine disorders, and idiopathic. In both OA and NOA, pregnancy may be achieved through in vitro fertilization associated to intracytoplasmic sperm injection (ICSI) [2, 3].

The goals of surgical sperm retrieval are threefold: (1) to retrieve an adequate number of sperm both for immediate use and cryopreservation, (2) to obtain the best quality sperm possible, and (3) to minimize damage to the reproductive tract as to not jeopardize future attempts of sperm retrieval and testicular function. Several surgical methods have been developed to retrieve epididymal and testicular sperm from azoospermic men. Either percutaneous (PESA) [69] or microsurgical epididymal sperm aspiration (MESA) [2] can be successfully used to retrieve sperm from the epididymis in men with obstructive azoospermia. TESA can be used to retrieve sperm from the testes both in men with OA who fail PESA as well as in those with NOA [70]. Testicular sperm extraction (TESE) using single or multiple open biopsies [71, 72], and more recently microsurgery (micro-TESE), is indicated for men with NOA [4, 71–74]. Sperm can be easily obtained from infertile men with OA, whereas individuals exhibiting NOA have historically been the most difficult to treat.

Preoperative Planning and Patient Evaluation

It is important to distinguish whether the lack of sperm in the ejaculate is from an obstructive or nonobstructive process since the choice of the retrieval method is based on the type of azoospermia. History, physical examination, and hormonal analysis (FSH, testosterone) are undertaken to define the type of azoospermia. Together, these factors provide a ~90% prediction of its type (obstructive or nonobstructive) [75]. Men with obstructive azoospermia usually have normal testes and endocrine profile. Occasionally, the epididymis or the seminal vesicles are enlarged, or a cyst may be palpable on rectal examination. The presence of a low-volume (<1.5 mL) acidic (pH < 7.0) azoospermic ejaculate with absent or low fructose and epididymal thickening is pathognomonic of obstructive azoospermia due to either congenital bilateral absence of the vas deferens or EDO; the differential diagnosis would be the presence of the vas in the latter. Approximately two thirds of men with CAVD have mutations of the cystic fibrosis transmembrane conductance regulator (CFTR) gene. Failure to identify a CFTR abnormality in a man with CBAVD does not rule out the presence of a mutation, since some are undetectable by routine testing methods. In such cases, the female partner should be offered CF testing before proceeding with treatments that utilize the sperm because of the high risk of the male being a cystic fibrosis (CF) carrier. If a CFTR gene mutation is identified (approximately 4% of female partners are carriers), testing should be offered to the male as well and counseling is recommended before proceeding with sperm retrieval and ICSI due to the risk of the transmission of cystic fibrosis to the off-spring [75, 76]. Azoospermic men with idiopathic obstruction and men with a clinical triad of chronic sinusitis, bronchiectasis, and obstructive azoospermia (Young syndrome) may be at higher risk for CF gene mutations as well.

The serum FSH is a critical factor in determining whether a diagnostic testicular biopsy is needed to differentiate the type of azoospermia in men with normal semen volume. Elevated FSH and small testis are indicative of testicular failure (NOA); therefore, a testicular biopsy is not necessary for diagnostic purposes [76]. However, if sperm retrieval is being considered, a biopsy may be performed to determine whether spermatozoa are likely to be retrievable by future TESA or extraction. The absence of sperm in a biopsy specimen taken from a man with NOA, however, does not absolutely predict whether sperm are present elsewhere within the testicle [4, 77]. Conversely, men with FSH levels and semen volume within normal ranges may have either nonobstructive or obstructive azoospermia [78]. In such cases, there is no noninvasive method to differentiate obstructive from NOA, and a testicular biopsy is usually required to provide a definitive diagnosis. Testicular biopsy can be performed by a standard open incision technique or by percutaneous methods. Histology evaluation of testicular specimens may indicate the presence of normal spermatogenesis in cases of OA, while hypospermatogenesis, maturation arrest or Sertoli cell-only syndrome is seen in NOA ones.

All men with primary testicular failure of unknown origin should be offered karyotyping and Y microdeletion testing. The frequency of karyotypic abnormalities is reported to be 10–15% in men with NOA, and Klinefelter syndrome accounts for approximately two-thirds of the cases [79]. Genetic testing may provide prognostic information for sperm retrieval [75]. In contrast to patients with either partial or complete AZFc deletion, in whom sperm can be found within the testis, the chance of finding sperm in men with complete AZFa or AZFb deletions is unlikely [80, 81]. Genetic counseling should be offered to the male whenever a genetic abnormality is detected prior to performing ICSI with his sperm.

Sperm retrieval from the epididymis is indicated in obstructive cases only. Testicular sperm retrieval can be performed either in OA and NOA cases. In OA, testicular retrievals are carried out after failed epididymal retrieval or as a primary retrieval procedure in cases of absent epididymis or intense epididymal fibrosis. In NOA, testicular sperm retrievals are the only option to collect sperm.

Anesthesia

Sperm retrieval techniques can be safely performed using local, regional, or general anesthesia. In the authors' practice, percutaneous sperm retrievals are carried out under local anesthesia alone or in association with intravenous bolus infusion of a short-acting hypnotic agent (propofol). In both cases, a 10–15 mL solution of 2% lidocaine hydrochloride is injected around the spermatic cord near the external inguinal ring. In cases of using intravenous anesthesia, local injection of the anesthetic is performed after patient unconsciousness is achieved. Microsurgical sperm retrievals are performed under either local anesthesia, as described above, in association with continuous infusion of propofol using a syringe-drive automated-pump device, or epidural anesthesia.

Techniques

Percutaneous sperm retrievals can be carried out with short duration anaesthesia, and are associated with less postoperative discomfort. They are easily repeatable and less expensive than open macro- or microsurgical techniques. Moreover, the procedures do not require microsurgery training. Microsurgical techniques, on the other hand, are associated with better quality and higher numbers of sperm retrieved per attempt, which optimizes the opportunity to cryopreserve sperm for future ICSI procedures.

Percutaneous Sperm Retrieval

Typically, percutaneous sperm retrieval is performed on an outpatient basis using a needle attached to a syringe. The standard procedures are described below. Minor technical modifications have been added, but irrespective of the technique the main goal is to aspirate either epididymal fluid or testicular parenchyma for diagnostic or therapeutic purposes. Loupe magnification may be used to avoid injuring small vessels seen through the scrotal skin.

- *Epididymal Sperm Aspiration (PESA)*. The epididymis is stabilized between the index finger, thumb, and forefinger while the testis is held with the palm of the hand. A 26-gauge needle attached to a 1-mL tuberculin syringe is inserted into the epididymis through the scrotal skin (Fig. 8.5a). Negative pressure is created, and the tip of the needle is gently moved in and out within the epididymis until fluid enters the syringe. The amount of epididymal fluid obtained during aspiration is often minimal (~0.1 mL), except in cases of CAVD in which 0.3–1.0 mL may be aspirated. The needle is withdrawn from the epididymis, and the aspirate is flushed into a 0.5–1.0 mL 37°C sperm medium. The tube containing the epididymal aspirate is transferred to the laboratory for microscopic examination. PESA is repeated at a different site of the same epididymis (from cauda up to the caput) and/or at the contralateral side until adequate number of motile sperm is retrieved. If PESA fails in retrieving motile sperm for ICSI, TESA is performed at the same operative time.
- *Testicular Sperm Aspiration (TESA)*. The epididymis is stabilized between the index finger, thumb, and forefinger while the anterior scrotal skin is stretched. A 18-gauge needle attached to a 20-mL syringe is connected to a syringe holder

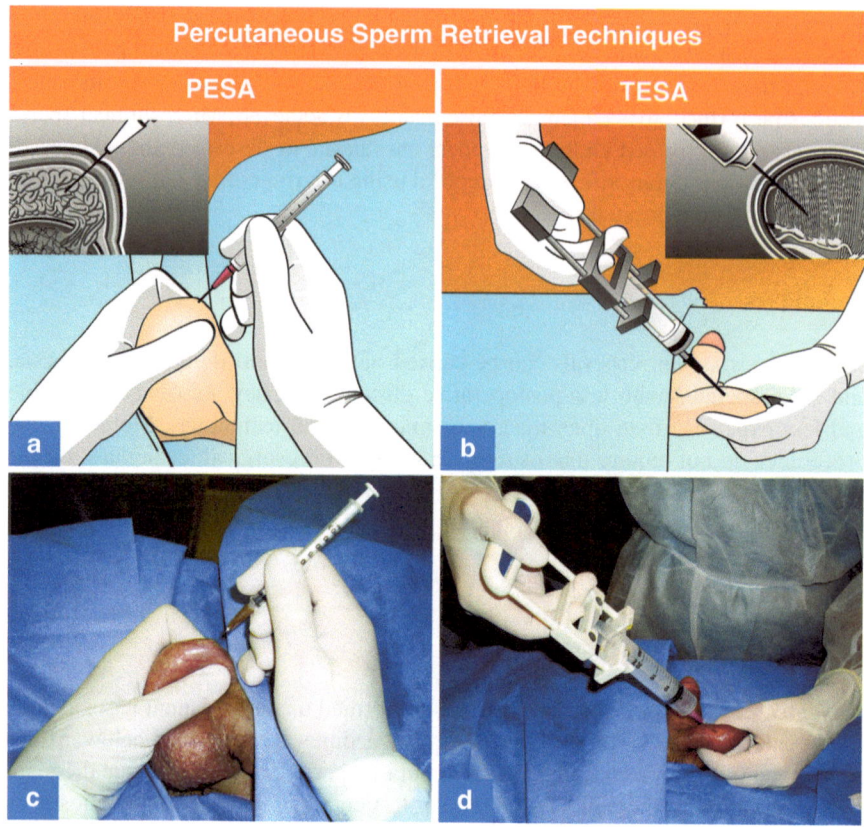

Fig. 8.5 Percutaneous sperm retrieval techniques [schematic representation (**a**) and (**b**) and intra-operative photographs (**c**) and (**d**)]. (**a**) Percutaneous epididymal sperm aspiration (PESA). Epididymis is stabilized between the index finger, thumb, and forefinger. A needle attached to a tuberculin syringe is inserted into the epididymis through the scrotal skin, and fluid is aspirated. (**b**) Testicular sperm aspiration (TESA). A 20-mL needled syringe connected to a holder is percutaneous inserted into the testis. Negative pressure is created and the tip of the needle is moved within the testis to disrupt the seminiferous tubules and sample different areas

and is inserted through the stretched scrotal skin into the anteromedial or antero-lateral portion of the superior testicular pole, in an oblique angle toward the medium and lower poles (Fig. 8.5b). Negative pressure is created by pulling the syringe holder while the tip of the needle is moved in and out within the testis in an oblique plane to disrupt the seminiferous tubules and sample different areas. When a small piece of testicular tissue is aspirated, the needle is gently with-drawn from the testis while the negative pressure is maintained. A pair of micro-surgery forceps is used to grab the seminiferous tubules that exteriorize from the scrotal skin, thus aiding in the removal of the specimen. The specimen is flushed into a tube containing 0.5–1.0 mL warm sperm medium and is transferred to the laboratory for microscopic examination. TESA or TESE may be performed at the contralateral testis if insufficient or no sperm are obtained.

Microsurgical Sperm Retrieval

The microsurgical approach allows direct visualization of epididymal and seminiferous tubules with high magnification. These techniques have been associated with retrieval of higher sperm numbers and of better quality in MESA and higher retrieval success rates in micro-TESE. MESA does not compromise the success of future reconstructive procedure, if desired, since the damage to the epididymal tubule is minimal. The amount of testicular parenchyma removed in micro-TESE is low compared to open biopsy, which is particularly important to preserve testicular androgen production in men with NOA who already have compromised testicular function.

- *Epididymal Sperm Aspiration* (*MESA*). A transverse incision (2-3 cm) is made through the anesthetized scrotal layers, and the testis is exteriorized. The epididymis is examined and its tunica incised. An enlarged tubule is dissected and opened with sharp microsurgical scissors. Fluid exuding from the tubule is aspirated with a silicone tube or blunted needle attached to a 1-mL tuberculin syringe (Fig. 8.6). The aspirate is flushed into a 0.5–1.0 mL 37°C sperm medium. The tube containing the epididymal aspirate is transferred to the laboratory for microscopic examination. MESA is repeated at a different site of the same epididymis (from cauda up to the caput) and/or at the contralateral side until adequate number of motile sperm is retrieved. If MESA fails to retrieve motile sperm, TESA or TESE may be performed at the same operative time.
- *Testicular Sperm Extraction* (*micro-TESE*). The testis is delivered in the same fashion as described for MESA. A single, large, midportion incision is made in an avascular area of the tunica albuginea under 6–8× magnification, and the testicular parenchyma is widely exposed (Fig. 8.6a). Dissection of the testicular parenchyma is carried out at ×16–25 magnification searching for enlarged seminiferous tubules. The superficial and deep testicular regions may be examined, if needed, and microsurgical-guided testicular biopsies are performed by removing enlarged tubules which are more likely to harbor active spermatogenesis (Fig. 8.6b–d). If enlarged tubules are not seen, then any tubule different than the remaining ones in size is excised. If all tubules are identical in appearance, random micro-biopsies (at least three at each testicular pole) are performed. Testicular tissue specimens are placed at an outer-well dish containing sperm media. Specimens are washed grossly to remove blood clots and are sent to the laboratory for processing and search for sperm. The albuginea and scrotal layers are closed using nonabsorbable and absorbable sutures, respectively.

Conventional Testicular Open-Biopsy Sperm Extraction (TESE)

Single or multiple open testicular biopsies may be taken to obtain sperm in both OA and NOA, but mainly in cases of NOA. TESE can be also used as a diagnostic tool to obtain testicular parenchyma for histopathology analysis and search of sperm prior to the ICSI cycle. A transverse 2-cm incision is made through the anesthetized scrotal skin, cremaster, and parietal tunica vaginalis. Conventional TESE is carried

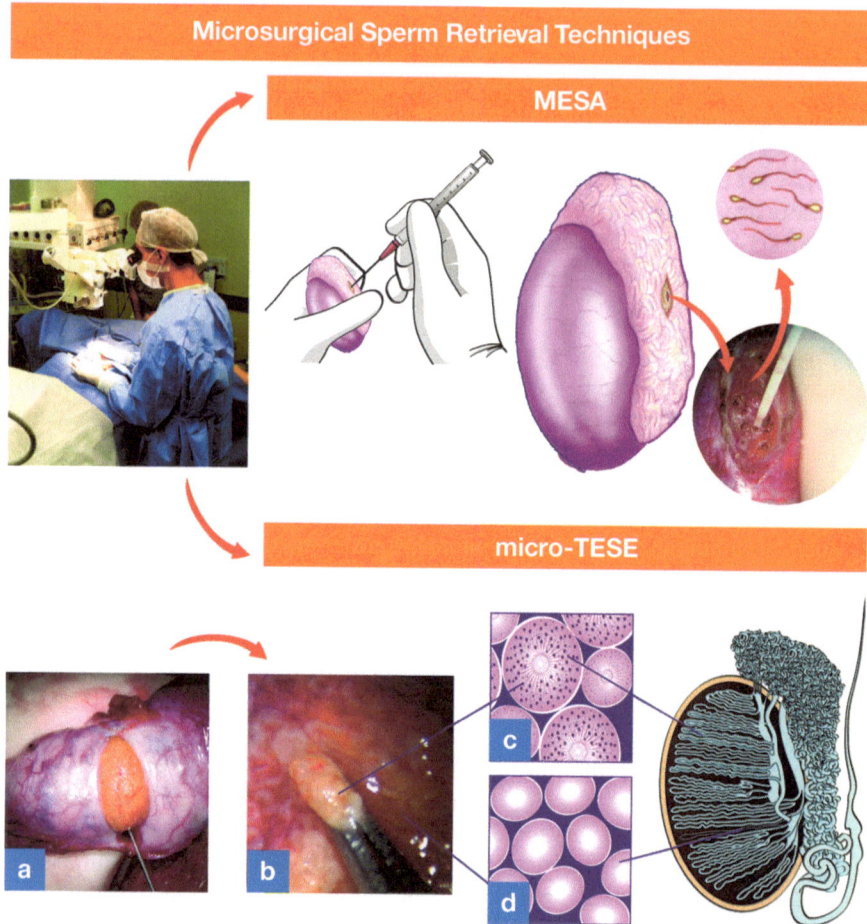

Fig. 8.6 Microsurgical sperm retrieval techniques. Operating microscope and microsurgical technique are used throughout the procedures. On the top: microsurgical epididymal sperm aspiration (MESA). After exposure of testis and epididymis, a dilated epididymal tubule is dissected and opened. Fluid is aspirated, diluted with sperm medium, and sent to the laboratory for examination. On the bottom: microsurgical testicular sperm extraction (micro-TESE). (**a**) After the testicle is exteriorized, a single and large incision is made in an avascular area of the albuginea to expose the seminiferous tubules. (**b**) Dilated tubules are identified and removed with microforceps (intraoperative photograph at ×25 magnification). (**c**) Illustration of the histopathology cross section of a dilated seminiferous tubule with active spermatogenesis. (**d**) Illustration of the histopathology cross section of a thin tubule with Sertoli cell-only syndrome

out without magnification. A small self-retaining eyelid retractor is placed to improve exposure of the tunica albuginea since the testis is not exteriorized. The tunica albuginea is incised for approximately 0.5–1 cm. Gentle pressure is made onto the testis to extrude testicular parenchyma out of the small incision. A fragment of approximately 5×5×5 mm is excised with sharp scissors and placed promptly in sperm culture medium. The specimen is sent to the laboratory for processing and microscopic examination. The albuginea is closed using nonabsorbable sutures. TESE can be repeated in a different testicular pole if the multiple biopsies approach is selected.

Postoperative Care

Patients are discharged at the same day and can return to normal activities 1 and 3 days after percutaneous and open techniques, respectively. Scrotal ice packing and supporter is recommended to control edema and alleviate pain. Patients should restrain from ejaculation and strenuous physical activity for approximately 7–10 days. Oral analgesics are prescribed, but pain complaint is often minimal.

Expert Commentary

Varicocele Repair

The surgical treatment of varicocele should aim to achieve the highest improvement in the male fertility status with lower complication rates. Increase in the likelihood of spontaneous pregnancy after treatment is difficult to ascertain due to a variety of factors that include the lack of a uniform posttreatment follow-up interval and the female factor parameters, such as age and reproductive health. Therefore, we believe that the ultimate treatment goal is to improve the male fertility status regardless of the method to be used for conception (unassisted or assisted). The ideal surgical technique should aim for ligation of all internal and external spermatic and cremasteric veins, with preservation of spermatic arteries and lymphatics. This only can be achieved by using the inguinal or subinguinal microsurgical techniques. The urologist who opts to treat varicocele using microsurgery should obtain appropriate training. It is also important to have adequate microsurgical instruments and a binocular operating microscope with foot-control zoom magnification. Microsurgical varicocelectomy, either using inguinal or subinguinal approaches, requires more skill as compared to other surgical modalities because a higher number of internal spermatic vein channels and smaller-diameter artery are seen at the level of the inguinal canal. However, the routine use of microsurgery during varicocele repair may aid the urologist to master his/her microsurgical skills, which will be of great benefit when performing more demanding and less frequent microsurgical procedures, such as vasovasostomies and vasoepididymostomies. In our practice, varicocelectomy is performed on both sides at the same operative time in the presence of bilateral palpable varicocele. When a clinically palpable varicocele is identified in one side, the contralateral cord is examined using a pencil-probe Doppler (9 MHz) stethoscope to determine if a subclinical varicocele exists. If so, it is treated at the same time as the coexistent clinical varicocele. This is based on the observation that altered blood flow after varicocelectomy may unmask an underlying venous anomaly and result in clinical varicocele formation [82, 83]. Loupe magnification may be used to facilitate the ligation of the dilated varicose veins; however, it is often insufficient for proper identification of both testicular arteries and lymphatics. In our early experience with loupe-assisted varicocele repair, papaverine instillation was needed in most cases to aid in the identification of arterial pulsations.

In our hands, the subinguinal microsurgical varicocelectomy using the operating microscope is the method of choice to treat varicocele-associated infertility. In a group of 384 treated individuals, the mean operative time was 113 and 90 minutes, and the number of veins ligated was 11 and 6, in unilateral and bilateral varicocelectomies, respectively. We do not use intraoperative Doppler to identify testicular arteries. Artery identification is based on microscopic examination using 10–16× magnification. Only occasionally papaverine instillation is used to facilitate positive identification of arterial pulsation. Using this approach, we were able to identify at least one artery in 97.6% of the cases. Recurrence was reported in 4 cases (1.0%), and no hydrocele formation occurred. Improvement ($\geq 15\%$ change from baseline preoperative values) in at least one semen parameter (count, motility, and morphology) was observed in 68.5% of the individuals. Spontaneous pregnancies were achieved in 58 couples (33.7%) whose male partners had been treated in a follow-up period of 18 months.

Reconstructive Surgery of the Vas Deferens and Epididymis

Both microsurgical reconstruction and sperm retrieval combined with IVF/ICSI are effective treatments for infertility due to obstructive azoospermia. A choice between the two must be based not only on the needs and preferences of the individual couple but also on the couple's clinical profile taking into account the cause of azoospermia and any coexisting factors in the female partner. Consequently, both partners should be evaluated thoroughly before making a specific treatment recommendation. Cost issues also play a role in the decision-making process since ART is seldom reimbursed by health insurance companies in most countries. Most importantly, infertility clinics and doctors should not limit couple's options for treatment based on their own technical limitations but always provide all treatment options available for that particular case scenario.

In experienced hands, reconstructive surgery of the male reproductive tract can be highly successful. Microsurgical techniques are clearly superior compared to macrosurgical or loupe-assisted anastomoses [35, 84]. Sperm return to the ejaculate after microsurgery in 50–95% of patients, and 30–75% of couples can be expected to achieve pregnancy without assisted reproductive techniques (ART). The likelihoods of sperm appearance in the semen and of pregnancy after microsurgical vasectomy reversal are inversely related to the duration of time since vasectomy [35]. Other factors that affect success rates include the gross appearance of vas fluid at the time of surgery, the presence or absence of sperm in the vas fluid and their quality, the length of the remaining segment adjacent to the epididymis, the age of the female partner, and the experience of the microsurgeon.

Currently, several programs offer microsurgical training for urology residents. Short-term microsurgery courses are of limited value; however, they can help urologists acquire the initial skills needed to use microsurgery in a routine basis. It is important to emphasize that microsurgical procedures for male infertility may be very demanding; therefore, one should only embark on performing either vasovasostomies or vasoepididymostomies after mastering microsurgical skills in the microsurgery laboratory using animals or synthetic models. Among several predictors for a successful microsurgical reconstruction of the male reproductive system, surgeon's skills are the most relevant for treatment outcomes. Surgeon's skills are crucial when vasoepididymostomies are needed, which frequently cannot be anticipated. Therefore, mastering both vasovasostomy and vasoepididymostomy techniques allows for real-time decision-making without compromising clinical results. Even with the advent of robotic surgery and its application in the infertility field with an expectation to "level the playing field" for surgeons with modest experience, training is still necessary.

Microsurgical vasovasostomy (VV) is the method of choice for vasectomy reversal. We prefer the end-to-end modified one-layer anastomosis using a vas clamp in such cases. Our approach is to use the intussusception technique whenever vasoepididymostomy (VE) is required. The reasons are that these techniques are less time-consuming and yield similar patency rates compared to other approaches. If no fluid effluxes from the testicular vasal end, VV is still our preferred approach in cases the if epididymis is soft on palpation and vasectomy interval is less than 15 years. VE is left for cases in which thick toothpaste-like and no-sperm vasal fluid is noted, particularly in vasectomy with vasectomy intervals greater than 15 years. The surgical principles for a successful anastomosis are (1) adequate mucosa-to-mucosa approximation, (2) watertight and tension-free anastomosis, (3) adequate blood supply and healthy mucosa and muscularis, and (4) atraumatic anastomotic technique. It is not advisable to perform varicocele repair at the same time of vasectomy reversal. In vasectomized men, vasal veins are often compromised which would jeopardize venous return after ligation of internal and external spermatic veins. If necessary, varicocelectomy may be performed 6 months later when new venous and arterial channels are formed around the anastomosis. Although vasectomy reversal can be performed after percutaneous epididymal aspiration (PESA), we advise our patients that reconstructive surgery is likely to be unsuccessful in such cases. Therefore, if an undecided patient ultimately opts for sperm retrieval coupled with ICSI, we prefer to retrieve sperm from the testis without jeopardizing the chances of a future reconstruction.

In our case series involving 180 vasectomy reversals, overall patency following the modified one-layer vasovasostomy ($N = 126$) and the intussusception vasoepididimostomy ($N = 54$) techniques were 79 and 44%, respectively. Spontaneous pregnancy rates were respectively 42% and 33% in a mean follow-up period of 15 months. Three out of five men with patent anastomosis achieved normal semen analysis postoperatively. We consider that the reconstructive procedure failed when no sperm is found in the semen analysis by 6 months after vasovasostomy or by 18 months after vasoepididymostomy. In our case series, late obstructions after patency occurred in 2% and 25% after vasovasostomies and vasoepididymostomies, respectively. Interestingly, all patients who had late obstructions were cigarette smokers and/or had obstruction intervals greater than 8 years. In our case series, most pregnancies occurred between 8 and 13 months postoperatively (range 3–24 months).

Transurethral Resection of Ejaculatory Ducts

Resection of the ejaculatory ducts is a hazardous procedure. The typical patient with EDO is young and has a small prostate. Therefore, TURED is carried out very close to the bladder neck, rectum, and sphincter. If a midline cyst is present, resection is performed to completely unroof the cyst. If not, the prostatic side of the verumontanum is resected until a dilated portion of the ejaculatory duct is seen. Resection is performed with pure cutting to avoid thermal injury to the proximal ejaculatory duct. We feel more comfortable placing a finger in the patient rectum to prevent rectal injury during resection and having methylene blue injected through the vasotomy site. Resection is completed by positive identification of free dye efflux into the urethra.

In our series involving 25 patients with complete or partial obstructions, TURED results varied according to the etiology of obstruction, congenital, or acquired. Semen quality improvement (ejaculate volume, sperm count, and motility) was observed in 85% of the patients in the congenital group. Spontaneous pregnancy was obtained in 60% of these patients an average of 7 months postoperatively. In the group of patients with secondary EDO, seminal improvement was detected in only 30% of the individuals, and only one spontaneous pregnancy was achieved. Two individuals (one in each group conceived via assisted reproduction techniques). Complication rates were similar in both groups (35%) and included reflux of urine to the unroofed cyst cavity with consequent impairment of the semen parameters, retrograde ejaculation, and one case of epididymitis with obstruction. Rectal injury or incontinence was not reported in our case series.

Sperm Retrieval Techniques

The adoption of strict criteria to diagnose OA is crucial for obtaining high success retrieval rate in the range of 90–100% using percutaneous techniques. Using PESA, our approach is to perform the first aspiration at the corpus epididymis, then proceed up to the caput if necessary since aspirates from the cauda are usually rich in poor-quality senescent spermatozoa, debris, and macrophages. Most cases of PESA failures are not necessarily technical failures because immotile spermatozoa are found. However, in certain cases of epididymal fibrosis due to multiple PESA attempts or postinfection, PESA may be ineffective to retrieve sperm. In these cases, PESA can be attempted at the contralateral epididymis, or TESA can be applied successfully if there is normal spermatogenesis. Some authors advocate that MESA allows the collection of larger and cleaner quantities of sperm than PESA, but this debate seems trivial. In our series of 142 men with OA, cumulative successful retrieval rates of PESA and/or TESA was 97.9%, and an adequate number of motile sperm for cryopreservation was obtained in approximately one-third of the cases [85]. In rare circumstances, we perform MESA for sperm retrieval in OA men with coagulation disorders. Successful sperm retrieval (SRR) is obtained in over 85% of the cases using PESA alone, but more than one aspiration is required in several cases. In cases of failed PESA, TESA is adequate to obtain sperm in practically all cases. Motile spermatozoa is obtained in approximately 73% of the cases after the first or second PESA aspirations, and TESA is carried out as a rescue procedure after failed PESA in about 14% of the individuals. In our series, success in sperm retrieval using percutaneous techniques and pregnancy outcomes by ICSI were similar in the vasectomy, CBAVD, and postinfectious etiology categories [85]. Either epididymal or testicular spermatozoa retrieved from these men exhibits similar reproductive potential. In our series of OA, live birth rates by ICSI were 40.2%. Also, our data indicated that ICSI outcomes using fresh epididymal and testicular spermatozoa retrieved from men with OA are comparable to those obtained with ejaculated sperm [86]. We routinely freeze epididymal and testicular spermatozoa which are left over from the ICSI cycle.

In cases of NOA, our approach is to retrieve sperm by TESA only in the favorable prognosis cases such as the ones with a previously successful TESA attempt or those with testicular biopsy result showing hypospermatogenesis. If TESA fails, however, we neither perform a second aspiration in the same testis, at the same operative time, nor convert it to an open procedure to avoid the risk of hematoma and testicular injury. Extensive bleeding is often seen during a rescue TESE after a failed TESA, and enlarged seminiferous tubules are difficult to identify even using the operating microscope. In these occasions, we opt to perform TESA or TESE at the contralateral testis. For NOA patients without previous diagnostic testicular biopsy or TESA attempt, our choice is to perform sperm extraction using micro-TESE. In the IVF laboratory, it is far less technically demanding and labor intensive to extract spermatozoa from small volume specimens than large pieces of testicular tissue that must be dissected, red blood cells lysed, and the rare spermatozoa searched for in a tedious fashion under an inverted microscope. TESE/micro-TESE may be scheduled either for the day of oocyte collection or the day before. In a previous study, we observed that optimal fertilization with ICSI using surgically retrieved sperm had been obtained when the time interval from hCG administration to microinjection did not exceed 44 h [87]. Testicular tissue sperm processing, searching, and selection of viable spermatozoa for ICSI may take several hours in NOA cases. Our laboratory takes approximately 11.6 min to handle a single testicular spermatozoon from processing to microinjection in NOA, and only 5.5 min in OA. In other words, the average time required to perform ICSI in a typical NOA treatment cycle involving 8–12 metaphase-II oocytes is approximately 2 h. For these reasons, we elect to perform micro-TESE on the day before oocyte collection when a busy next day IVF laboratory workload is anticipated.

According to our experience involving approximately 200 individuals with NOA, SRR rate was 55.7% and sperm could be obtained in similar rates in all etiology categories of cryptorchidism, orchitis, genetic, radio-/chemotherapy, and idiopathic. Testicular histopathology results were predictive of sperm collection using both TESA and micro-TESE [74, 77]. SRR by TESA was 100% and 82.3% in our group of NOA presenting with either hypospermatogenesis or a history of previous successful TESA attempt. Using micro-TESE, SRR rates were significantly higher than TESA in cases of SCO and maturation arrest (39.2% vs. 22.8%) [77]. Both methods yielded similar SRR of 100% in cases of hypospermatogenesis. According to our data, the chances of retrieving spermatozoa (odds ratio [OR] = 43.0; 95% confidence interval [CI]: 10.3–179.5) and of achieving a live birth by ICSI (OR = 1.86; 95% CI: 1.03–2.89) were significantly increased in couples whose male partner had obstructive rather than NOA [88]. These findings indicate that the reproductive potential of infertile men undergoing ART is related to the type of azoospermia.

Five-Year View

Varicocele Repair

In a recent systematic review comparing different surgical modalities to treat varicocele for male infertility [30], it was concluded that open microsurgical inguinal or subinguinal varicocelectomy techniques resulted in higher spontaneous pregnancy rates and fewer recurrences and postoperative complications than laparoscopic, radiologic embolization and macroscopic inguinal or retroperitoneal varicocelectomy techniques. Postoperative complications vary with surgical techniques. Hydrocele formation is the most common complication of varicocelectomy, with the incidence ranging from 0% to 10%. The lowest and highest reported hydrocele formation rates are seen in the microsurgical and in the high retroperitoneal series, respectively. Recurrences range from 0% to 35% varying with varicocelectomy techniques. Overall recurrence rates are low for microsurgical varicocelectomy and high for retroperitoneal and macrosurgical inguinal approaches [30]. Accidental testicular artery ligation during microsurgical varicocelectomy has been reported in about 1% of the cases, and it may cause testicular atrophy [89]. It has been recently demonstrated that the concomitant use of intraoperative vascular Doppler during microsurgical varicocelectomy allows more arterial branches to be preserved, and more internal spermatic veins are likely to be ligated [90]. Table 8.2 summarizes treatment results, postoperative recurrence, hydrocele formation, and spontaneous pregnancy rates among different techniques.

Varicocelectomy studies report significant improvements in one or more semen parameters in approximately 65% of men [91]. The mean time for semen improvement and spontaneous pregnancy after surgery is approximately 5 and 7 months,

Table 8.2 Treatment results for varicocele repair in infertile men. Postoperative recurrence, hydrocele formation, and spontaneous pregnancy rates among different techniques[a]

Technique	Recurrence rate (%)	Hydrocele formation rate (%)	Spontaneous pregnancy rate (%)
Retroperitoneal high ligation [30, 32]	7–35	6–10	25–55
Laparoscopic [30, 32]	2–7	0–9	14–42
Macroscopic inguinal [30, 32]	0–37	7	34–39
Microscopic inguinal or subinguinal [15, 30, 32, 93]	0–0.3	0–1.6	33–56

[a]Values are expressed as range

respectively [92]. However, it is still unknown why fertility potential is not always improved after varicocelectomy. Studies evaluating predictors for successful varicocele repair indicate that infertile men either with higher preoperative semen parameters or undergoing varicocele repair for large varicoceles are more likely to show postoperative semen parameters improvement [91, 93]. It was also shown that men who achieved a postoperative total motile sperm count greater than 20 million and decreased sperm DNA fragmentation after surgical varicocelectomy were more likely to initiate a pregnancy either spontaneously or via assisted conception [94, 95]. The distribution of antioxidant enzyme genes genotype of infertile men with varicocele has been recently determined. It has been suggested that genetic polymorphisms in the glutathione S-transferase T1 gene may affect individual response to varicocelectomy [96]. Conversely, reduced preoperative testicular volume, elevated serum FSH levels, diminished testosterone concentrations, subclinical varicocele, as well as the presence of Y chromosome microdeletions seem to be negative predictors for fertility improvement after surgery [27, 97].

It is recommended to treat bilateral clinical varicoceles at the same operative time [15]. The management of infertile men with a unilateral clinical varicocele and a subclinical one at the contralateral side, on the other hand, is a matter of debate. Zheng et al. found that bilateral varicocelectomy had no benefit over the left clinical varicocelectomy [98]. However, the authors used a retroperitoneal approach for vein ligation which has been shown to be associated with high recurrence rate. Elbendary et al., in a prospective trial, observed that the magnitude of change in sperm count and motility, and the spontaneous pregnancy rates were significantly higher in the group of men who had bilateral varicocele repair [99].

It is still debatable whether varicoceles can cause or contribute to azoospermia. A recent meta-analysis reported appearance of sperm in ejaculates of 39% of azoospermic individuals whose varicoceles had been treated [28]. In the aforesaid study, testicular histopathology results were predictive of success. Postoperatively, appearance of sperm in the ejaculates was increased 9.4-fold in patients with biopsy-proven hypospermatogenesis (HS) or maturation arrest (MA) than in Sertoli cell-only syndrome. Although the use of motile ejaculated sperm is preferred for ICSI [86], persistent azoospermia after varicocele repair is still a potential problem and sperm extraction before ICSI will be inevitable for many individuals. In these circumstances, successful sperm retrieval rates of 60% have been reported using testicular microdissection (micro-TESE) sperm extraction [100]. It has been suggested that varicocele repair may maximize the chances of retrieving sperm for ICSI in azoospermic men with clinical varicoceles [101].

In cases that a clinical palpable varicocele coexists with impaired semen quality, its surgical repair has been shown to be the best treatment option [11]. Recent meta-analyses demonstrated a beneficial effect of varicocelectomy on the fertility status of infertile men with clinical varicocele [11, 102, 103]. Overall, sperm concentration, motility, and morphology are increased by 9.7 million/mL, 10% and 3%, respectively, after varicocelectomy [104]. Sperm DNA integrity is also increased after varicocele repair [95, 105, 106]. Spontaneous pregnancy rates are higher in men with treated (33–36%) as compared to untreated varicoceles (15–20%) [11, 103]. Our group has recently demonstrated that treatment of clinical varicoceles may improve the outcomes of ICSI in couples with varicocele-related infertility [12]. In our study, the chances of live birth were significantly increased by 1.9-fold, while the chances of miscarriage were reduced by 2.3-fold if the varicocele had been treated before assisted conception.

Reconstructive Surgery of the Vas Deferens and Epididymis

Over the past two decades, treatment options for couples with reconstructible obstructive azoospermia had a marked improvement. Refinements in microsurgical reconstruction as well as advances in ART, specifically sperm retrieval techniques for ICSI, have led to improved outcomes and cost-effectiveness. According to the most recent data, microsurgical reconstruction of the vas remains a cost-effective, reliable, and effective means of restoring fertility in the majority of men who have previously undergone vasectomy when the reconstruction is performed by an experienced microsurgeon [107–111]. However, data comparing surgical reconstruction versus sperm retrieval/ICSI are neither randomized nor homogenous. Therefore, a comprehensive understanding of the factors that can affect outcomes, overall cost, and the morbidity associated with each treatment modality, taking into account the institution providing the treatment, is recommended.

Overall, patency/pregnancy rates following microsurgical vasovasostomy and vasoepididimostomy are 92/55% and 78/40%, respectively [35, 38, 45, 48, 50, 57–60, 112] (Table 8.3). Most pregnancies occur within 24 months after surgery. Pregnancy rates are related to the time elapsed from vasectomy and reversal and female age. Although female partner's age obviously does not affect patency rates after vasectomy reversal, it does affect pregnancy rates (14% in women aged >40 years vs. 56% in those aged <39 years) [47]. Pregnancy rates are also lower after longer duration of vasal obstruction. Approximately 30–40% of couples achieve pregnancy following surgical reconstructions performed in obstruction intervals greater than 15 years as compared to >50% in shorter intervals [41, 48]. Vasectomy reversal has been shown to be feasible in patients who failed percutaneous epididymal aspiration (PESA). Marmar et al. showed that PESA procedures cause limited trauma to the epididymis, and up to 50% pregnancy rates may be obtained in

Table 8.3 Treatment results for vasovasostomy and vasoepididymostomy

Author	Patients (N)	Technique	Patency rate (%)	Pregnancy rate (%)
Vasovasostomy				
Belker et al. [35]	1,247	Modified one-layer	89	57
		Two-layer	86	51
Boorjian and Lipkin [38]	159	Two-layer	95	83
Chan and Goldstein [45]	1,048	Two-layer	99	54
Kolettis et al. [50]	34	Both	76	35
Vasoepididimostomy				
Silber [57]	139	End-to-end	78	56
Thomas [58]	137	End-to-side	79	50
Berger [59]	12	Triangulation intussusception	92	NR
Marmar [60]	9	Modified intussusception	78	22
Chan et al. [112]	68	Triangulation intussusception	84	40
Schiff et al. [48]	153	End-to-end	73	NR
		End-to-side	74	
		3-Suture intussusception	84	
		2-Suture intussusception	80	

Type of anastomosis, patency, and spontaneous pregnancy rates using different techniques

vasectomy reversal after PESA; however, success is higher for couples whose female partners have 37 years old or less [113].

As patency and pregnancy rates yielded by the existing technically demanding surgical procedures do not reach 100%, efforts continue to be made in order to widen the options for reconstructive repair. Several modifications have been suggested and include intussusception vasoepididymostomy anastomotic techniques, the use of novel biomaterials/sealants and absorbable and nonabsorbable stents, and the use of robotics [48, 56, 112, 114–117]. Recent modifications to the conventional vasoepididymostomy techniques simplified the anastomoses. In a prospective study, Chan et al. reported overall patency and pregnancy rates of 84% and 40% using the intussusception technique [114]. These findings were confirmed by Schiff et al. who reported patency and pregnancy rates of approximately 82% and 45%, respectively, using simplified intussusception techniques [48]. It is suggested that anastomoses are more watertight by using intussusception techniques; therefore, granuloma formation is decreased. Since pregnancy rates following vasoepididymostomy are below 50% and late failures occur in approximately 20% of the cases, it is tempting to retrieve sperm intraoperatively for cryopreservation, particularly in cases of difficult reconstruction. However, a recent cost-analysis study demonstrated that sperm harvesting and cryopreservation during vasectomy reversal is not cost-effective [51]. The rationale of using sealants around the anastomotic site is to decrease operative time and to simplify the procedure without compromising success rates. Fibrin sealant can stimulate the coagulation cascade producing a fibrin seal around the anastomosis. When mixed with thrombin and calcium, fibrinogen is converted to fibrin monomer which in turn is converted to a stable cross-linked fibrin polymer [115]. Ho et al. achieved 85% patency rates and 23% pregnancy rates using three transmural 9-0 sutures and fibrin glue in a mean follow-up of 6.2 months [115]. There are concerns, however, about the potential contact of the glue with the vas lumen, which may result in possible obstruction, and also about transmission of viral disease because fibrin glue is derived from pooled plasma [112]. The use of nonabsorbable polymeric stent has been reported only in animal model. Preliminary results showed 100% patency rates in a follow-up of 39–47 weeks, and the total sperm count was significantly higher in the stented group [116]. The use of robotics for microsurgical procedures is also a novel concept. The rationale to add this technology to the already existing armamentarium relies on the possibility of controlling the physiologic static tremor, enhancing visual magnification (up to 100× when using a digital microscopic camera), and improving the ergonomics [117]. Animal studies suggest that robotic-assisted vasectomy reversal is easier to perform and yields better pregnancy rates than microsurgical reversal [118]. In a preliminary experience in humans, Parekattil et al. reported shorter operative time and higher postoperative sperm count for robot-assisted vasectomy reversal as compared to the microsurgical technique [115]. However, the advantages of the robot over an experienced microsurgeon are yet to be proven in larger series. A robotic system costs more than 1 million dollar, and its annual maintenance surpasses U$100,000. These cost issues will certainly represent a barrier to the widely adoption of robotics into microsurgical urologic practice.

Transurethral Resection of Ejaculatory Ducts

EDO is a treatable cause of male infertility, but the diagnosis is difficult to make, particularly in cases of partial obstruction. Transrectal ultrasound is valuable but not specific. It is suggested that adjunctive procedures, such as magnetic resonance imaging, chromotubation, seminal vesicle aspiration, seminal vesicle scintigraphy, and ejaculatory duct manometry, are more sensitive for diagnosis [119–121]. Transurethral resection of ejaculatory ducts (TURED) remains the treatment of choice. However, less invasive approaches using balloon dilation coupled or not with transurethral incision of the ejaculatory ducts have been yielded with similar results with fewer complications than TURED [122, 123].

Sperm Retrieval Techniques

The best technique for sperm retrieval in men with obstructive and NOA is yet to be determined. To date, no randomized controlled trial has compared the efficiency of these strategies, and thus, current recommendations are based on cumulative evidence provided by descriptive, observational, and controlled studies [124]. Percutaneous epididymal aspiration can be performed without surgical scrotal exploration, repeatedly, easily, at low cost, without an operating microscope or expertise in microsurgery, under local anesthesia, and it is associated with minimal postoperative discomfort. Microsurgical aspiration has the advantage of retrieving larger number of sperm which facilitates cryopreservation, and it is associated with a reduced risk of hematoma [109]. Meta-analysis results demonstrated no significant difference in any outcome measure between the use of epididymal or testicular sperm in men with OA [125]. The etiology of the obstruction and the use of fresh or frozen-thawed epididymal/testicular sperm do not seem to affect ICSI outcomes in terms of fertilization, pregnancy, or miscarriage rates [85, 109, 126]. In cases of NOA, the efficiency of TESA for retrieving spermatozoa is lower than TESE [127–129], except in the favorable cases of men with previous successful TESA or testicular histopathology showing hypospermatogenesis. In these circumstances, SRR rates may be as high as 100% [77]. In a recent systematic review, the mean reported SRR for TESE was 49.5% [128]. TESE with multiple biopsies resulted in higher SRR than fine-needle aspiration, a variation of TESA, especially in cases of Sertoli cell-only (SCO) syndrome and maturation arrest [128]. In NOA, current evidence suggests that micro-TESE performs better than conventional TESE or TESA in cases of SCO, where tubules containing active focus of spermatogenesis can be positively identified using microsurgery. Sperm retrieval rates ranging from 35 to 77% have been reported with micro-TESE [74, 128–132]. To allow for adequate healing and the resumption of spermatogenesis, the minimum recommended interval between sperm retrieval procedures in NOA is 3–6 months [129–131].

Postoperative complications of sperm retrieval techniques include persistent pain, swelling, infection, hydrocele, and hematoma [127–134]. The development of intratesticular hematoma has been observed in most patients undergoing TESE with single or multiple biopsies based on postoperative ultrasound results but they often resolve spontaneously without compromising testicular function [132]. In the larger-volume standard testicular biopsy, the risk of transient or even permanent testicular damage (such as complete devascularization) can result in decreased serum testosterone levels [129, 131]. Less invasive techniques, such as TESA and micro-TESE, aim to reduce the incidence of short and long-term complications. Several studies have documented a lower frequency of complications following micro-TESE compared with the conventional technique [128–131, 133]. Using micro-TESE, proper identification of testicular vessels under the tunica albuginea is made prior to the placement of an incision in the albuginea. The use of optical magnification and microsurgery technique allows the preservation of intratesticular blood supply, as well as the identification of tubules more likely to harbor sperm production [131]. Therefore, efficacy of sperm retrieval is improved while the risks of large tissue removal are minimized. The small amount of tissue extracted also facilitates sperm processing [130]. In certain groups of patients such as those with Klinefelter syndrome, who already have diminished androgen production, a significant decrease on serum testosterone has been documented following micro-TESE [130]. However, testosterone levels return to the presurgical values in most Klinefelter men in a 12-month follow-up period. It is recommended that sperm retrieval should be performed by surgeons who have training in the procedures because of the potential serious postoperative complications [129].

It has been suggested that the clinical outcomes of ICSI using testicular sperm extracted by TESA or micro-TESE in NOA are significantly lower than those obtained with either ejaculated or epididymal/testicular sperm from men with OA [86, 88, 125]. Testicular spermatozoa of men with severely impaired spermatogenesis seems to have decreased fertility potential and have a higher tendency to carry deficiencies such as the ones related to the centrioles and genetic material, which ultimately affect the capability of the male gamete to activate the egg and trigger the formation and development of a normal zygote and a viable embryo [134]. From the limited data available, it is suggested that the sperm retrieval technique itself has no impact on ICSI success rates [128]. However, frozen-thawed surgically retrieved sperm from NOA men have significantly impaired reproductive potential than fresh ones [125, 134]. Meta-analysis results showed that fertilization rates by ICSI remained similar, but implantation was significantly higher (by 73%) with the use of fresh compared to frozen-thawed testicular sperm [135].

The question of whether or not ICSI using sperm retrieved from men with either OA or NOA might be associated with increased risk for birth defects is still unresolved. In vitro fertilization, in general, is associated with multiple gestation and an increased risk of congenital abnormalities (including hypospadias) [136]. ICSI, in particular, carries an increased risk of endocrine abnormalities, as well as epigenetic imprinting effects [136]. Although the absolute risk of any of these conditions remains low [136–139], current data is limited and study populations are heterogenic. It is therefore recommended that well-defined groups of ICSI with ejaculated sperm, ICSI with epididymal sperm and ICSI with testicular sperm, and a control group of naturally conceived children are closely followed up.

Key Issues

- Varicocele treatment is indicated for men with clinically palpable varicocele and abnormal semen parameters. Open microsurgical inguinal or subinguinal techniques are considered the best treatment modalities because they result in higher spontaneous pregnancy rates and fewer recurrences and postoperative complications than laparoscopic, radiologic embolization and macroscopic inguinal or retroperitoneal varicocelectomy techniques. There are no absolute predictive factors for a successful varicocele repair, and existing evidence does not support the recommendation for treating infertile men with subclinical varicocele.
- Surgical repair of varicocele improves semen parameters and functional markers of oxidative stress and DNA integrity. The chance for either spontaneous or assisted conception is increased after repair of clinical varicoceles. Recovery of spermatogenesis can be achieved after repair of clinical varicocele in infertile men with NOA. Testicular histopathology is predictive of success, and men with maturation arrest and hypospermatogenesis are more likely to ejaculate motile spermatozoa after surgery. Also, the chance of retrieving testicular sperm for ICSI is optimized in non-obstructed azoospermic men with treated clinical varicocele.
- Men with obstructive azoospermia may father children either by surgical correction of the obstruction, which may allow the couple to conceive naturally, or retrieval of sperm directly from the epididymis or testis, followed by ICSI.
- Best results with reconstructive surgery of the male reproductive tract are achieved by surgeons who have the necessary microsurgical training and ongoing

experience with the procedures. Ideally, procedures should be performed by surgeons who have the capability to perform both vasovasostomy and vasoepididymostomy because, in many cases, the need of the latter cannot be anticipated.

- In experienced hands, microsurgical vasectomy reversal is highly successful. Sperm return to the ejaculate in 70–95% of the patients after surgery, and 30–75% of couples can be expected to achieve unassisted pregnancy. Patency and pregnancy after microsurgical vasectomy reversal are inversely related to the interval of obstruction since vasectomy. Other factors that affect success rates include the intraoperative appearance of vasal fluid, the presence or absence of sperm in the vasal fluid and their quality, the length of the remaining segment adjacent to the epididymis, the age of the female partner, and the experience of the microsurgeon.
- Vasoepididymostomy should be performed only by those having the requisite training and experience in reproductive microsurgery. When treatment requires a complex reconstruction of the male reproductive tract, cryopreservation of retrieved sperm should be considered because surgery may not be successful.
- EDO is a potentially treatable cause of male infertility, and TURED is the treatment of choice. After TURED, sperm return to the ejaculate in approximately 50–75% of the men, and approximately 20% of couples achieve spontaneous pregnancy. However, results are highly variable and depend on the etiology (acquired or congenital) and type (partial or complete) of obstruction. Complications of TURED occur in approximately 20% of men, including hematuria, hematospermia, urinary tract infection, epididymitis, and a watery ejaculate due to reflux of urine.
- In obstructive azoospermia, sperm production is normal and gametes can be easily retrieved from epididymis or testes in most cases, irrespective of the technique. PESA or TESA are simple and efficient methods for retrieving epididymal or testicular spermatozoa in men with OA. In NOA, TESE with or without magnification (micro-TESE) is the preferred approach, and sperm can be retrieved in approximately 50% of the cases. The use of microsurgery during TESE may improve the efficacy of sperm extraction with significantly less tissue removed, which ultimately facilitates sperm processing. Testicular histology results, if available, may be useful to predict the chances to retrieve sperm in men with NOA. However, sperm can be obtained even in the worst case scenario except in the cases of Y chromosome infertility with complete AZFa and/or AZFb microdeletions.
- The goals of sperm retrieval are to obtain the best quality sperm possible, to retrieve adequate numbers of sperm for immediate use and cryopreservation, and to minimize damage to the reproductive tract. In both OA and NOA, sperm retrieval technique itself seems to have no impact on IVF/ICSI success rates. The reproductive potential of infertile men undergoing ART is related to the type of azoospermia. The chances of retrieving spermatozoa and of achieving a live birth by ICSI are increased in couples whose male partner had obstructive rather than NOA. Children conceived using sperm retrieved from men with OA and NOA should be followed up because it is still unclear if there is an increased risk of birth defects when ICSI is carried out with non-ejaculated sperm.

Acknowledgments The authors are indebted to Mrs. Fabiola Bento for her editorial assistance and to Dr. Marcelo Coccuza for providing his personal observations regarding reconstructive surgery.

References

1. Vital and Health Statistics, series 23, no.26, CDC. http://www.cdc.gov. Accessed 10 Dec 2009.
2. Silber S, Nagy ZP, Liu J, et al. Conventional in-vitro fertilization versus intracytoplasmic sperm injection for patients requiring microsurgical sperm aspiration. Hum Reprod. 1994;9:1705–9.
3. Devroey P, Liu J, Nagy ZP, et al. Pregnancies after testicular extraction (TESE) and intracytoplasmic sperm injection (ICSI) in non-obstructive azoospermia. Hum Reprod. 1995;10:1457–60.
4. Schlegel PN. Testicular sperm extraction: microdissection improves sperm yield with minimal tissue excision. Hum Reprod. 1999;14:131–5.
5. Goldstein M, Eid JF. Elevation of intratesticular and scrotal skin surface temperature in men with varicocele. J Urol. 1989;142:743–5.
6. Chehval MJ, Purcell MH. Varicocelectomy: incidence of external vein involvement in the clinical varicocele. Urology. 1992;39:573–5.
7. Nistal M, Gonzalez-Peramato P, Serrano A, et al. Physiopathology of the infertile testicle. Etiopathogenesis of varicocele. Arch Esp Urol. 2004;57:883–904.
8. Agarwal A, Prabakaran S, Allamaneni SS. Relationship between oxidative stress, varicocele and infertility: a meta-analysis. Reprod Biomed Online. 2006;12:630–3.
9. World Health Organization. The influence of varicocele on parameters of fertility in a large group of men presenting to infertility clinics. Fertil Steril. 1992;57:1289–93.
10. Jarow JP. Effects of varicocele on male fertility. Hum Reprod Update. 2001;7:59–64.
11. Marmar JL, Agarwal A, Prabaskan S, et al. Reassessing the value of varicocelectomy as a treatment for male subfertility with a new meta-analysis. Fertil Steril. 2007;88:639–48.
12. Esteves SC, Oliveira FV, Bertolla RP. Clinical outcomes of intracytoplasmic sperm injection in infertile men with treated and untreated clinical varicocele. J Urol. 2010;184:1241–586.
13. Redmon JB, Carey P, Pryor JL. Varicocele-the most common cause of male factor infertility? Hum Reprod Update. 2002;8:53–8.
14. Esteves S. Infertilidade masculina. In: Rhoden EL, editor. Urologia no consultório. 1ªth ed. Porto Alegre: Artmed Editora; 2009. p. 470–500.
15. Libman J, Jarvi K, Lo K, Zini A. Beneficial effect of microsurgical varicocelectomy is superior for men with bilateral versus unilateral repair. J Urol. 2006;176:2602–5.
16. Gat Y, Bachar GN, Zukerman Z, et al. Physical examination may miss the diagnosis of bilateral varicocele: a comparative study of 4 diagnostic modalities. J Urol. 2004;172:1414–7.
17. Geatti O, Gasparini D, Shapiro B. A comparison of scintigraphy, thermography, ultrasound and phlebography in grading of clinical varicocele. J Nucl Med. 1991;32:2092–7.
18. Yamamoto M, Hibi H, Hirata Y, et al. Effect of varicocelectomy on sperm parameters and pregnancy rate in patients with subclinical varicocele: a randomized prospective controlled study. J Urol. 1996;155:1636–8.
19. Kantartzi PD, Goulis ChD, Goulis GD, et al. Male infertility and varicocele: myths and reality. Hippokratia. 2007;11:99–104.
20. Esteves SC, Glina S. Recovery of spermatogenesis after microsurgical subinguinal varicocele repair in azoospermic men based on testicular histology. Int Braz J Urol. 2005;31:541–8.
21. Steckel J, Dicker AP, Goldstein M. Relationship between varicocele size and response to varicocelectomy. J Urol. 1993;149:769–71.
22. Marmar JL. The pathophysiology of varicoceles in the light of current molecular and genetic information. Hum Reprod Update. 2001;7:461–72.
23. Marks JL, McMahon R, Lipshultz LI. Predictive parameters of successful varicocele repair. J Urol. 1986;136:609–12.

24. Yoshida K, Kitahara S, Chiba K, et al. Predictive indicators of successful varicocele repair in men with infertility. Int J Fertil. 2000;45:279–84.
25. Cayan S, Lee D, Black LD, et al. Response to varicocelectomy in oligospermic men with and without defined genetic infertility. Urology. 2001;57:530–5.
26. Pryor JL, Kent-First M, Muallem A, et al. Microdeletions in the Y chromosome of infertile men. N Engl J Med. 1997;336:534–9.
27. Kondo Y, Ishikawa T, Yamaguchi K, et al. Predictors of improved seminal characteristics by varicocele repair. Andrologia. 2009;41:20–3.
28. Weedin JW, Khera M, Lipshultz LI. Varicocele repair in patients with nonobstructive azoospermia—a meta-analysis. J Urol. 2010;183:2309–15.
29. Esteves SC. Editorial comment. J Urol. 2010;183:2315.
30. Cayan S, Shavakhabov S, Kadioglu A. Treatment of palpable varicocele review in infertile men: a meta-analysis to define the best technique. J Androl. 2009;30:33–40.
31. Sautter T, Sulser T, Suter S, et al. Treatment of varicocele: a prospective randomized comparison of laparoscopy versus antegrade sclerotherapy. Eur Urol. 2002;41:398–400.
32. Al-Kandari AM, Shabaan H, Ibrahim HM, et al. Comparison of outcomes of different varicocelectomy techniques: open inguinal, laparoscopic, and subinguinal microscopic varicocelectomy: a randomized clinical trial. Urology. 2007;69:417–20.
33. Hopps CV, Lemer ML, Schlegel PN, et al. Intraoperative varicocele anatomy: a microscopic study of the inguinal versus subinguinal approach. J Urol. 2003;170:2366–70.
34. Anderson JE, Warner L, Jamieson DJ, et al. Contraception. 2010;82:230–5.
35. Belker AM, Thomas AJ, Fuchs EF, et al. Results of 1469 microsurgical vasectomy reversals by the Vasovasostomy Study Group. J Urol. 1991;145:505–11.
36. Vasectomia no Brasil. Veja online; http://veja.abril.com.br/041000/p_084.html. Accessed 3 Oct 2010.
37. Lipshultz LI, Rumohr JA, Bennet RC. Techniques for vasectomy reversal. Urol Clin N Am. 2009;36:375–832.
38. Boorjian S, Lipkin M, Goldstein M. The impact of obstructive interval and sperm granuloma on outcome of vasectomy reversal. J Urol. 2004;171:304–6.
39. Parekattil SJ, Kuang W, Agarwal A, et al. Model to predict if a vasoepididymostomy will be required for vasectomy reversal. J Urol. 2005;173:1681–4.
40. Hernandez J, Sabanegh ES. Repeat vasectomy reversal after initial failure. J Urol. 1999;161:1153–6.
41. Bolduc S, Fischer MA, Deceunik G, et al. Factors predicting overall success: a review of 74 microsurgical vasovasostomies. Can Urol Assoc J. 2007;1:388–91.
42. Carbone Jr DJ, Shah A, Thomas Jr AJ, Agarwal A. Partial obstruction, not antisperm antibodies, causing infertility after vasovasostomy. J Urol. 1998;159:827–30.
43. Chawla A, O'Brien J, Lisi M, et al. Should all urologists performing vasectomy reversal be able to perform vasoepididymostomy if required? J Urol. 2004;172:829–30.
44. Eggert-Kruse W, Christmann M, Gerhard I, et al. Circulating antisperm antibodies and fertility prognosis: a prospective study. Hum Reprod. 1989;4:513–20.
45. Chan PT, Goldstein M. Superior outcomes of microsurgical vasectomy reversal in men with the same female partners. Fertil Steril. 2004;81:1371–4.
46. Hinz S, Rais-Bahrami S, Kempkensteffen C, et al. Fertility rates following vasectomy reversal: importance of age of the female partner. Urol Int. 2008;81:416–20.
47. Gerrard Jr ER, Sandlow JI, Oster RA, et al. Effect of female partner age on pregnancy rates after vasectomy reversal. Fertil Steril. 2007;87:1340–4.
48. Schiff J, Chan P, Li PS, et al. Outcome and late failures compared in 4 techniques of microsurgical vasoepididymostomy in 153 consecutive men. J Urol. 2005;174:651–5.
49. Sharlip I. Absence of fluid during vasectomy reversal has no prognostic significance. J Urol. 1996;155:365–9.
50. Kolettis PN, Burns JR, Nangia AK, et al. Outcomes for vasovasostomy performed when only sperm parts are present in the vasal fluid. J Androl. 2006;27:565–7.

51. Boyle KE, Thomas Jr AJ, Marmar JL, et al. Sperm harvesting and cryopreservation during vasectomy reversal is not cost effective. Fertil Steril. 2006;85:961–4.
52. Sharlip ID. Microsurgical vasovasostomy: modified one-layer technique. In: Goldstein M, editor. Surgery of male infertility. 1st ed. New York: WB Saunders; 1995. p. 67–76.
53. Belker AM. Microsurgical vasovasostomy: two-layer technique. In: Goldstein M, editor. Surgery of male infertility. 1st ed. New York: WB Saunders; 1995. p. 61–76.
54. Goldstein M. Vasovasostomy: surgical approach, decision making, and multilayer microdot technique. In: Goldestein M, editor. Surgery of male infertility. 1st ed. New York: WB Saunders; 1995. p. 46–60.
55. Fleming C. Robot-assisted vasovasostomy. Urol Clin N Am. 2004;31:769–72.
56. Parekattil SJ, Cohen MS. Robotic surgery in male infertility and chronic orchialgia. Curr Opin Urol. 2010;20:75–9.
57. Silber S. Microscopic vasoepididymostomy: specific microanastomosis to the epididymal tubule. Fertil Steril. 1978;30:565–71.
58. Thomas Jr AJ. Vasoepididymostomy. Urol Clin North Am. 1987;14:527–38.
59. Berger RE. Triangulation end-to-side vasoepididymostomy. J Urol. 1998;159:1951–3.
60. Marmar JL. Modified vasoepididymostomy with simultaneous double needle placement, tubulotomy and tubular invagination. J Urol. 2000;163:483–6.
61. Chan PT, Li PS, Goldstein M. Microsurgical vasoepididymostomy: a prospective randomized study of 3 intussusception techniques in rats. J Urol. 2003;169:1924–9.
62. Netto Jr NR, Esteves SC, Neves PA. Transurethral resection of partially obstructed ejaculatory ducts: seminal parameters and pregnancy outcomes according to the etiology of obstruction. J Urol. 1998;159:2048–53.
63. Meacham RB, Hellerstein DK, Lipshultz LI. Evaluation and treatment of ejaculatory duct obstruction in the infertile male. Fertil Steril. 1993;59:393–7.
64. Carter SS, Shinohara K, Lipshultz LI. Transrectal ultrasonography in disorders of the seminal vesicles and ejaculatory ducts. Urol Clin N Am. 1989;16:773–90.
65. Hellerstein DK, Meacham RB, Lipshultz LI. Transrectal ultrasound and partial ejaculatory duct obstruction in male infertility. Urology. 1992;39:449–52.
66. Jones TR, Zagoria RJ, Jarow JP. Transrectal US-guided seminal vesiculography. Radiology. 1997;205:276–8.
67. Jarow JP, Espeland MA, Lipshultz LI. Evaluation of the azoospermic patient. J Urol. 1989;142:62–5.
68. Farley S, Barnes R. Stenosis of ejaculatory ducts treated by endoscopic resection. J Urol. 1973;109:664–6.
69. Craft I, Tsirigotis M, Bennett V, et al. Percutaneous epididymal sperm aspiration and intracytoplasmic sperm injection in the management of infertility due to obstructive azoospermia. Fertil Steril. 1995;63:1038–42.
70. Craft I, Tsirigotis M. Simplified recovery, preparation and cryopreservation of testicular spermatozoa. Hum Reprod. 1995;10:1623–7.
71. Okada H, Dobashi M, Yamazaki T, et al. Conventional versus microdissection testicular sperm extraction for nonobstructive azoospermia. J Urol. 2002;168:1063–7.
72. Tsujimura A, Matsumiya K, Miyagawa Y, et al. Conventional multiple or microdissection testicular sperm extraction: a comparative study. Hum Reprod. 2002;17:2924–9.
73. Ramasamy R, Lin K, Gosden LV, et al. High serum FSH levels in men with nonobstructive azoospermia does not affect success of microdissection testicular sperm extraction. Fertil Steril. 2009;92:590–3.
74. Esteves SC, Verza Jr S, Gomes AP. Successful retrieval of testicular spermatozoa by microdissection (micro-TESE) in nonobstructive azoospermia is related to testicular histology. Fertil Steril. 2006;86:S354.
75. Schlegel PN. Causes of azoospermia and their management. Reprod Fertil Dev. 2004;16: 561–72.
76. Sharlip ID, Jarow J, Belker AM, et al. Report on evaluation of the azoospermic male. AUA Best Practice Policy and ASRM Practice Committee Report. American Urological Association, April 2001.

77. Esteves SC, Verza S, Prudencio C, Seol B. Sperm retrieval rates (SRR) in nonobstructive azoospermia (NOA) are related to testicular histopathology results but not to the etiology of azoospermia. Fertil Steril. 2010;94(Suppl):S132.

78. Male Infertility Best Practice Policy Committee of the American Urological Association, Practice Committee of the American Society for Reproductive Medicine. Report on evaluation of the azoospermic male. Fertil Steril. 2006;86 Suppl 1:S210–215.

79. De Braekeleer M, Dao TN. Cytogenetic studies in male infertility: a review. Hum Reprod. 1991;6:245–50.

80. Brandell RA, Mielnik A, Liotta D, et al. AZFb deletions predict the absence of spermatozoa with testicular sperm extraction: preliminary report of a prognostic genetic test. Hum Reprod. 1998;13:2812–5.

81. Hopps CV, Mielnik A, Goldstein M, et al. Detection of sperm in men with Y chromosome microdeletions of the AZFa, AZFb and AZFc regions. Hum Reprod. 2003;18:1660–5.

82. Nagler HM, Luntz RK, Martinis FG. Varicocele. In: Lipshultz LI, Howards SS, editors. Infertility in the Male. 3rd ed. St Louis: Mosby; 1997. p. 336–59.

83. Dhabuwala CB, Hamid S, Moghisi KS. Clinical versus subclinical varicocele: improvement in fertility after varicocelectomy. Fertil Steril. 1992;57:854–7.

84. Jee SH, Hong YK. One-layer vasovasostomy: microsurgical versus loupe-assisted. Fertil Steril. 2010;94(6):2308–11.

85. Esteves SC, Verza S, Prudencio C, Seol B. Success of percutaneous sperm retrieval and intracytoplasmic sperm injection (ICSI) in obstructive azoospermic (OA) men according to the cause of obstruction. Fertil Steril. 2010;94(Suppl):S233.

86. Verza Jr S, Esteves SC. Sperm defect severity rather than sperm source is associated with lower fertilization rates after intracytoplasmic sperm injection. Int Braz J Urol. 2008;34:49–56.

87. Schneider DT, Gomes AP, Verza Jr S, et al. Optimal time interval for intracytoplasmic sperm injection after administration of human chorionic gonadotrophin in severe male factor infertility. Fertil Steril. 2006;86:S155.

88. Prudencio C, Seol B, Esteves SC. Reproductive potential of azoospermic men undergoing intracytoplasmic sperm injection is dependent on the type of azoospermia. Fertil Steril. 2010; 94(Suppl):S232–3.

89. Chan PT, Wright EJ, Goldstein M. Incidence and postoperative outcomes of accidental ligation of the testicular artery during microsurgical varicocelectomy. J Urol. 2005;173:482–4.

90. Cocuzza M, Pagani R, Coelho R, et al. The systematic use of intraoperative vascular Doppler ultrasound during microsurgical subinguinal varicocelectomy improves precise identification and preservation of testicular blood supply. Fertil Steril. 2010;93:2396–9.

91. Schlesinger MH, Wilets IF, Nagler HM. Treatment outcome after varicocelectomy. A critical analysis. Urol Clin North Am. 1994;21:517–29.

92. Colpi GM, Carmignani L, Nerva F, et al. Surgical treatment of varicocele by a subinguinal approach combined with antegrade intraoperative sclerotherapy of venous vessels. BJU Int. 2006;97:142–5.

93. Shindel AW, Yan Y, Naughton CK. Does the number and size of veins ligated at left-sided microsurgical subinguinal varicocelectomy affect semen analysis outcomes? Urology. 2007;69:1176–80.

94. Matkov TG, Zenni M, Sandlow J, et al. Preoperative semen analysis as a predictor of seminal improvement following varicocelectomy. Fertil Steril. 2001;75:63–8.

95. Smit M, Romijn JC, Wildhagen MF, et al. Decreased sperm DNA fragmentation after surgical varicocelectomy is associated with increased pregnancy rate. J Urol. 2010;183: 270–4.

96. Jeng SY, Wu SM, Lee JD. Cadmium accumulation and metallothionein overexpression in internal spermatic vein of patients with varicocele. Urology. 2009;73:1231–5.

97. Cocuzza M, Cocuzza MA, Bragais FM, Agarwal A. The role of varicocele repair in the new era of assisted reproductive technology. Clinics (Sao Paulo). 2008;63:395–404.

98. Zheng YQ, Gao X, Li ZJ, et al. Efficacy of bilateral and left varicocelectomy in infertile men with left clinical and right subclinical varicoceles: a comparative study. Urology. 2009;73: 1236–40.

99. Elbendary MA, Elbadry AM. Right subclinical varicocele: how to manage in infertile patients with clinical left varicocele? Fertil Steril. 2009;92:2050–3.

100. Schlegel PN, Kaufmann J. Role of varicocelectomy in men with nonobstructive azoospermia. Fertil Steril. 2004;81:1585–8.

101. Inci K, Hascicek M, Kara O, et al. Sperm retrieval and intracytoplasmic sperm injection in men with nonobstructive azoospermia, and treated and untreated varicocele. J Urol. 2009;182:1500–5.

102. Meng MV, Greene KL, Turek PJ. Surgery or assisted reproduction? A decision analysis of treatment costs in male infertility. J Urol. 2005;174:1926–31.

103. Ficarra V, Cerruto MA, Liguori G, et al. Treatment of varicocele in subfertile men: the cochrane review—a contrary opinion. Eur Urol. 2006;49:258–63.

104. Agarwal A, Deepinder F, Cocuzza M, et al. Efficacy of Varicocelectomy in Improving Semen Parameters: new meta-analytical approach. Urology. 2007;70:532–8.

105. Zini A, Blumenfeld A, Libman J, et al. Beneficial effect of microsurgical varicocelectomy on human sperm DNA integrity. Hum Reprod. 2005;20:1018–21.

106. Moskovtsev SI, Lecker I, Mullen JB, et al. Cause-specific treatment in patients with high sperm DNA damage resulted in significant DNA improvement. Syst Biol Reprod Med. 2009;55:109–15.

107. Lee R, Li PS, Goldstein M, Tanrikut C, et al. A decision analysis of treatments for obstructive azoospermia. Hum Reprod. 2008;23:2043–9.

108. Robb P, Sandlow JI. Cost-effectiveness of vasectomy reversal. Urol Clin North Am. 2009;36:391–6.

109. Male Infertility Best Practice Policy Committee of the American Urological Association, Practice Committee of the American Society for Reproductive Medicine. Report on the management of infertility due to obstructive azoospermia. Fertil Steril. 2008;90 Suppl 3:S121–4.

110. Malizia BA, Hacker MR, Penzias AS. Cumulative live-birth rates after in vitro fertilization. N Engl J Med. 2009;360:236–43.

111. Hsieh MH, Meng MV, Turek PJ. Markov modeling of vasectomy reversal and ART for infertility: how do obstructive interval and female partner age influence cost effectiveness? Fertil Steril. 2007;88:840–6.

112. Chan PT, Brandell RA, Goldstein M. Prospective analysis of outcomes after microsurgical intussusceptions vasoepididymostomy. BJU Int. 2005;96:598–601.

113. Marmar JL, Sharlip I, Goldstein M. Results of vasovasostomy or vasoepididymostomy after failed percutaneous epididymal sperm aspirations. J Urol. 2008;179:1506–9.

114. Kolettis PN. Restructuring reconstructive techniques—advances in reconstructive techniques. Urol Clin N Am. 2008;35:229–34.

115. Ho KLV, Witte MN, Bird ET, et al. Fibrin glue assisted 3-suture vasovasostomy. J Urol. 2005;174:1360–363.

116. Vrijhof EJ, De Bruine A, Zwinderman A, et al. The use of newly designed nonabsorbable polymeric stent in reconstructing the vas deferens: a feasibility study in New Zealand white rabbits. BJU Int. 2005;95:1081–5.

117. Parekattil SJ, Atalah HN, Cohen MS. Video technique for human robot-assisted microsurgical vasovasostomy. J Endourol. 2010;24:511–4.

118. Schiff J, Li PS, Goldstein M. Robotic microsurgical vasovasostomy and vasoepididymostomy in rats. Int J Med Robot. 2005;1:122–6.

119. Eisenberg ML, Walsh TJ, Garcia MM, et al. Ejaculatory duct manometry in normal men and in patients with ejaculatory duct obstruction. J Urol. 2008;180:255–60.

120. Orhan I, Duksal I, Onur R, et al. Technetium Tc 99 m sulphur colloid seminal vesicle scintigraphy: a novel approach for the diagnosis of the ejaculatory duct obstruction. Urology. 2008;71:672–6.

121. Onur MR, Orhan I, Firdolas F, et al. Clinical and radiological evaluation of ejaculatory duct obstruction. Arch Androl. 2007;53:179–86.

122. Lawler LP, Cosin O, Jarow JP, et al. Transrectal US-guided seminal vesiculography and ejaculatory duct recanalization and balloon dilation for treatment of chronic pelvic pain. J Vasc Interv Radiol. 2006;17:169–73.
123. Manohar T, Ganpule A, Desai M. Transrectal ultrasound- and fluoroscopic-assisted transurethral incision of ejaculatory ducts: a problem-solving approach to nonmalignant hematospermia due to ejaculatory duct obstruction. Endourol. 2008;22:1531–5.
124. Van Peperstraten A, Proctor ML, Johnson NP, et al. Techniques for surgical retrieval of sperm prior to ICSI for azoospermia. Cochrane Database Syst Rev. 2006;3:CD002807.
125. Nicopoullos JD, Gilling-Smith C, Almeida PA, et al. Use of surgical sperm retrieval in azoospermic men: a meta-analysis. Fertil Steril. 2004;82:691–701.
126. Kamal A, Fahmy I, Mansour R, et al. Does the outcome of ICSI in cases of obstructive azoospermia depend on the origin of the retrieved spermatozoa or the cause of obstruction? A comparative analysis. Fertil Steril. 2010;94(6):2135–40.
127. Hauser R, Yogev L, Paz G, et al. Comparison of efficacy of two techniques for testicular sperm retrieval in nonobstructive azoospermia: multifocal testicular sperm extraction versus multifocal testicular sperm aspiration. J Androl. 2006;27:28–33.
128. Donoso P, Tournaye H, Devroey P. Which is the best sperm retrieval technique for nonobstructive azoospermia? A systematic review. Hum Reprod Update. 2007;13:539–49.
129. Carpi A, Sabanegh E, Mechanick J. Controversies in the management of nonobstructive Azoospermia. Fertil Steril. 2009;91:963–70.
130. Schiff JD, Palermo GD, Veeck LL, et al. Success of testicular sperm injection and intracytoplasmic sperm injection in men with Klinefelter syndrome. J Clin Endocrinol Metab. 2005;90:6263–7.
131. Ramasamy R, Yagan N, Schlegel PN. Structural and functional changes to the testis after conventional versus microdissection testicular sperm extraction. Urology. 2005;65:1190–4.
132. Carpi A, Menchini Fabris F, Palego F, et al. Fine-needle and large needle percutaneous aspiration biopsy of the testicle in men with nonobstructive azoospermia: safety and diagnostic performance. Fertil Steril. 2005;83:1029–33.
133. Turunc T, Gul U, Haydardedeoglu B, et al. Conventional testicular sperm extraction combined with the microdissection technique in nonobstructive azoospermic patients: a prospective comparative study. Fertil Steril. 2010;94(6):2157–60. Epub 20 Feb 2010.
134. Tesarik J. Paternal effects on cell division in the human preimplantation embryo. Reprod Biomed Online. 2005;10:370–5.
135. Schlegel PN, Liotta D, Hariprashad J, et al. Fresh testicular sperm from men with nonobstructive azoospermia works best for ICSI. Urology. 2004;64:1069–71.
136. Alukal JP, Lamb DJ. Intracytoplasmic sperm injection (ICSI)—what are the risks? Urol Clin North Am. 2008;35:277–88.
137. Knoester M, Helmerhorst FM, Vandenbroucke JPM, et al. Artificial Reproductive Techniques Follow-up Project. Cognitive development of singletons born after intracytoplasmic sperm injection compared with in vitro fertilization and natural conception. Fertil Steril. 2008;90:289–96.
138. Belva F, Henriet S, Liebaers I, et al. Medical outcome of 8-year-old singleton ICSI children and a spontaneously conceived comparison group. Hum Reprod. 2007;22:506–15.
139. Woldringh GH, Besselink DE, Tillema AH, et al. Karyotyping, congenital anomalies and follow-up of children after intracytoplasmic sperm injection with non-ejaculated sperm: a systematic review. Hum Reprod Update. 2010;16:12–9.

Chapter 9
Microsurgery for Male Infertility: The AIIMS Experience

Rajeev Kumar

The All India Institute of Medical Sciences (AIIMS), New Delhi, is a government funded tertiary care medical institution that provides medical education, undertakes research and provides medical care at nominal costs. All citizens, and even non-citizens, can avail themselves of the services. Academically, it is consistently ranked the best among over 300 medical colleges in the country. The institution is equipped with state-of-the-art technologies including two da Vinci®(Intuitive Surgicals, CA) surgical robots. The low cost along with exceptional facilities results in a high demand for services and leads to significant waiting periods for most elective surgical procedures. Understanding this basic nature of the institution is essential to understanding the development and experience of microsurgery for male infertility at AIIMS.

Infertility is a major social issue in the Indian culture. Parenthood is considered an essential function in life with immense social pressure on married couples to have children. The stigma surrounding infertility is such that couples prefer seeking treatment through discreet unqualified practitioners who offer quick cures rather than visit a public hospital. Coupled with the low per capita income and lack of adequate health insurance, social issues have a major impact on the management of male infertility at AIIMS.

First, there is significant delay in seeking treatment for the male partner. In a survey, we found that 8–10% of all patients presenting to the urology clinic had infertility, the average age of the male partner at presentation to us was 27 years, the mean duration of infertility was 6.2 years, 88% had previously consulted medical practitioners, and 84% had received medical therapy, most often of unknown nature (unpublished data). Interestingly, in no case did we find the male presenting to us on his own, without a referral from the physician evaluating the wife. This delayed presentation increases the need for early intervention and quick results.

R. Kumar, MCh
Department of Urology, All India Institute of Medical Sciences,
Ansari Nagar, New Delhi 110029, India
e-mail: rajeev02@gmail.com

S.J. Parekattil, A. Agarwal (eds.), *Male Infertility for the Clinician*,
© Springer Science+Business Media New York 2013

The second major impact of the social conditions is the need for cost-effective interventions. There is no financial support for undergoing in vitro fertilization (IVF), which continues to be expensive. Patients are willing to accept even minimal success rates if surgery can help prevent IVF. Less than 2% of our patients choose IVF over microsurgical reconstruction.

Evaluation and Etiologies

Evaluation of the infertile male aims at identifying the etiology, reversibility, and potential underlying medical conditions that may have manifest as infertility. Microsurgery is currently offered for bypassing an obstruction in the epididymis or the vas deferens and for correction of a varicocele. The evaluation and investigations are tailored to diagnose suitability for microsurgery and maximize successful outcomes.

All men provide a detailed history of their condition. A history of previous vasectomy, hernia surgery, retroperitoneal surgery, hydroceles/scrotal surgery, and tuberculosis suggests obstructive azoospermia. Low volume ejaculate is determined from direct questioning of "few drops" versus a "spoonful," while a history of orchitis, radiation or chemotherapy would indicate testicular failure. Previous conceptions, work environment, and smoking histories are recorded. The physical examination is used to confirm the presence of vas deferens, testicular size, epididymis, secondary sexual characteristics and record any abnormalities in the genitalia. Examination for varicocele is performed in the erect and supine positions. Since all men come to us with a referral from another physician, most carry a semen analysis report that is used for focusing further evaluation. At least two semen samples are used to categorize the abnormality.

Congenital bilateral absence of the vas deferens (CBAVD) is diagnosed clinically in the majority of patients. A combination of low volume ejaculate, absent vas on palpation, hemi-epididymis, and acidic azoospermia are considered sufficient evidence [1]. Patients with a low volume ejaculate and a palpable vas undergo transrectal ultrasound (TRUS) for determining dilatation of the seminal vesicles and ejaculatory ducts secondary to an ejaculatory duct obstruction. A post-ejaculate urine examination for sperms is performed to rule out retrograde ejaculation if the TRUS findings are inconclusive. These men are generally not considered candidates for microsurgical reconstruction.

Men with normal volume azoospermia, normal secondary sexual characteristics, normal size testis, and palpable vas deferens are evaluated to determine suitability for microsurgery. The primary aim in these men is to differentiate obstructive from nonobstructive azoospermia. Unless a history suggestive of testicular insult is present, these men undergo estimation of serum follicle stimulating hormone levels (FSH) and fine needle aspiration cytology of both the testis (FNAC). Normal testicular spermatogenesis in such men is considered diagnostic of obstruction. FNAC is performed using a 23 G butterfly needle attached to a 10 ml syringe, with multiple passes into the testis through a single skin puncture. A minimum of 2,000 cells are evaluated on an air-dried slide stained with the May–Grunwald–Giemsa stain. Similar to biopsy histology, these are reported as normal spermatogenesis, hypo-spermatogenesis, maturation arrest, or only Sertoli cells seen [2]. We rely on the FNAC reports to determine normal sperm production and do not perform diagnostic biopsies [3]. The FSH levels are used to prognosticate the outcome and an evalua-tion of outcomes when the FSH and FNAC are discordant is currently being performed.

We are able to determine the etiology of obstruction in less than one in five of men diagnosed with obstructive azoospermia [4]. This is in stark contrast to the under 20% incidence of idiopathic cases in most reported series of microsurgical recon-struction [5, 6]. Vasectomy reversals form a very small proportion of men undergoing microsurgery for infertility at our center primarily because vasectomy is an uncom-mon method of contraception among Indian couples. Vasectomy reversals, on the other hand, form the commonest indications for microsurgery in western populations [5, 6]. We believe that the most common cause of obstruction in our population is undiagnosed genital infection [4]. Three conditions specific to this population are tuberculosis, filariasis, and small pox.

Tuberculosis

Tuberculosis (TB) continues to be a significant public health problem in develop-ing countries. Genital tuberculosis is an extrapulmonary form of tuberculosis seen most often in men in the reproductive age group [7]. The epididymis is one of the favored sites for genital TB and may be the primary site of involvement in over three-fourths of cases [8]. The propensity for involvement of the epididymis prob-ably stems from the high vascularity of the globus minor [9]. Other sites that may be involved include the prostate, seminal vesicles, and the penile shaft [10]. The pathophysiology of TB induced infertility is most often obstructive. Obstruction may arise either directly by the granulomatous lesions or due to distortion of normal architecture and scarring [11].

Evaluation for TB requires a high degree of suspicion. Most men do not provide a definitive history of past TB and physical signs may be minimal. Involvement of scrotal structures most often presents with normal volume azoospermia. This may be accompanied by palpable nodules within the epididymis or a beaded feel to the vas deferens. Rarely, scrotal abscesses or sinuses may be present. Involvement of the prostate/seminal vesicles and the ejaculatory ducts is usually contiguous. It may manifest as low volume azoospermia due to an obstruction of the ejaculatory ducts. A tissue diagnosis may be attempted but does not always yield positive results and such men may be classified as idiopathic obstruction. Discrete obstruction of the ejaculatory ducts may be treated with a transurethral resection of the ejaculatory ducts [10]. Involvement of the vas and the epididymis with nodules is rarely ame-nable to microsurgical reconstruction. If discrete nodules in the vas are felt, an attempt may be made at vasovasal anastomosis, bypassing the obstructing nodule. Unfortunately, the outcomes of surgery in such patients are usually poor and they are rarely correctable.

Filariasis

Filarial involvement of the lymphatic system can involve the scrotum and the epididymis. Filariasis is endemic in a large part of north-central India. Infertility due to filariasis is probably a result of inflammatory scarring and, at times, iatrogenic following interventions to treat filarial hydroceles. A number of studies have described the association between filariasis and male infertility [12, 13]. The most common clinical manifestation of scrotal filariasis is hydrocele. While the hydrocele itself may not cause infertility, this is often associated with dense adhesions around the epididymis and tunical calcifications. The tunica vaginalis is extremely thickened and the underlying tubules of the epididymis are often thin and flimsy [4]. The adhesions and scarring may be so dense that identification of the epididymis itself is not feasible, making it prone to injury during corrective hydrocele surgery. We generally discourage men who have had previous hydrocele surgeries from attempting microsurgical reconstruction because of the poor outcomes in such men.

Small Pox

Despite the eradication of small pox from India in the 1970s, we still occasionally come across men in their early 40s with clinical stigmata of the disease. Small pox resulted in obstructive azoospermia with a much higher incidence than would be expected from population studies [14]. Microsurgical reconstruction in these men is often gratifying because the disease tended to affect the terminal part of the epididymis, allowing a vaso-epididymostomy in the more proximal dilated tubules.

Microsurgical Procedures

Microsurgical reconstruction is offered at AIIMS for vasectomy reversal, vaso-epididymal obstruction, and varicoceles (Table 9.1). All procedures are performed as day-care surgery under regional or light general anesthesia. An operating microscope with face-to-face attachments for surgeon and assistant along with an offset arm with facility for camera attachment and transmission is used. There has been a steady evolution in case selection and techniques over the years and this has been accompanied by an improvement in outcomes.

Table 9.1 Common surgeries and their indications	Vasoepididymostomy
	Idiopathic
	Inflammatory
	Tuberculosis
	Filarial
	Unknown
	Post-vasectomy
	Vasovasostomy
	Post-vasectomy
	Inflammatory nodules
	Trauma
	Hernia surgery
	Hydrocele surgery
	Varicocelectomy
	Clinically palpable varicocele

Table 9.2 Evolution in vasoepididymostomy technique	Early 1990s: 6-0/7-0 sutures, non-mucosal anastomosis
	Poor expertise in microsurgery
	Limited equipment
	Late 1990s: Berger's technique [15] of three suture intussusception
	Thicker needles, inadequate space for three needles
	Early 2000s: Marmar's technique [16] of two suture intussusception
	Thicker needles
	Thin tubules
	Current: Modified, longitudinal technique of two suture intussusception [18]

Vaso-Epididymal Anastomosis

Scrotal explorations for vaso-epididymal anastomosis form the most common microsurgical procedure performed. Nearly all such procedures are performed for men with idiopathic obstruction. An obstruction is suspected in men with normal volume azoospermia with palpable vas deferens and normal spermatogenesis on testicular FNAC. These men are counseled about the options of scrotal exploration and IVF. A presumptive prognosis for success of reconstruction is provided based on age, testicular size, serum FSH, and presence of scrotal pathology.

In the 1990s, we used to perform a non-mucosal anastomosis between the vas deferens and the epididymal tubules, often with large 6-0 or 7-0 sutures. This was primarily due to a lack of microsurgical expertise. The results of this "fistula" technique were universally poor with a rare patient reporting patency. Two publications toward the end of the last century resulted in major changes in our approach (Table 9.2). Berger's paper on the triangulation intussusception technique of end-to-side vasoepididymostomy was the first of these publications [15]. The use of three double-armed sutures instead of multiple independent sutures for the inner layer, coupled with our increasing familiarity with an operating microscope allowed us to attempt this technique in a number of patients with some success. A major problem that we faced with this approach was with the size of needles for the 10-0 suture. The 10-0 double-armed polyamide suture available to us was swaged on 200-μm needles. Placing three such needles in the small epididymal tubule proved difficult and we would often manage to get only two sutures in place.

Marmar's article in 2000 on the two-suture technique of vasoepididymostomy proved to be the turning point in our approach to this procedure [16]. It was simpler to perform and afforded excellent results. We began using this technique in 2002 and have been using our modifications of it since then [17, 18].

In 2003, Chan et al. published a comparative report on three different intussusception techniques in rats and concluded longitudinal placement of sutures in the epididymal tubule resulted in higher patency rates [19]. Difficulty in placing our thicker needles transversely in the tubules had led us to this modification in our patients at about the same time and we commented on our findings in a reply to their publication [20].

Our Surgical Technique

During the initial part of our experience, we performed microsurgical reconstruction unilaterally. Prior to using the two-suture technique, our results had been poor and we wished to keep one side untouched in case the patient wished to seek treatment for our failure elsewhere. Our initial microscope had a relatively high minimal height and the height of the operating table and the eyepiece of the microscope made it impossible to sit and operate. Thus, all our microsurgeries were performed with the surgeon standing up. This initial practice has been continued and we still perform all such surgeries standing up even after changing our microscope in 2009 to a Zeiss Opmi Vario® (*Carl Zeiss Micro Imaging GmbH, Germany*) with an S-88 stand. Our basic microsurgical instruments set consists of curved and straight micro-needle holders without ratchet, curved microscissors, straight iris scissors, Jeweler's toothed, and non-toothed microforceps with a platform to assist suture tying and Adson's toothed and non-toothed forceps. We do not use clamps for holding the epididymis or the vas deferens.

With the patient supine, a longitudinal incision is made in the scrotum at its antero-lateral edge toward the upper end of the testis. The incision is deepened to expose the tunica vaginalis, which is incised to deliver the testis. Any adhesions within the tunical layer are divided to expose the anterior surface of the epididymis. The surface is inspected for calcifications/nodules and visibly dilated tubules. In patients with a previous hydrocelectomy, the tunical layer is obliterated and an attempt is made, by feel, to identify the epididymis and incise layers of tissue above it to expose the epididymal tunic. The spermatic cord is palpated posterior-lateral to the testis to confirm the presence of the vas deferens and get a visual impression of its diameter. Occasionally, in men with a more distal obstruction, the vas may feel dilated and thick fluid in the lumen may be visible through its wall.

Before dividing the vas deferens, we inspect the epididymis through its tunica to identify dilated tubules. In men with clearly dilated tubules, we proceed to preparing the vas. However, if the epididymis does not show any dilated tubules and feels flabby in its entire length, we make an incision in the epididymal tunic and observe the individual tubules under the microscope. If there still appears to be a doubt about the presence of obstruction, one of the distal loops of the tubule is incised and the fluid is examined for sperms. If sperms are confirmed, a more proximal site is selected for the anastomosis.

The vas is isolated from the remaining cord structures with blunt dissection, maintaining a mesentery of blood vessels to the vas in its entire length. The junction of the convoluted and straight vas is identified and a small segment of the vas at this site is elevated from its mesentery on a small hemostat. Using a sharp straight knife, the vas is hemisectioned at this level and inspected for any fluid that may suggest a more distal block. A 24 G angiocatheter is carefully inserted into the lumen of the distal vas and flushed slowly with up to 20 cm^3 of saline. Free flow of saline with no regurgitation is used as an indicator of distal patency and the section of the vas is completed. If there is resistance to flow of saline, a 3-0 polyamide suture is threaded into the lumen to determine the level of block. If the block is at a short distance, the vas is exposed to the expected site of block and a fresh vasotomy is made at that site and the procedure repeated. For more distant blocks, a formal vasography is performed.

Once distal patency of the vas is confirmed, further mobilization of the mesentery is performed, keeping a good amount of tissue and blood vessels around the vas. The periadventitial tissue is held gently with a hemostat until the first seromuscular sutures are placed.

The epididymis is reinspected and its tunica incised over the most visibly dilated tubules. Individual loops of the tubule are gently separated from their surrounding alveolar tissue until the selected tubule bulges above the rest. In our earlier cases, the sutures were placed transversally in the loop in a manner that they could be tied without crossing over of the sutures [19, 20] (Fig. 9.1). In our more recent cases, we place the sutures longitudinally, again in a manner such that they can be tied to each other without crossing over [17] (Fig. 9.2).

The end of the vas is maneuvered to the site of the tunical incision. An 8-0 polyamide suture is placed from outside-in at the 5 o'clock position in the seromuscular layer of the vas. The needle is then passed through the epididymal tunic from inside out and tied. The procedure is repeated with another suture at the 7 o'clock position. The direction of placement of these sutures is important in that placing the suture along the direction of the vas helps provide traction to the needle as it enters the thick vas. Placement inside-out on the epididymal tunic allows the needle to lift the tunic from the underlying tubules, preventing inadvertent injury to the tubules.

Once the vas is secured to the epididymis, the needle of a 10-0 polyamide double-armed suture is placed in the loop of the epididymal tubule. The needle is inserted at the end closer to the vas and exits at the opposite end. This needle may be placed transversally or longitudinally in the loop depending on the selected procedure. A second similar suture is placed, parallel to the first. The tubule between the two

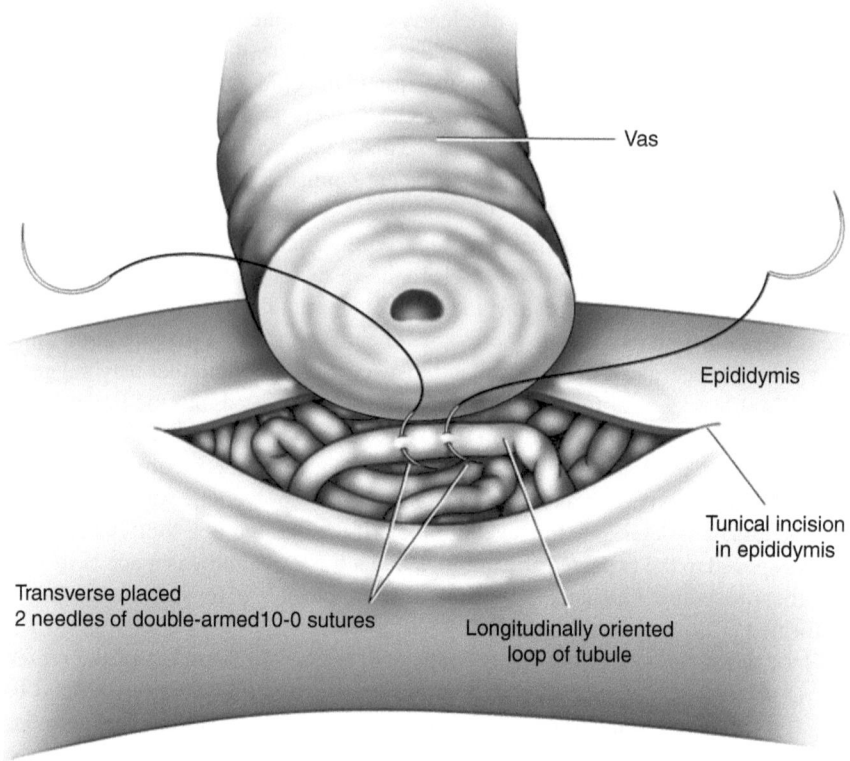

Vas

Epididymis

Tunical incision
in epididymis

Transverse placed
2 needles of double-armed10-0 sutures

Longitudinally oriented
loop of tubule

Fig. 9.1 Transverse suture placement in the epididymal tubule for a vasoepididymostomy

needles is incised using a microknife. It is important to ensure that the length of this
incision does not extend beyond the entry and exit points of the two sutures [18].
Fluid from the tubules is directly collected on a sterile microslide for examination
under a light microscope. The procedure is continued if sperms are seen in the fluid.
The needles are pulled through and kept separate from each other. The other ends of
the sutures with their needles are now closer to the vas and are placed first into the
vas lumen. These needles are placed at the 5 o'clock and 7 o'clock positions in the
vas from inside the lumen, out through the muscular layer but not the full thickness
of the vas. The two needles away from the vas are now placed similarly into the vas
lumen at the 1 o'clock and 11 o'clock positions ensuring that the sutures are not
entangled. The needles exiting at 7 o'clock and 11 o'clock in the vas belong to the
same suture as do the 5 o'clock and 1 o'clock needles. The two needles of each
suture are held together and pulled to "hitch" up the tubule into the vas lumen. Both
ends of the same suture are then tied to each other, intussuscepting the loop into the
vas lumen. Additional 8-0 polyamide sutures are placed in the anterior layer of the
vas and the epididymal tunic to secure the anastomosis. Two to three 8-0 polyamide
sutures are also placed proximally in the serosal layer of the vas and the epididymal

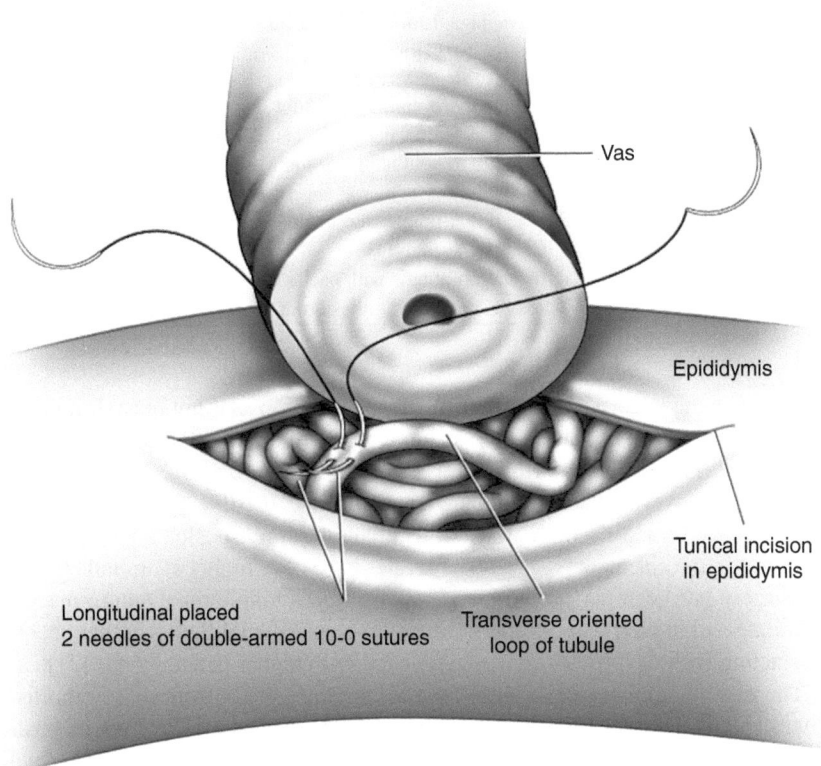

Fig. 9.2 Longitudinal suture placement in the epididymal tubule for a vasoepididymostomy

tissue to protect the anastomosis from cremasteric contractions. In case there are no sperms in the epididymal fluid, the sutures are removed and the procedure repeated at a more proximal site. All patients receive 3–5 days of antibiotics and are reviewed for suture removal after a week. A semen analysis is performed at 6 weeks and repeated every 3 months until patency is demonstrated. Patients who do not have a patent anastomosis by 1 year are advised to begin evaluation for IVF though they are counseled that delayed patency may occur even at 18 months. The modifications in our technique are described in Table 9.3.

Outcomes

Despite our stringent inclusion criteria for a VEA, we are able to perform an anastomosis in only about 60% of all explorations [4]. Even among men where we are able to find sperms within the epididymis, in some the tubules are extremely thin with minimal dilatation. In such cases, particularly where the sperms are found only

Table 9.3 Modifications to the vasoepididymostomy technique

1. Vas fixed to epididymal tunic prior to tubular sutures
   Advantage: Limited manipulations required once the mucosal sutures are in place
   Disadvantage: Vas sutures need to be taken down if there are no sperms in the epididymal fluid
2. Mucosal sutures placed sequentially, not simultaneously
   Difficult to hold both 200-µm needles together in the micro-needle holder
3. Use of 200-µm needles on 10-0 suture instead of 70-µm
   Cost and availability
4. Incision of tubule with needles in situ
   Avoids inadvertent division of the suture material

in tubules in the head, a single tubule mucosal anastomosis is not feasible and a non-mucosal anastomosis between the vas lumen and epididymal tunic with an incision in the tubules needs to be performed.

Among cases where a single tubule anastomosis is feasible, our success rates, on average, have been 50% in the form of a patent anastomosis, documented by return of sperms in the ejaculate [17, 18]. These rates have been higher at around 80% when the surgery has been performed bilaterally using the longitudinal suture placement technique and in men with motile sperms in the epididymal fluid. Further, technical satisfaction with the procedure was associated with higher patency rates [21].

There are a number of reasons why our outcomes differ from those reported by other centers. The most important among these is an unclear etiology of obstruction. Most of our patients have primary infertility and the diagnosis of obstruction at the vasoepididymal junction is one of exclusion. Another potential reason is the use of thicker needles on the sutures. The 200-µm needles that we use are five times less expensive than the standard 70-µm needles and this difference is often a major concern for our patients. Our attempts at preserving one side and operating unilaterally may also be causative since our outcomes among bilateral procedures have been much better. Finally, short follow-up of patients is a problem that plagues all our procedures. It is well known that patency may become apparent many months after a procedure but most of our patients provide only one or at most two semen samples after the surgery. This may also be related to the previously discussed issues of social pressure and need for early outcomes. A number of these men possibly opt for assisted reproduction soon after the surgery, not willing to wait for a successful surgery.

Vasovasal Anastomosis

Vasectomy is an uncommon form of contraception in India, accounting for fewer than 5% of all contraceptive methods [22]. A decision to undergo a vasectomy is usually taken after careful thought and requests for reversal are rare. The most frequent reason for seeking a reversal is the loss of a child [23]. This statistic has two important implications. First, the stress on success is likely to be greater in this group of patients than in those who already have living children and second, most patients are interested in early patency during which they may father a child without significant concern about delayed closures. The low volumes of procedures also mean that there is inadequate training of surgeons. These factors have been instrumental in our attempts at simplifying the surgical technique of vasectomy reversal.

Our Surgical Technique

A semen analysis is obtained in all men seeking vasectomy reversal to confirm azo- ospermia. No additional investigations are requested if the testicular size is normal and both vas are palpable. A longitudinal incision is placed in the scrotal skin, as for the VEA procedure. The testis and the spermatic cord are delivered out of the scro- tum and the site of vasectomy is identified. A Babcock forceps is used to hold the vas deferens above and below the site of vasectomy and a short segment of the vas is stripped of its adventitial tissue. The distal vas is sharply divided and flushed with saline to test for patency, similar to the procedure previously described for a vaso- epididymostomy. The proximal end of the vas is then divided and the fluid exam- ined for sperms. In the absence of any fluid, a gentle barbotage of the proximal vas is performed with saline and this fluid is then examined. If no fluid or sperms are demonstrable, the epididymis is examined to look for a secondary block and a vaso- epididymostomy is considered.

The adventitial tissue of the two ends of the vas is held with the tip of small hemostats to appose them to each other. Two 8-0 polyamide sutures are placed at the 5 and 7 o'clock positions in the seromuscular layers of the two ends and tied. The suture ends are left long and held in rubber shod hemostat clamps. The hemo- stats applied to the adventitia are removed. A double-armed 10-0 polyamide suture is placed, inside out at 6 o'clock in the mucosa of the distal vas and the second needle is placed at the corresponding position of the proximal vas. The suture is tied. Three additional 10-0 polyamide sutures are placed at the 3, 9, and 12 o'clock positions in the mucosa of both ends of the vas. These three sutures are tied sequentially once all have been placed. Two additional 8-0 polyamide sutures are placed in the seromuscular layer (Fig. 9.3). Additional sutures may be placed in the seromuscular layer or the adventitia to stabilize the anastomosis [24]. The postoperative advice and follow-up are as described for the vasoepididymostomy procedure.

Outcomes

Vasectomy reversals have traditionally been a very satisfying procedure with excellent patency rates, usually above 90% [25]. Our own practice of vasectomy

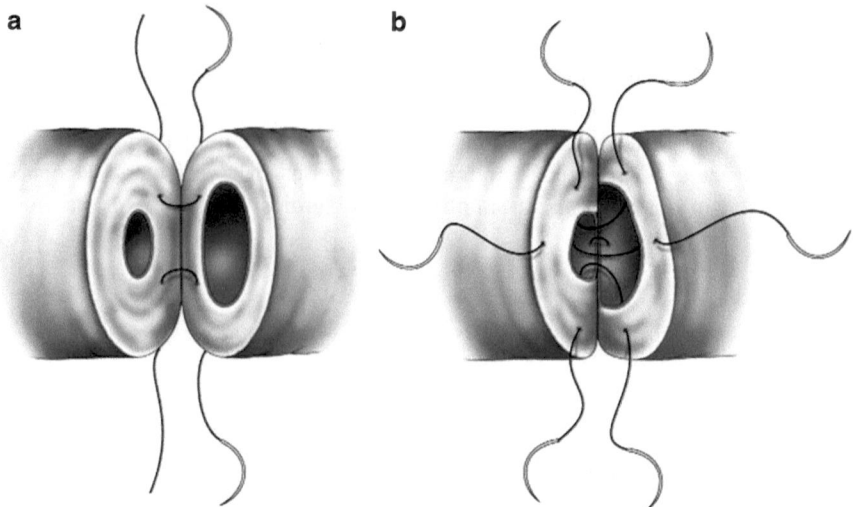

Fig. 9.3 Suture placement technique for a 4 × 4 vasovasostomy

reversals has been sporadic with fewer than 8–10 cases per year. The results were felt to be good but a detailed record is not available. Since 2008, we began using the 4 × 4 technique described above exclusively following a study protocol. We have found this technique simple to perform with excellent outcomes. All eight patients described in our recent report have a patent anastomosis [24]. Cases performed after the last accrual in this report are also patent. One of the potential problems with this technique is the possibility of sperm leakage and delayed closure. While this is certainly a theoretical possibility, as we stated earlier, most of our patients are keen on an immediate patency with little interest in delayed results. This procedure is simple and may be performed by a greater number of surgeons than the more difficult microdot technique. We feel the simplicity of the procedure with excellent early results, but unknown long-term outcomes may be an acceptable trade off with the more difficult techniques that have proven long-term outcomes.

Microsurgical Varicocelectomy

We maintain a high threshold for case selection for varicocelectomy. Only men with clinically palpable varicoceles are accepted. This policy began even before the AUA and ASRM guidelines were published but were reinforced by these guidelines [26, 27]. Surgery is performed for the side where the varicocele is palpable and a Doppler of the scrotum is requested only where a clinical examination is doubtful.

Our Surgical Technique

The external inguinal ring is identified by insinuating a finger through the scrotal skin into the inguinal region. A 2 cm transverse incision is made in the skin overlying the external ring. Under magnification, this incision is deepened to expose the spermatic cord. The tissue around the cord and over the external ring is separated and a small incision is made in the external ring to make it wider. This incision is directed along the inguinal canal. The cord is held with a Babcock's forceps and, under the microscope, is freed from the bed and surrounding tissues. The cord is then brought out onto the surface. The fossa is examined for any visibly dilated veins that are ligated and divided. The cord is held on the surface over a hemostat. The superficial layers of the spermatic fascia are divided longitudinally, closer to the cranial end of the cord. The artery is identified and isolated. All visible veins are individually identified and ligated and divided. The cord is then taken onto the surgeon's nondominant hand and scanned inside and outside the spermatic fascia to confirm that all major veins have been divided. We do not deliver the testis into the wound or ligate the gubernacular vessels.

Outcomes

We have previously reported our outcomes for subinguinal varicocelectomy [26]. Briefly, one-third of patients are able to father a child through natural conception after the surgery and a majority will show improvements in seminal parameters. The procedure has resulted in downgrading the ART techniques required in a number of patients who have undergone this procedure [28].

Training and Credentials

Andrology and microsurgery procedures are performed as a part of the standard urological services available to all patients. Urology residents, during their 3 years of training, are posted to assist in these surgical procedures. There are no fellowship programs in male infertility or andrology and few would return for dedicated specialized training in microsurgery. This results in very little postresidency acquisition of skills or even skills maintenance because the numbers of procedures performed in urologic practice in the community is very limited.

Five-Year View and Key Issues

The major issues concerning microsurgery for male infertility in our practice are lack of awareness and inadequate training facilities. The general perception among treating gynecologists and IVF specialists is that the outcomes of surgical intervention are poor. We are focusing our energies toward improving this outlook by delivering lectures and publishing our results so that a greater number of men with obstructive azoospermia may be counseled about surgical options. With regards surgical training, the opportunities still remain limited, primarily due to inadequate infrastructure and individuals performing these surgeries. Over the next few years, we hope to train a significant number of urologists in microsurgical techniques so that these may become available at more centers.

Another important aspect of our practice is the inability to diagnose the etiology of obstruction in the majority of cases. While infection remains the most likely suspect, we have been unable to document this. We have initiated studies to evaluate etiology using molecular methods and hope to be able to reach some conclusion over the next 5 years.

Conclusions

The diseases responsible for male infertility and for cases undergoing exploration for microsurgical reconstruction at AIIMS possibly differ from those reported in most Western literature. The largest majority of cases explored are for primary infertility with obstruction of unknown etiology. This has resulted in lower percentage of patients with a successful outcome. However, the socioeconomic factors around infertility management in our country dictate an attempt at reconstruction even when the expected outcomes are poor. In patients with favorable prognostic factors, the outcomes are generally good.

References

1. Kumar R, Thulkar S, Kumar V, Jagannathan NR, Gupta NP. Contribution of investigations to the diagnosis of congenital vas aplasia. ANZ J Surg. 2005;5:807–9.
2. Meng MV, Cha I, Ljung BM, Turek PJ. Testicular fine-needle aspiration in infertile men: correlation of cytologic pattern with biopsy histology. Am J Surg Pathol. 2001;25:71–9.
3. Kumar R, Gautam G, Gupta NP, Aron M, Dada R, Kucheria K, et al. Role of testicular fine-needle aspiration cytology in infertile men with clinically obstructive azoospermia. Nat Med J Ind. 2006;19:18–9.
4. Kumar R. Surgery for azoospermia in the Indian patient: why is it different? Indian J Urol. 2011;27(1):98–101.
5. Schiff J, Chan P, Li PS, Finkelberg S, Goldstein M. Outcome and late failures compared in 4 techniques of microsurgical vasoepididymostomy in 153 consecutive men. J Urol. 2005;174:651–5.
6. Chan PT, Brandell RA, Goldstein M. Prospective analysis of outcomes after microsurgical intussusception vasoepididymostomy. BJU Int. 2005;96:598–601.
7. Viswaroop B, Johnson P, Kurian S, Chacko N, Kekre N, Gopalakrishnan G. Fine-needle aspiration cytology versus open biopsy for evaluation of chronic epididymal lesions: a prospective study. Scand J Urol Nephrol. 2005;39:219–21.

8. Orakwe JC, Okafor PI. Genitourinary tuberculosis in Nigeria; a review of thirty-one cases. Niger J Clin Pract. 2005;8:69–73.
9. Lenk S, Schroeder J. Genitourinary tuberculosis. Curr Opin Urol. 2001;11:93–8.
10. Kumar R. Reproductive tract tuberculosis and male infertility. Indian J Urol. 2008;24:92–5.
11. Kumar R, Hemal AK. Bilateral epididymal masses with infertility. ANZ J Surg. 2004;74: 391.
12. Ekwere PD. Filarial orchitis: a cause of male infertility in the tropics–case report from Nigeria. Cent Afr J Med. 1989;35:456–60.
13. Eyquem A, Heuze D, Schwartz J, Languillat G. Implications of heterophile antigens in immunological infertility in males. Arch Androl. 1978;1:241–8.
14. Phadke AM, Samant NR, Dewal SD. Smallpox as an etiologic factor in male infertility. Fertil Steril. 1973;24:802–4.
15. Berger RE. Triangulation end-to-side vasoepididymostomy. J Urol. 1998;159:1951–3.
16. Marmar JL. Modified vasoepididymostomy with simultaneous double needle placement, tubulotomy and tubular invagination. J Urol. 2000;163:483–6.
17. Kumar R, Gautam G, Gupta NP. Early patency rates following the two-stitch invagination technique of vasoepidiymal anastomosis for idiopathic obstruction. BJU Int. 2006;97:575–7.
18. Kumar R, Mukherjee S, Gupta NP. Intussusception vasoepididymostomy with longitudinal suture placement for idiopathic obstructive azoospermia. J Urol. 2010;183:1489–92.
19. Chan PT, Li PS, Goldstein M. Microsurgical vasoepididymostomy: a prospective randomized study of 3 intussusception techniques in rats. J Urol. 2003;169:1924–9.
20. Kumar R. Re: microsurgical vasoepididymostomy: a prospective randomized study of 3 intussusception techniques in rats. J Urol. 2004;171:810–1.
21. Gautam G, Kumar R, Gupta NP. Factors predicting the patency of two-stitch invagination vasoepididymal anastomosis for idiopathic obstruction. Indian J Urol. 2005;21:112–5.
22. Dhillon BS, Chandhiok N, Kambo I, Saxena NC. Induced abortion and concurrent adoption of contraception in the rural areas of India (an ICMR task force study). Indian J Med Sci. 2004;58:478–84.
23. Jina RP, Kumar V. Recanalisation of vas. J Indian Med Assoc. 1979;72:30–2.
24. Kumar R, Mukherjee S. "4 × 4 vasovasostomy": a simplified technique for vasectomy reversal. Indian J Urol. 2010;26(3):350–2.
25. Belker AM, Thomas Jr AJ, Fuchs EF, Konnak JW, Sharlip ID. Results of 1,469 microsurgical vasectomy reversals by the Vasovasostomy Study Group. J Urol. 1991;145:505–11.
26. Kumar R, Gupta NP. Subinguinal microsurgical varicocelectomy: evaluation of results. Urol Int. 2003;71:361–7.
27. Sharlip ID, Jarow JP, Belker AM, Lipshultz LI, Sigman M, Thomas AJ, Schlegel PN, Howards SS, Nehra A, Damewood MD, Overstreet JW, Sadovsky R. Best practice policies for male infertility. Fertil Steril. 2002;77:873–82.
28. Kumar R, Gupta NP. Varicocele and the urologist. Indian J Urol. 2006;22:98–104.

Chapter 10
Advanced Techniques
for Vasoepididymostomy

Wayland Hsiao and Marc Goldstein

The first vasoepididymostomy (VE) was reported in 1902 by Dr. Edward Martin at the University of Pennsylvania. His technique involved slashing across multiple epididymal tubules and anastomosis of the vas to the epididymal tunic in a side-to-side manner with four fine silver wires [1, 2]. Patency depended on the formation of a fistula. In 1909, Martin reported in a series of 11 patients with epididymal obstruction a patency rate of 64% and a pregnancy rate of 27% [3]. He proved that vasoepididymostomy was technically feasible and his approach is the foundation on which subsequent work was based.

With advances in surgical technique and the development of microsurgical techniques, modern vasoepididymostomy allows us to accurately approximate the mucosa of a single epididymal tubule to the mucosa of the vasal lumen [4]. With this increased precision, we have been able to achieve even higher patency and pregnancy rates [5, 6]. Microsurgical vasoepididymostomy, however, is the most technically demanding procedure in all of microsurgery. In virtually no other operation are results so dependent upon technical perfection. Thus, microsurgical vasoepididymostomy should only be attempted by an experienced microsurgeon who performs a sufficient volume of microsurgery.

W. Hsiao, MD (✉)
Department of Urology, Emory University, 1365 Clifton Road,
NE Building B, Suite 1400 Atlanta, GA 30322, USA
e-mail: whsiao@emory.edu

M. Goldstein, MD
Cornell Institute for Reproductive Medicine, New York Presbyterian Hospital/
Weill Cornell Medical Center, Weill Cornell Medical College
of Cornell University, 525 East 68th Street,
580, New York, NY 10021, USA
e-mail: mgoldst@med.cornell.edu

S.J. Parekattil, A. Agarwal (eds.), *Male Infertility for the Clinician*,
© Springer Science+Business Media New York 2013

Vasoepididymostomy

Vasoepididymostomy is indicated in patients with obstructive azoospermia, and the decision to perform a vasoepididymostomy rather than a vasovasostomy is an intra-operative decision. During vasectomy reversal, the testicular end of the vas is cut and the intravasal fluid is evaluated both grossly as well as with the aid of a 400× bench microscope. The presence of thick toothpaste like fluid devoid of sperm, scant fluid in a patient without a sperm granuloma, or scant fluid with no spermato-zoa seen on barbitage, constitute indications for vasoepididymostomy. For non-vasectomy-related obstruction, vasoepididymostomy is indicated when a testis biopsy reveals complete spermatogenesis and transaction of the proximal vas reveals no sperm even with barbitage.

The evolution of modern single tubule vasoepididymostomy techniques has pro-gressed from the original end-to-end anastomoses described by Silber, end-to-side anastomoses described by Wagenknecht and Fogdestam, and end-to-side intussus-ception anastomoses first described by Berger. In all of these, the initial exposure and setup are similar. A high vertical scrotal incision is made about 3–4 cm in length aimed toward the external ring of the inguinal canal. In cases with inade-quate length of the vas, the incision can be extended over the external ring and inguinal dissection of the vas performed. After incision through the skin and dartos fascia, the testicle is delivered with the tunica vaginalis intact. Using a Babcock clamp, the vas is isolated and surrounded with a Penrose drain. The operating microscope is brought into the field. The junction of the straight and convoluted vas is identified and isolated. The vas is then dissected free of its investing sheath and blood vessels under the operating microscope to expose a clean segment of bare vas. The bare segment of vas is hemitransected with a 15° ultrasharp knife until the lumen is visualized. The vasal fluid is then sampled using a bench microscope at 400× magnification. If no spermatozoa are seen then an additional 0.1–0.2 ml of fluid is injected into the testicular end and that fluid is expressed back out by squeez-ing the testis and epididymis and the fluid examined under the bench microscope. Absence of vasal sperm on microscopic exam in a man with either a normal testis biopsy or a positive antisperm antibody assay [7] confirms the diagnosis of epididy-mal obstruction.

At this point, the abdominal end of the vas is checked for patency by cannulating the abdominal end of the vas with a 24-gage angiocather and injecting 1 ml of lac-tated ringers. Smooth injection without resistance or backflow confirms patency of the abdominal end of the vas. If further confirmation is desired, then a Foley cathe-ter can be inserted after injecting indigo carmine and the color of the urine inspected. Green urine or blue urine confirms the patency of the abdominal vas as well as the ejaculatory ducts.

Once epididymal obstruction is confirmed and the need for a vasoepididymos-tomy verified, the vas is prepared for anastomosis by complete transection using an ultrasharp knife drawn through a slotted 2, 2.5, or 3 mm nerve holding clamp. This gives the surgeon a perfect 90° cut of healthy vasal tissue. The cut surface of the testicular end of the vas deferens is inspected using 15–25 power magnification and should look like a bullseye with the three vasal layers distinctly visible. A healthy white mucosal ring should be seen which springs back immediately after gentle dilation. This layer is surrounded by muscularis which should appear smooth and homogeneous. A gritty-looking muscularis layer may indicate the presence of scar/fibrosis. Healthy bleeding should be noted from both the cut edge of the mucosa and the surface of the muscularis. If the blood supply is poor or the muscularis is gritty, the vas is recut until healthy tissue is found. The vasal artery and vein are ligated with 6-0 vicryl. Small bleeders are controlled with a microbipolar forceps set at low power. At this point, the tunica vaginalis is opened and the epididymis is inspected.

In patients with previous vasectomy, there are some minor variations, but the overall approach is similar. In these patients, the testicular and abdominal ends of the vas are identified and dissected free. The abdominal end is transected and checked for patency. After confirmation of abdominal end patency, the testicular end is then inspected, sectioned, and intravasal fluid microscopically inspected. Serial sectioning and microscopic evaluation are performed until either sperm are seen or one has reached the convoluted vas. Once, sectioning has progressed well into the convoluted vas and barbitage reveals no spermatozoa, the need for vasoepididymostomy is confirmed. The tunica vaginalis is opened and the epididymis is inspected under the operating microscope. At this point, it is time to determine the site of anastomosis.

End-to-End Anastomosis

This is the original microsurgical technique introduced by Silber and it is the first technique to allow the anastomosis of a specific epididymal tubule to the vas. At its introduction, it was far superior to any method previously described. In this technique, the epididymis is dissected down to it junction with the convoluted vas. The epididymis is then serially sectioned until a large rush of fluid is noted (Fig. 10.1), indicating that the area of obstruction has been bypassed. The single tubule with gushing fluid is identified and anastomosed to the vas with 3–5 interrupted 10-0 nylon sutures. The outer layer of the vas is anastomosed to the tunica of the epididymis with 9-0 nylon sutures (Fig. 10.2).

The advantages of this technique include the ability to dissect off the epididymis and rotate it to gain additional length if there are issues with short vasal length. A major disadvantage of this technique is that the outer diameter of the epididymal tunica is far larger than the outer diameter of the vas deferens, making a water-tight closure exceedingly difficult. Also, given that the blood supply is invariably affected during transaction, it becomes more difficult to clean, blood-free sperm for cryopreservation than it is with the end-to-side technique.

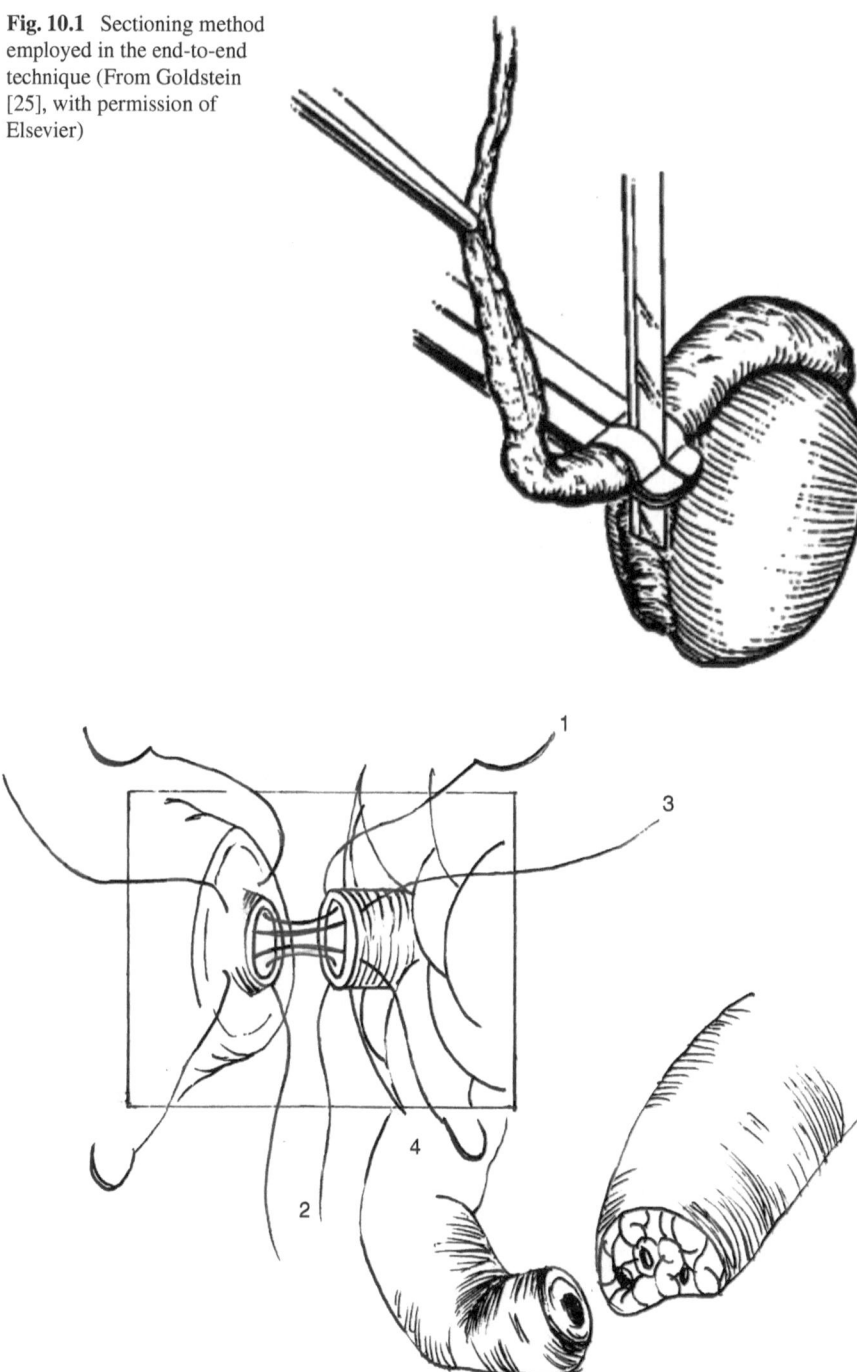

Fig. 10.1 Sectioning method
employed in the end-to-end
technique (From Goldstein
[25], with permission of
Elsevier)

Fig. 10.2 End-to-end anastomosis showing anastomosis of a single epididymal tubule to the vasal
lumen. Note that the outer vasal layers are then anastomosed to the tunica of the epididymis (From
Goldstein [25], with permission of Elsevier)

Fig. 10.3 Example of dilated epididymal tubules seen under the operating microscope

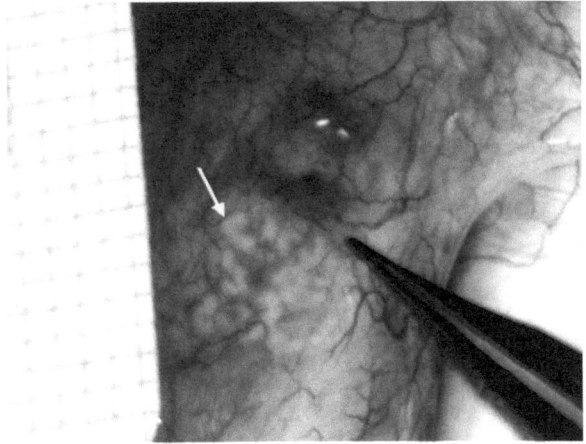

End-to-Side Techniques

End-to-side techniques of vasoepididymostomy improved on the end-to-end technique and have the advantage of being relatively bloodless and less traumatic to the delicate epididymis [8–11]. It requires minimal dissection of the tubule and allows the surgeon to easily tailor the size of the opening in the epididymal tubule. Also, this method allows for the preservation of the epididymal branches of the testicular artery. Thereby, if another vasovasostomy is required, the blood supply to the intervening segment of vas can be preserved. In cases where the integrity of the testicular artery is in doubt (previous orchiopexy, previous varicocelectomy, or hernia repair), preservation of the deferential artery may be required for the maintenance of testicular blood supply.

The selection of an anastomotic site is a bit more involved with the end-to-side technique when compared with the end-to-end technique. After the vas has been prepared, the tunica vaginalis is opened and the testis delivered. Inspection of the epididymis under the operating microscope may reveal a clearly delineated demarcation above which epididymal tubules are markedly dilated and below which the tubules are collapsed. Often, a discrete yellow sperm granuloma is noted, above which the epididymis is indurated and the tubules dilated and below which the epididymis is soft and the tubules collapsed (Fig. 10.3). If the level of obstruction is not clearly delineated a 70-μm tapered needle from the 10-0 nylon microsuture is used to puncture the epididymal tubule beginning as distal as possible and fluid sampled from the puncture site until sperm are found. At that level, the puncture is sealed with microbipolar forceps and the anastomosis is performed proximal to the puncture site.

An anastomotic site is selected where the epididymal tubules are clearly dilated. An avascular area is grasped with jeweler's forceps and the epididymal tunica tented upwards. A 3–4 mm buttonhole is made in the tunica with microscissors to match the outer diameter of the vas. The epididymal tubules are then gently dissected until dilated loops of tubules are clearly exposed.

At this point an opening is made in the tunica vaginalis and the vas deferens end is brought through and secured to the tunic with 2–3 interrupted 6-0 prolene sutures to ensure that the vasal lumen reaches the opening in the epididymal tunica without tension and with some length to spare. The posterior edge of the epididymal tunica is then approximated to the posterior edge of the vas muscularis and adventitia with 2–3 interrupted suture of double-armed 9-0 nylon. At the end of this step, the vasal lumen should be in close approximation to the epididymal tubule selected as the site for anastomosis. The proper positioning of the vasal segment as well as proper setup are critical to the creation of a long-lasting tension-free anastomosis.

Anastomotic Technique

Once setup for the anastomosis is complete, the surgeon has a choice of anastomotic techniques which vary by the number of sutures placed, the order of suture placement, and intussusception of the tubule. We will discuss the classic end-to-side anastomosis as well as the various intussusception techniques.

Original End-to-Side

The classic end-to-side approach involves creation of a longitudinal incision along the selected epididymal tubule. This is done under 25–32× magnification. The intra-tubular fluid is microscopically inspected with the bench microscope. If no sperm are seen on microscopic exam, then the tubule is closed with a 10-0 suture and the overlying tunica closed with 9-0 nylon. A more proximal location is then identified and the setup for anastomosis is repeated. If sperm are found on microscopic inspection, it is safe to continue with the procedure. The extruded epididymal fluid is aspirated into glass capillary tubes and flushed into media for cryopreservation [12]. Diluted indigo carmine is applied to the field to highlight the edges of the epididymal tubule as well as the mucosal edges of the vas segment. Of note, we have previously shown that methylene blue and radiographic contrast are toxic to spermatozoa, while diluted indigo carmine is not [13]. Thus, it is our preference to use indigo carmine diluted 50% with lactate ringers for all vasograms and for emphasis of the mucosal edges.

Constant irrigation with saline or lactated ringers is required to keep the delicate epididymal tubule open and to visualize the edges. The posterior mucosal edge of the cut epididymal tubule is approximated to the posterior edge of the vasal mucosa with 2 interrupted sutures of 10-0 nylon double-arm sutures with 70-µm diameter tapered needles. After these mucosal sutures are tied, the anterior mucosal anastomosis is completed with 2–4 additional 10-0 interrupted sutures. The outer muscularis and adventitia of the vas is then approximated to the cut edge of the epididymal tunica with 6–10 additional interrupted sutures of 9-0 nylon double armed with 100-µm diameter needles. The vasal sheath is secured to the epididymal tunica with 3–5 sutures of 9-0 nylon allowing for a straight course without kinks. The tunica

Fig. 10.4 Triangle of needles formed during the triangulation end-to-side intussusception technique introduced by Berger

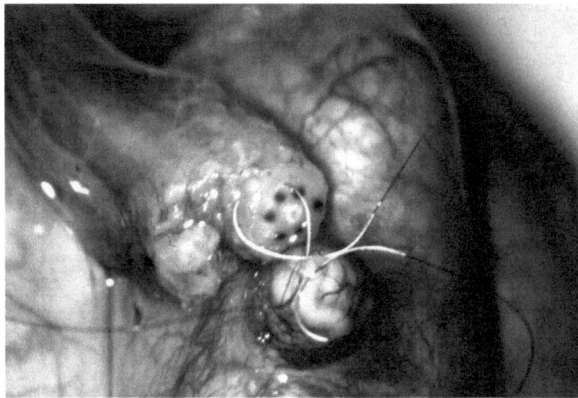

vaginalis is then closed with 5-0 Vicryl and the dartos reapproximated with absorbable suture. The skin is closed in a subcuticular fashion.

End-to-Side Intussusception Technique

The next advance in vasoepididymostomy techniques came with the development of intussusception techniques. This method was first introduced by Berger in 1998 [14]. The setup is identical to that for the classic procedure. After the vas is fixed to the opening in the epididymal tunica, six microdots are placed on the cut surface of the vas to mark the sites of needle exit. The microdot technique ensures precise suture placement by exact mapping of each planned suture. The microdot method separates the planning from the placement of sutures [15]. Much as a civil engineer is consulted before workmen commence construction on a bridge, the microdot method allows the surgeon to completely focus on each individual task at hand. This results in substantially improved accuracy in suture placement as well as better suture spacing. Next, the epididymal tubule selected for anastomosis is dissected until it is free of surrounding tissue and displays prominently. Indigo carmine is applied to highlight the tubule. Using double-arm 10-0 nylon sutures with 70μm tapered needles, three sutures are placed in the epididymal tubule in a triangular configuration. The needles are left in situ, creating a triangle of needles (Fig. 10.4). It must be remembered that the needle of the 10-0 suture is 70 μm in diameter while the suture material itself is only 17 μm. Thus, if the needles are pulled through prematurely, epididymal fluid and sperm would immediately leak though the suture hole causing the tubules to collapse, making placement of subsequent sutures and opening the tubules more difficult. Leaving the needles in situ also prevents accidentally cutting sutures when making the opening in the epididymal tubule.

After all three needles are properly placed, Berger originally described using a 9-0 cutting needle to lift the tubule and tear an opening in it. We prefer a 15°

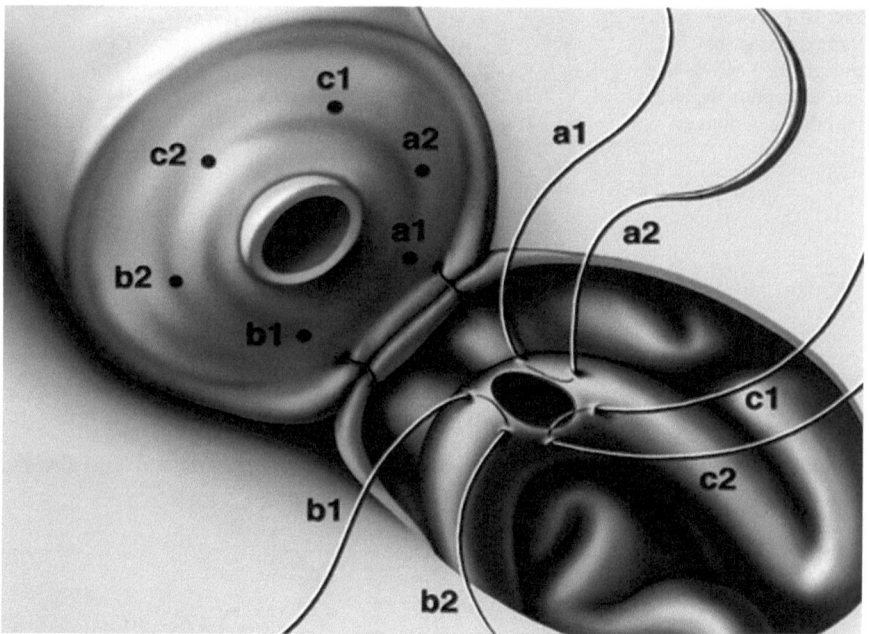

Fig. 10.5 End-to-side triangulation intussusception technique introduced by Berger (From Goldstein [25], with permission of Elsevier)

microknife to make an opening is made in the epididymal tubule in the center of the triangle. The three needles are then pulled though. The six needles are now laid out to avoid tangling. The extruded fluid is inspected under the microscope for sperm. If sperm are seen, then the six needles are passed inside out the vas deferens exiting through the six previously placed microdots (Fig. 10.5). The sutures are then tied and intussuscepting the epididymal tubule into the vas lumen and thereby creating a watertight closure. Intussusception also allows the flow of fluid from the epididymal tubule into the vas to push the edges epididymal tubule against the vasal mucosa, further reinforcing the watertight nature of this anastomosis. The edges of the vas are then closed with interrupted 9-0 nylon sutures (Fig. 10.6). Limitations of the triangulation technique include the need for a relatively large tubule for the three needles to fit. Thus, this technique is not suitable for anastomosis to the efferent ductules or the proximal caput epididymis where the tubule is smaller.

Two-Stitch Variation of Vasoepididymostomy

This is our currently preferred method of VE which allows for a two–stitch intussuscepted anastomosis. In this technique, four microdots are made on the vasal end. Two needles from two separate 10-0 double-arm sutures are then placed

Fig. 10.6 Closure of the epididymal tunica should be done with 9-0 nylon sutures with particular attention paid to avoid incorporating any underlying tubules into the closure (From Goldstein [25], with permission of Elsevier)

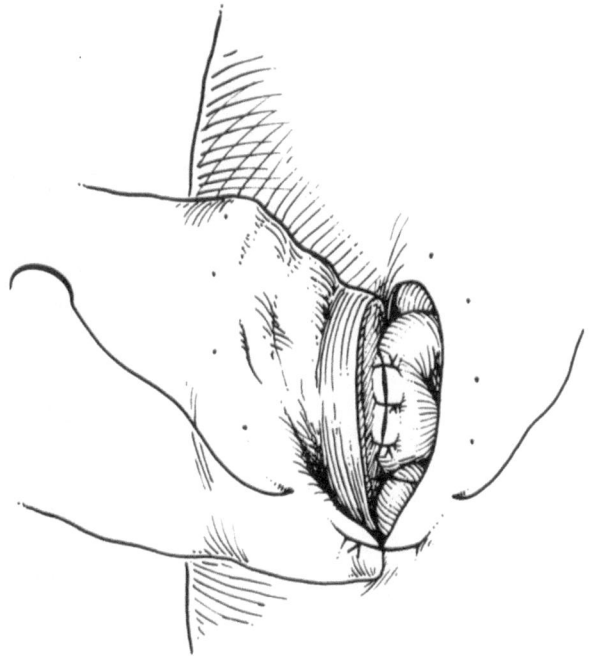

longitudinally in the tubule with care not to pull the needles completely through. The opening in the epididymal tubule is then made with a 15° microknife between the needles. After microscopic confirmation of the presence of spermatozoa, the needles are passed. The four needles are then passed through the vasal lumen and exiting the microdots (inside to outside). A 9-0 suture is placed to pull the anterior vas and adventitia toward the opening in the epididymal tubule bringing the vas mucosa into close approximation to the opening in the epididymal tubule. The lumen is irrigated with heparinized saline just prior to tying the mucosal sutures. Finally, the mucosal sutures are tied down (Fig. 10.7), allowing for the intussusception of the epididymal tubule. The outer layer is closed with interrupted 9-0 nylon sutures careful to not inadvertently incorporate any epididymal tubules when placing these sutures (Fig. 10.8). Again, by not passing the needles, one keeps a distended tubule which makes suture placement more accurate and reliable. Variations in this technique include mounting two needles in a single needle holder and placing them simultaneously transversely in the tubule as suggested by Marmar.

Of note, the cost of double-arm sutures can be high. In response to this, we have developed a single-arm technique of VE which we have found to be almost as effective as its double-arm counterpart [16]. It begins with the standard setup for VE. We then place four microdots in the vasal end. Two 10-0 single-arm nylon sutures are then passed through the microdots and exiting the vasal lumen (outside to inside). After this, the same two sutures are placed longitudinally in the selected tubule and

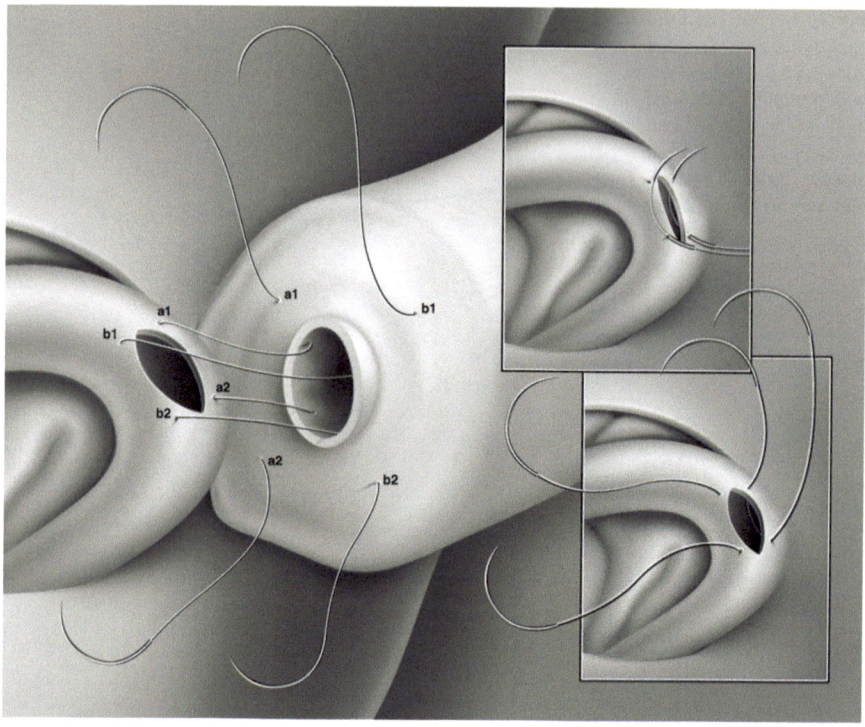

Fig. 10.7 Longitudinal intussuscepted vasoepididymostomy technique. Mucosal suture placement (From Goldstein [25], with permission of Elsevier)

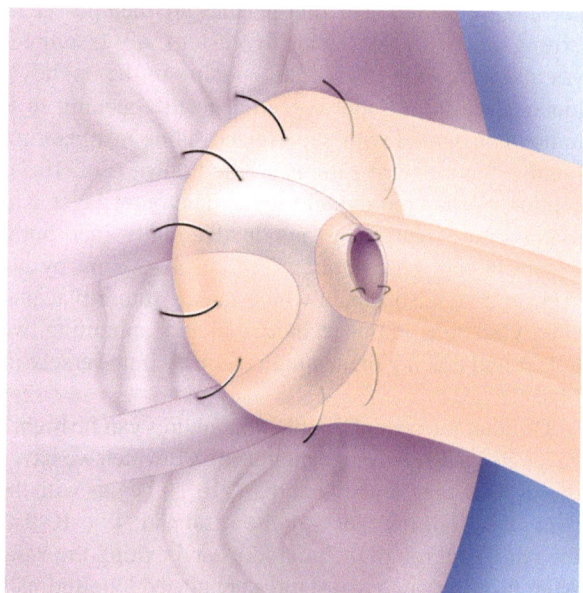

Fig. 10.8 Completed anastomosis for longitudinal intussuscepted technique (From Goldstein [25], with permission of Elsevier)

Fig. 10.9 Technique of single-arm vasoepididymostomy technique. Needles are passed outside in on the vas deferens. The needles are then passed longitudinally in the selected epididymal tubule and the cut made in the epididymal tubule. The needles are then passed and then placed inside out in the vas deferens (From Goldstein [25], with permission of Elsevier)

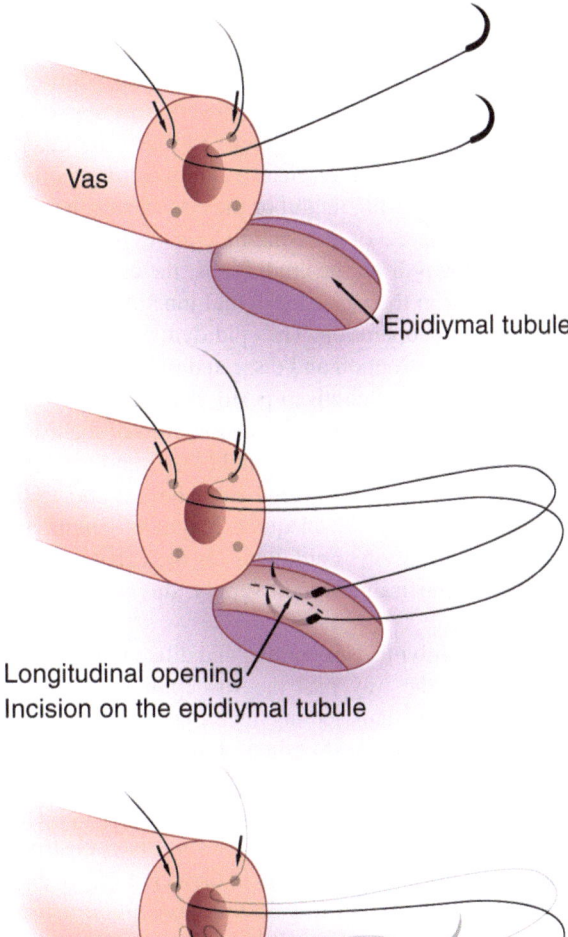

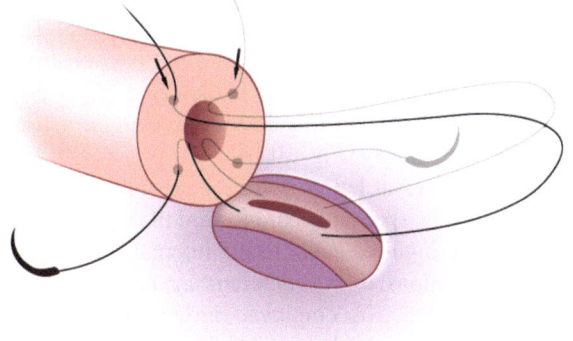

the needles are not completely passed. After opening the tubule and confirming the presence of spermatozoa, the needles are pulled through and the needles passed through the vasal lumen and exiting the microdot (inside to outside) (Fig. 10.9). The sutures are then tied allowing the intussusceptions of the epididymal tubule. The outer sheath of the vas deferens is then approximated to the tunic of the epididymis with 2–4 interrupted 9-0 nylon sutures, removing all tension from the anastomosis.

Techniques When Vasal Length Is Severely Compromised

One of the most common problems that arise during vasoepididymostomy is inadequate vasal length, often due to a very destructive vasectomy. When there is inadequate length of the vas deferens to reach the dilated epididymal tubule without tension, a number of surgical techniques may be employed involving any of the following: increasing length of the epididymis, increasing the vasal length, fixation of the testis, or use of the contralateral vas deferens.

To gain length on the epididymis, the cauda and corpus epididymis can be dissected down to the vasoepididymal junction and then dissected off the testes as in the end-to-end operation. The epididymis is encircled with a small Penrose drain at the level of obstruction and dissected off of the testis up to the level of obstruction, yielding sufficient length to perform the anastomosis. Usually an avascular plane can be found right on the tunica albuginea of the testis between the epididymis and testis and injury to the epididymal blood supply can be avoided. The inferior and, if necessary, middle epididymal branches of the testicular artery are ligated and divided to free up an adequate length of epididymis. The superior-epididymal branches entering the epididymis at the caput are always preserved and since the epididymis has a dual blood supply, this is adequate blood supply for the entire epididymis.

If the epididymis is indurated and dilated throughout its length, the epididymis is dissected all the way past the vasoepididymal junction. This dissection is often facilitated by first dissecting the convoluted vas to the vasoepididymal junction from below, and then, after encircling the epididymis with a Penrose drain, dissecting the epididymis to the vasoepididymal junction from above. In this way, the entire vasoepididymal junction can be freed up. This will allow preservation of maximal epididymal length in cases of distal obstruction near the vasoepididymal junction. After the epididymis is dissected off of the testis and flipped-up, a two-stitch longitudinal end-to-side intussusception anastomosis can be performed as described previously (Fig. 10.10).

Increasing vasal length can be done with extensive blunt dissection of the vas deferens off the spermatic cord toward the inguinal ring. Dissection can also be carried into the inguinal canal to the internal ring with a finger sweeping motion. In extreme situations, the vas deferens can be rerouted medial to the vessels similar to the Prentiss maneuver employed during difficult orchiopexies [17]. An opening in the floor of the inguinal canal is made and the vas rerouted medially under the floor of the canal and right over the pubis.

It is also possible to perform an orchiopexy positioning the testicle in a horizontal or even upside down configuration to decrease the length needed. One must be careful to make sure the cord has no kinks in it and that the stitches do not damage the blood supply to the testis.

In cases where there is a unilateral atrophic testis or the contralateral testis is missing, it is possible to perform a crossed transseptal vasoepididymostomy. This is even more attractive if there is an ipsilateral hernia repair or where there is a second obstruction in the inguinal or abdominal vas. In this procedure, the contralateral vas

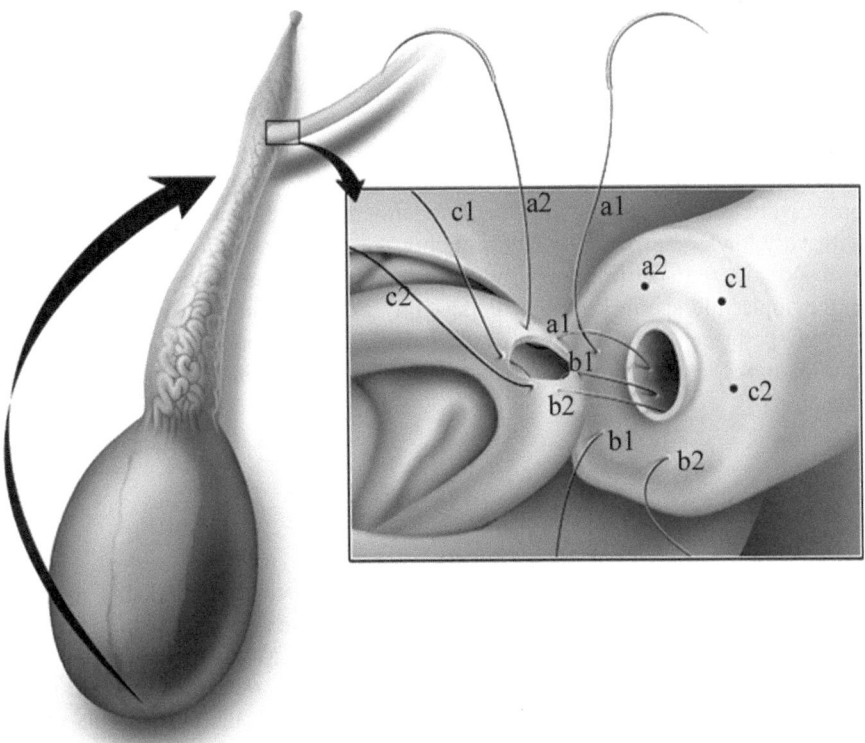

Fig. 10.10 Technique of dissecting the corpus and cauda epididymis to gain further length in cases of short vasal length. This is most helpful when the entire epididymis is dilated (From Goldstein [25], with permission of Elsevier)

is harvested as close to the vasoepididymal junction as possible. If vasal length is still inadequate, then the testicle can be pexed in the contralateral scrotal compartment to facilitate a tension-free anastomosis.

Long-Term Follow-up Evaluation and Results

Microsurgical vasoepididymostomy in the hands of experienced skilled microsurgeon will result in the appearance of sperm in the ejaculate in 50–85% of men. Classic end-to-side or older end-to-end methods result inpatency rates about 70% with a 43% pregnancy rate with a follow-up of 2 years [5, 18]. With intussusception techniques, patency rates are 70–90% with pregnancy rates of 40–45% [6, 14, 19–22]. Regardless of technique, pregnancy rates are higher the more distal the anastomosis is performed [23]. Therefore, one should always strive to make the anastomosis as distal as possible on the epididymis.

Another vexing problem is that of late anastomotic failure. With the older end-to-end or end-to-side methods, at 14 months after surgery 25% of initially patent anastomoses have shut down [12]. With intussusception techniques, the late shut down rates appear to be less than 10%, but long-term follow-up with these techniques have not yet been reported. Nevertheless, we recommend banking sperm both intraoperatively [24] and as soon as motile sperm appear in the ejaculate post-operatively after vasoepididymostomy, regardless of technique employed. In men with very low counts or poor sperm quality postoperatively and men who remain azoospermic, the sperm intraoperatively cryopreserved can be used for IVF with intracytoplasmic sperm injection. Persistently azoospermic men without cryopreserved sperm can opt for either a redo-vasoepididymostomy and/or microscopic epididymal sperm aspiration combined with IVF and intracytoplasmic sperm injection.

Expert Commentary

The modern evolution of vasoepididymostomy has been a remarkable journey. Since Martin's first attempts over 100 years ago, we have continued to make significant strides in the refinement of this surgical technique. Most recently, adoption of microsurgical techniques and intussusception methods of vasoepididymostomy have made this surgery progressively more effective. With the introduction of the two-stitch longitudinal intussusception method, anastomoses have become simpler and easier to teach with a decreasing risk of technical error.

Modern IVF–ICSI has opened up reproductive options for those couples desiring fertility. This has caused some to question the need for advanced reconstructive reproductive tract surgery. However, in the hands of experienced microsurgeons, vasoepididymostomy is a safe, effective method of reconstruction for patients who do not want to undergo IVF or desire multiple children. In addition, vasoepididymostomy skills are crucial to have because of the possibility of finding secondary epididymal obstruction at the time of vasectomy reversal. It is of our opinion that any reproductive surgeon what performs vasal reconstruction must be capable of performing a vasoepididymostomy.

Five-Year View

While vasoepididymostomy is already associated with good outcomes we look forward to the future. Further technical refinements will most likely focus on the simplification of the vasoepididymostomy procedure, decreasing operative times and making the procedure more accessible to more surgeons. These developments will come from microsurgical models and animal models.

On the other hand, refinements in molecular genetics will continue to elucidate the pathophysiology of idiopathic infertility and allow us to identify those patients that will most benefit from advanced surgical reconstruction. The focus of this research must be on translation of these genetic preoperative predictors into treatments that increase postoperative success.

Key Issues

- Good anastomoses relies on healthy tissue and an accurate watertight mucosa to mucosa opposition in a tension-free anastomosis; setup is key.
- Anastomotic techniques include: end-to-end, end-to-side, and end-to-side intussuscepted.
- Vasal length can be increased on the epididymal end or the vasal end or both. If these two maneuvers prove insufficient, orchiopexy should be considered as well as a crossed septal vasoepididymostomy in cases of unilateral testicular atrophy or absence.
- Our preferred anastomosis is the two-suture longitudinal, end-to-side intussuscepted technique.
- We have developed a single-arm version of vasoepididymostomy, which is useful when double-arm sutures are difficult to obtain.
- Vasoepididymostomy is the most challenging of all microsurgery and should only be performed by surgeons with sufficient training and adequate volume of microsurgery.

Acknowledgments Dr. Hsiao is supported by a grant from the Frederick J. and Theresa Dow Wallace Fund of the New York Community Trust.

References

1. Jequier AM. Edward Martin (1859–1938). The founding father of modern clinical andrology. Int J Androl. 1991;14(1):1–10.
2. Martin E, Carnett JB, Levi JV, et al. The surgical treatment of sterility due to obstruction at the epididymis; together with a study of the morphology of human spermatozoa. Univ Pa Med Bull. 1902;15:2.
3. Martin E. The operation of epididymo-vasostomy for the relief of sterility. Ther Gaz. 1909;1–19.
4. Silber SJ. Microscopic vasoepididymostomy: specific microanastomosis to the epididymal tubule. Fertil Steril. 1978;30(5):565–71.
5. Schlegel PN, Goldstein M. Microsurgical vasoepididymostomy: refinements and results. J Urol. 1993;150(4):1165–8.
6. Chan PT, Brandell RA, Goldstein M. Prospective analysis of outcomes after microsurgical intussusception vasoepididymostomy. BJU Int. 2005;96(4):598–601.

7. Lee R, Goldstein M, Ullery BW, Ehrlich J, Soares M, Razzano RA, et al. Value of serum antisperm antibodies in diagnosing obstructive azoospermia. J Urol. 2009;181(1):264–9.

8. Wagenknecht LV, Klosterhalfen H, Schirren C. Microsurgery in andrologic urology. I. Refertilization. J Microsurg. 1980;1(5):370–6.

9. Krylov VS, Borovikov AM. Microsurgical method of reuniting ductus epididymis. Fertil Steril. 1984;41(3):418–23.

10. Fogdestam I, Fall M, Nilsson S. Microsurgical epididymovasostomy in the treatment of occlusive azoospermia. Fertil Steril. 1986;46(5):925–9.

11. Thomas Jr AJ. Vasoepididymostomy. Urol Clin North Am. 1987;14(3):527–38.

12. Matthews GJ, Schlegel PN, Goldstein M. Patency following microsurgical vasoepididymostomy and vasovasostomy: temporal considerations. J Urol. 1995;154(6):2070–3.

13. Sheynkin YR, Starr C, Li PS, Goldstein M. Effect of methylene blue, indigo carmine, and Renografin on human sperm motility. Urology. 1999;53(1):214–7.

14. Berger RE. Triangulation end-to-side vasoepididymostomy. J Urol. 1998;159(6):1951–3.

15. Goldstein M, Li PS, Matthews GJ. Microsurgical vasovasostomy: the microdot technique of precision suture placement. J Urol. 1998;159(1):188–90.

16. Monoski MA, Schiff J, Li PS, Chan PT, Goldstein M. Innovative single-armed suture technique for microsurgical vasoepididymostomy. Urology. 2007;69(4):800–4.

17. Prentiss RJ, Weickgenant CJ, Moses JJ, Frazier DB. Surgical repair of undescended testicle. Calif Med. 1962;96:401–5.

18. Pasqualotto FF, Agarwal A, Srivastava M, Nelson DR, Thomas Jr AJ. Fertility outcome after repeat vasoepididymostomy. J Urol. 1999;162(5):1626–8.

19. Kolettis PN, Thomas Jr AJ. Vasoepididymostomy for vasectomy reversal: a critical assessment in the era of intracytoplasmic sperm injection. J Urol. 1997;158(2):467–70.

20. Schiff J, Chan P, Li PS, Finkelberg S, Goldstein M. Outcome and late failures compared in 4 techniques of microsurgical vasoepididymostomy in 153 consecutive men. J Urol. 2005;174(2):651–5. quiz 801.

21. Marmar JL. Modified vasoepididymostomy with simultaneous double needle placement, tubulotomy and tubular invagination. J Urol. 2000;163(2):483–6.

22. Brandell AR, Goldstein M. Reconstruction of the male reproductive tract using the microsurgical triangulation technique for vasoepididymostomy. J Urol. 1999;161(Suppl):350.

23. Silber SJ. Role of epididymis in sperm maturation. Urology. 1989;33(1):47–51.

24. Matthews GJ, Goldstein M. A simplified method of epididymal sperm aspiration. Urology. 1996;47(1):123–5.

25. Goldstein M. Surgical management of male infertility. In: Wein AJ, editor. Campbell-Walsh urology, 9th ed. St. Louis: WB Saunders; 2006.

Chapter 11
Grafting Techniques for Vasectomy Reversal

Henry M. Rosevear and Moshe Wald

Surgical reconstruction of the vas deferens is performed to remove an obstructive lesion that is present along its course. Obstruction can exist at various parts of the vas deferens and can be the result of a prior vasectomy, congenital anomaly, inflammation secondary to a urogenital tract infection, trauma, or a surgical misadventure during prior inguinal, pelvic, or scrotal surgery. While no official reporting system exists in the United States to monitor the number of vasectomies performed each year, a survey in 2002 estimated this to be 526,501, which is approximately consistent with data reported in 1991 and 1995 [1, 2]. An estimated 2–6% of all men, and up to 11% of men aged 20–24 at the time of vasectomy, request a vasectomy reversal [3]. It has been estimated that between 30,000 and 80,000 vasectomy reversals are performed annually in the USA, though as with vasectomies, reporting requirements are not standardized so the exact number is unknown [4].

Congenital anomalies which can lead to obstruction of the vas deferens include congenital absence of the vas deferens, which is commonly associated with cystic fibrosis [5]. Partial vasal agenesis and congenital prostatic cysts can also lead to obstruction of the vas deferens [6, 7]. One example of a genetic disorder which can lead to obstructive azoospermia is Young's syndrome, which is characterized by chronic sinusitis and bronchiectasis as well as obstructive azoospermia [8]. In Young's syndrome, the obstruction usually occurs at the junction of the caput to corpus epididymis due to inspissated secretions. Inflammatory causes of obstruction are rare in the antibiotic era but include tuberculous epididymitis, gonorrheal urethritis progressing to obstructive epididymitis, and chlamydial epididymitis [9].

The success of a vasectomy reversal depends on several factors, only some of which can be controlled at the time of surgery. Factors which are independent of the method of reversal but which may influence subsequent conception include age and fertility

H.M. Rosevear, MD (✉) • M. Wald, MD
Department of Urology, University of Iowa, 200 Hawkins Drive, 3RCP,
Iowa City, IA 52242-1089, USA
e-mail: henry-rosevear@uiowa.edu; moshe-wald@uiowa.edu

S.J. Parekattil, A. Agarwal (eds.), *Male Infertility for the Clinician*,
© Springer Science+Business Media New York 2013

potential of the patient's partner, length of obstructive interval, presence of antisperm antibodies, and high intravasal and epididymal pressure after the original obstruction [10–13]. Some factors which influence the success of the reversal are directly related to the technique chosen and include rate of stricture or scar development and granuloma formation [14]. The most commonly cited reason for these specific complications is an anastomosis made under tension, devascularization of the wall of the vas deferens, or a technical problem with the anastomosis leading to sperm leakage [15].

The current gold standard to surgically correct an obstructed vas deferens is a microscope-assisted two-layered vasovasostomy, but this has not always been so [16, 17]. Given the complex and time-consuming nature of this operation, new surgical techniques including robotics, modifications, and tools are continuously being explored. Some of these techniques include the use of fibrin glue, laser soldering, absorbable and nonabsorbable stents, and artificial conduits with or without specific growth factors added [18]. This chapter highlights the development of surgical grafting techniques for vasectomy reversal, including the use of stents and grafts, as well as the current clinical application of these devices and areas where further research is required.

Grafting Techniques in Reconstruction of the Male Reproductive Tract

Stents

As previously stated, several factors related to the success of a vasectomy reversal can be controlled at the time of surgery. From the 1950s to the mid-1970s, macrosurgical techniques for vasovasostomy were common and accepted as the gold standard. This technique allowed a primary anastomosis of the vas deferens to be created but was plagued with, by today's standards, low patency and pregnancy rates. According to a survey of American Urological Association (AUA) members published in 1973, members at that time practicing vasovasostomy reported a 38 % patency rate and a 19.5% pregnancy rate [19]. It should be remembered that the microsurgical techniques which are common today were not developed until the mid-1970s, and, as such, stricture resulting in either partial or complete vasal obstruction was the most pressing technical complication of that period. To address this common complication, approximately 90 % of urologists performing vasovasostomies at that time employed stents, with either silver wire or nylon suture being the most commonly reported [19]. The reason for the widespread use of stents can also be found in the 1973 AUA survey. Members reported that the pregnancy rate for non-stented reversals was significantly lower, at 10.9 % compared to 19.9–26 % for stented procedures, depending on the stent used. Numerous techniques had been developed by 1973 which maximized both patency and pregnancy rates. The main variation between these techniques was the use of loupes for magnification and/or the use of stent [20].

In the lexicon of the modern urologist, a stent most commonly refers to the hollow silicon tube that is used in the ureter for treatment of either intrinsic or extrinsic ureteral obstruction. A vasovasostomy stent, as it was originally used, was quite different. A stent in that sense was any foreign body, usually a piece of suture, the purpose of which was to maintain patency of the lumen of the vas deferens during and immediately after a macrosurgical (either with or without the supplemental use of loupes) primary anastomosis of the vas deferens. The simple goal of the stent was to prevent obstruction at the anastomosis site either because of a poorly placed suture at the time of surgery or as prevention of stricture or scar formation in the immediate postoperative period. In one example of this technique, a short section of 2-0 nylon suture is used as a stent to bridge the anastomosis while 6-0 Prolene is used to actually complete the anastomosis [21]. In this technique, the nylon suture is removed before the operation is completed, and its purpose is to ensure that the vas deferens lumen remains patent during the procedure. In another variation on this theme, described by Dorsey, a zero monofilament suture is fed through a hollow needle introduced approximately 1 cm proximal to the site of the intended anastomosis [22]. This suture is then fed into the distal vas deferens. The anastomosis is then completed using 6-0 Ethiflex, and the proximal end of the stenting suture is brought through the scrotal skin and removed in 12–14 days. The goal of this stent in this technique is to ensure patency of the anastomotic site both during the procedure and in the immediate postoperative healing period. The success rates of these procedures were reported to be over 80% patency, which contrasts with the success rates reported in the 1973 AUA survey.

Even with the improvement in both patency and pregnancy rates reported by clinicians using stents during vasovasostomy, there were numerous known disadvantages of stents, especially with the use of exteriorized stents such as described by Dorsey [20]. The point of exit for the stent is a theoretical source of infection as well as a location where sperm can leave the lumen of the vas [20, 23]. Additionally, the location where the exteriorized stent left the lumen of the vas was identified in a publication by Fernandes as a common site of subsequent luminal obstruction (often instead of the primary anastomosis itself) [24]. To avoid the problem of an exteriorized stent, some groups have experimented with absorbable intravasal suture as a stent to bridge the anastomosis—the theoretical advantage being that these stents would slowly dissolve, maintaining the patency of the anastomosis both during the procedure itself and the postoperative healing period without need to be removed. In one experiment in a canine model, Montie et al. compared three groups: no stent, a Dexon intravasal stent, and a chromic intravasal stent [23]. Three to six months after the vasectomy reversal procedure, retrograde vasography was used to identify patency rates. Both absorbable stent groups had higher patency rates than the control (no stent) group, with the chromic group having the highest overall patency at 70 % vs. 60 % for the Dexon group and 50 % for the no stent group. This concept was tested in a human clinical model by Rowland and colleagues a few years later, who found that intravasal absorbable stents (using 3-0 chromic) had higher patency rates than a group using exteriorized silkworm gut stents (86 % vs. 67 %, respectively) [25].

In 1975, Silber reported the first use of microsurgical vasovasostomy in humans [26]. His work, along with independent work by Owen, led the way to the modern

Fig. 11.1 Hollow
polyglycolic acid stent
(0.5-mm outer diameter)
shown on a dime. (Used with
permission from Flam et al.
[30], with permission)

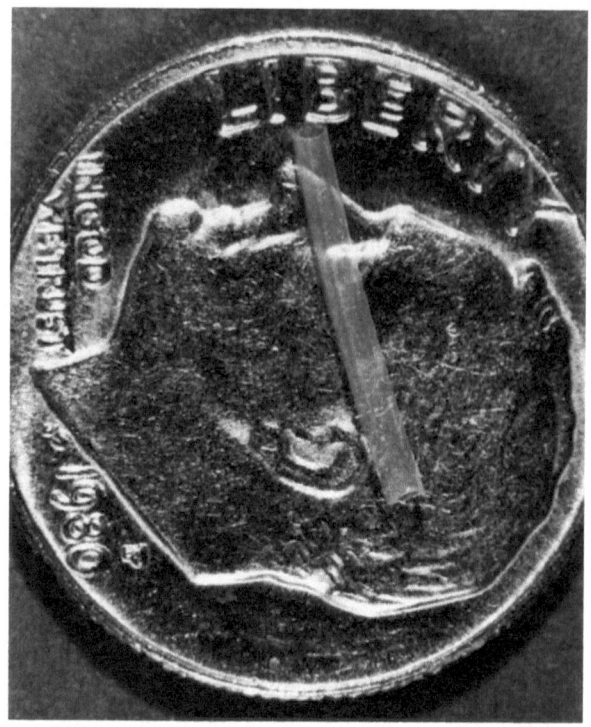

microsurgical two-layered anastomosis [26, 27]. From a historical standpoint, it should be noted that it was Silber and his group who found through histologic and electron microscopic work that stricture was more common than originally thought with macrosurgical anastomosis techniques [28]. Silber also popularized the two-layered closure based on his observation that this technique provided a better watertight mucosal approximation given the common discrepancies between proximal and distal luminal diameters of the vas deferens [29]. The techniques developed by these investigators have allowed the microsurgical two-layered vasovasostomy anastomosis to become the gold standard for vasectomy reversal, with success rates dependent on time since obstruction. These success rates may be as high as 97% patency and 76% pregnancy when the obstructive interval is less than 3 years, and 71% patency and 30% pregnancy after 15 years of obstruction [13].

The reproducible success of this new technique resulted in a dearth of research into alternative techniques for many years. Even with its success, Silber's microsurgical technique was not perfect. The downside was that microsurgical anastomosis was a time-consuming operation best done by surgeons with specialized training using expensive operating microscopes. This prompted research into new techniques that would simplify the technique while maintaining the high patency and pregnancy rates. In 1989, Flam et al. reported work in a rat model on a hollow, absorbable polyglycolic acid tube [30]. In their experiment, they inserted a 10-mm long by 0.5-mm outer diameter hollow stent into the lumen of the vas at the site of anastomosis on one side and completed the anastomosis with a single layer of suture (Fig. 11.1). On

Fig. 11.2 Absorbable
self-retaining polyglycolic
acid stent

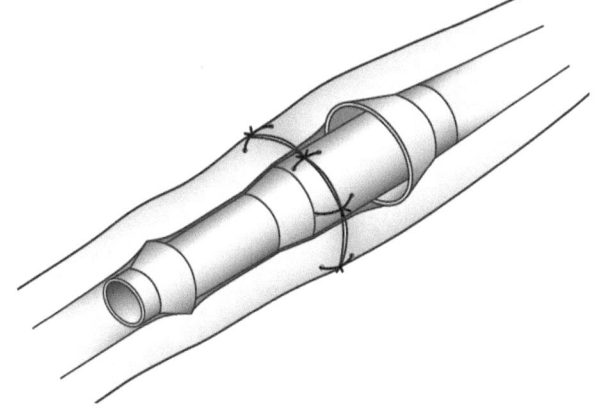

the contralateral side, they performed standard microsurgical anastomosis. They showed a trend toward improved patency in the stented vas deferens. Flam emphasized in his paper that sperm leakage at the site of the anastomosis could lead to secondary stricture and should be avoided. This work led to a clinical trial using absorbable intravasal stents conducted by Rothman and colleagues in 1996 [31]. This randomized study compared conventional two-layered microsurgical anastomosis to a modified approach using an absorbable polyglycolic acid stent without intraluminal sutures (Fig. 11.2). While the operative time was significantly reduced in the stented group (118 min vs. 137 min), both the patency and the pregnancy rates were lower in the stented groups (81% vs. 89% and 22% vs. 51%, respectively), and the authors concluded that intravasal stents should not be used.

More recently, Vrijhof et al. reported on a nonabsorbable stent in a rabbit model [14]. They theorized that the absorbable nature of the previously reported stents allowed strictures to develop at the site of the anastomosis once the stent had dissolved and that a nonreactive nonabsorbable stent would bypass this problem while simplifying the operation. Their stent was made of a biocompatible material designed to have both hydrophilic and hydrophobic characteristics. The stent also had a transverse ridge which was designed to minimize migration from the anastomotic site (Fig. 11.3). This group reported that all vasa were patent at the end of their study (39–47 weeks) and that total sperm count was higher in the stented group. No human data is available on this type of stent.

In the era of cost-conscious medicine, especially when many patients must pay out of pocket for vasectomy reversals, further research into efforts that simplify the present gold standard is appropriate with the caveat that patency and pregnancy rates should not be compromised. It is important to note that all of the absorbable and nonabsorbable stents which have been used to date in human studies have been well tolerated with no side effects and little to no inflammatory response.

In summary, stents were investigated as a method to improve patency rates in the era of macrosurgical vasovasostomy but were eclipsed by the application of the operating microscope to the field and the introduction of microsurgical two-layered vasovasostomy. Efforts to improve and simplify the microsurgical operation using

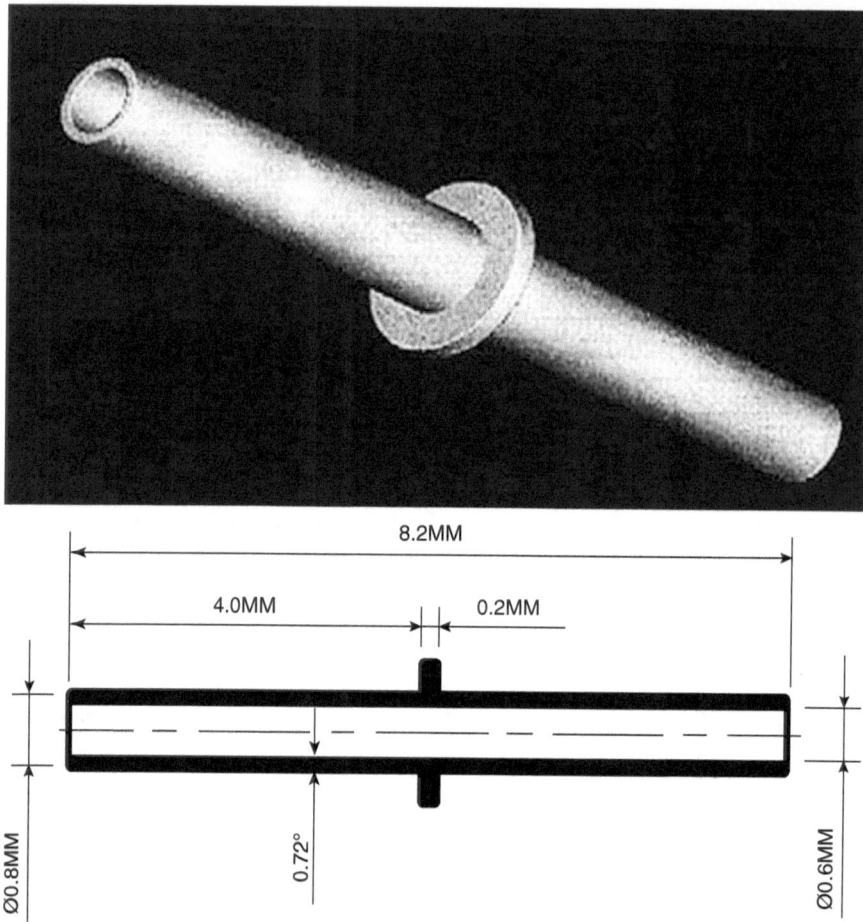

Fig. 11.3 Nonabsorbable polymeric stent with transverse ridge to minimize migration (From Vrijhof et al. [14], with permission)

absorbable stents have not improved overall patency or pregnancy rates. Recent efforts using nonabsorbable stents show promise in animal models but have not been tested in humans so their utility remains unproven. The ideal stent would, at a minimum, maintain the patency and pregnancy rates achieved through a conventional two-layer microsurgical anastomosis while decreasing the operative time, training, and cost required to achieve these results.

Conduits

The preferred method to bypass an obstructed portion of the vas deferens, regardless of the etiology of the obstruction, is surgical excision or exclusion of the obstructed segment and reanastomosis of the vas deferens using a microsurgical two-layered anastomosis. The goal of the operation is a watertight, tension-free, widely patent anastomosis. As described previously, numerous techniques have been suggested in an attempt to simplify this procedure while preserving its patency and pregnancy rates. The assumption in all of the previously described techniques is that the vas deferens could be sufficiently mobilized to allow a tension-free anastomosis. Unfortunately, cases exist where, due to the physical length of the obstruction, the vas deferens cannot be reconstructed in a watertight, tension-free manner. These cases present a clinical challenge because the resulting obstructive azoospermia is theoretically amenable to surgical correction. Presently, the only reproductive option available for these patients is surgical sperm retrieval. The technique of retrieving sperm from either the testicle or epididymis has been successfully reported in cases of obstructive azoospermia that is not surgically correctable but must be coupled with in vitro fertilization [32]. The hormonal manipulation, surgical interventions, risk of multiple gestations, and increased financial cost of in vitro fertilization make this solution less than ideal and creates an intriguing field of research into reconstruction of the male reproductive tract.

Grafting of the male reproductive tract theoretically can take one of three forms. The first option is to use transplanted vas deferens with all of the complications, both technical and immunological, associated with such a procedure. The second option is to replace the obstructed segment of vas deferens with a tubular structure, the sole purpose of which is to simply allow passage of sperm in a distal direction. An analogous clinical problem can be found in vascular surgery where surgeons often replace diseased segments of vessels with either endogenous grafts such as the long saphenous vein or exogenous grafts such as a Teflon-coated endovascular stent. The third option involves tissue engineering. Tissue engineering as it applies to reconstruction of the male reproductive system involves the concept of creating an artificial conduit which serves as a scaffolding for the regrowth of the vas deferens itself. In a different biological system, polymer scaffoldings have been shown to facilitate peripheral nerve regeneration in segments as long as 1 cm [33]. Regardless of the method chosen to graft over the obstructed segment of vas deferens, the goal is to reestablish continuity of the male reproductive tract, allowing sperm to be present in the ejaculate and eliminating the need for assisted reproductive techniques (ART). It should be noted that even small amounts of ejaculated sperm could be a significant improvement, as this may allow for less invasive forms of ART [34].

The first reported experiment on the use of grafts in reconstruction of the male reproductive tract was by Romero-Maroto and colleagues in 1989 [35]. This group reported successfully autotransplanting a pediculated segment of vas deferens from one side to the contralateral in rabbits. They reported good patency rates, but no data on pregnancies was noted. The clinical use of this technique is likely limited, as these subjects would likely be candidates for crossover vasovasostomies, a rare procedure with a high reported success rate [36], and given the questionable feasibility of harvesting a long vasal segment for reconstruction of the contralateral side.

Regarding the second option for grafting the male reproductive tract, Carringer et al. in 1995 reported patency rates in rats after either a vasal or vascular graft obtained from either the contralateral side of the same animal or from female rats,

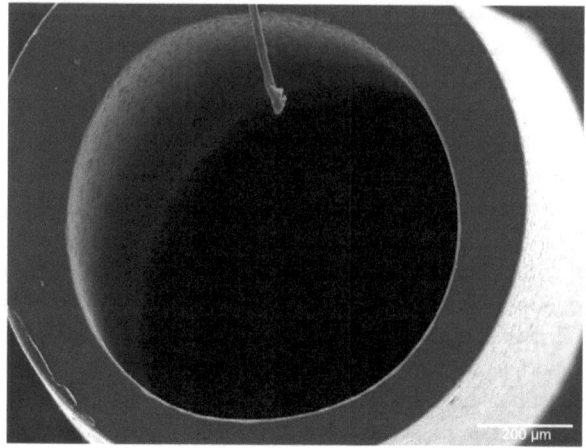

Fig. 11.4 Scanning electron microscope image of PDLA conduit. Bar = 200 μm (From Simons et al. [42], with permission)

respectively [37]. In this study, three different lengths of grafts were used (0.5, 1.0, and 1.5 cm), corresponding to approximately 10, 20, and 30% of the entire vas deferens length. Patency was confirmed by direct examination of the graft 4 weeks postoperatively. The authors found an overall patency rate of approximately 40% in both surgical groups (vasal and vascular graft) with higher rates in the shorter segments. Pregnancy rates were not evaluated. No human clinical trials have been reported using either of these techniques. Questions on long-term patency of extensive artificial grafts remain unanswered, even in animal models, and should be further investigated.

The lack of a suitable allograft in humans for vasal reconstruction has led to research on the potential for biocompatible degradable polymer scaffolding for tissue engineering. As mentioned earlier, this model has been successfully applied to the clinical problem of peripheral nerve regeneration [33]. Additions to this technology, including micro-patterned (grooved) inner lumens as well as target-specific growth factors, can increase the efficacy of this technology [38, 39]. The vas deferens is a good target for investigation because it has been shown to undergo spontaneous recanalization at the site of vasectomy [40].

Further evidence that may support tissue engineering of the vas deferens is the demonstration of elevated levels of selected growth factors at the vasectomy site in an animal model. Previous examination of vasectomy sites in rats using real-time polymerase chain reaction, enzyme-linked immunosorbent assay, and histopathological analysis demonstrated a 12-fold increase in platelet-derived growth factor beta and a ninefold increase in transforming growth factor beta [41].

Using the peripheral nerve regeneration model as a guide, biodegradable conduits made of D,L-lactide were studied for reconstruction of the reproductive tract in a rat model [42]. Biodegradable conduits with micro-patterned grooves on the inner surface were implanted in 47 rats following vasectomy (Fig. 11.4, scanning electron microscopy image). At 8 weeks postimplantation of the conduits, no evidence of recanalization was found. However, at 12 weeks, evidence of recanalization was

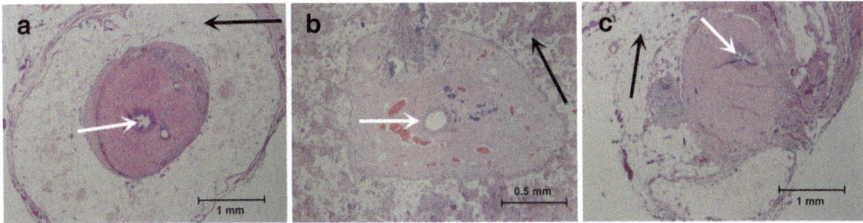

Fig. 11.5 (**a**) Evidence of microrecanalization at the midpoint of a 0.5-cm poly-(D,L-lactide) (PDLA) graft (magnification ×40). Bar = 1 mm. (**b**) Microcanal at the midpoint of a 0.5-cm PDLA graft (magnification ×200) Bar = 0.5 mm. (**c**) Microcanal at the interface zone of a 0.5-cm PDLA graft (magnification ×40). Bar = 1 mm. *All panels*: *white arrows* microcanals, *black arrows* graft (From Simons et al. [42], with permission)

noted in three of the remaining rats, with one showing a microcanal spanning the entire 0.5-cm conduit and the other two showing distinct epithelialized vas deferens microcanals at the conduit edges (Fig. 11.5) [42].

Following the demonstration of microrecanalization of the vas deferens in this biodegradable graft model, attempts were made to identify ways to maximize this response (unpublished data). Based on the identification of elevated growth factor levels at the site of vasectomy, the effect of local microparticle-delivered growth factors on the rate of vasal recanalization in a biodegradable conduit model was examined. Delivering growth factors to a specific location in the body over a sustained period of time is not a simple task. Effective supplementation of growth factors selectively at the site of the grafted vas deferens may be compromised by the fact that the ability of growth factors to perform their function depends on their tertiary structure, which is susceptible to degradation if it is not protected from the local environment. Thus, delivery of a locally sustained concentration of growth factors requires the use of microspheres. The goal of a microsphere is to sequester the biologically active molecule and allow a controlled, sustained release of the molecule. The exact timing of the sustained release is a function of the characteristics of the microsphere into which it is placed. With these considerations in mind, a poly-(D,L-lactide) material was chosen for construction of the microspheres. As the biodegradable conduits used in this study were constructed of the identical material, noncovalent binding was assumed to keep the microspheres near the conduit. Reconstruction of surgically induced vasal gaps using biodegradable conduits soaked in microspheres containing TGF-beta and PDGF revealed an increase in the number of new microcanals in the graft but not in their length at 12 weeks postoperatively.

In an effort to further optimize the conditions for vasal recanalization, methods to increase the vascularity of the reconstructed vas deferens were investigated, based on an observation suggesting that neovascularization increased with time at the conduit to vasal border (unpublished data). To bolster this neovascularization and potentially increase the rate of recanalization, the effect of oral sildenafil citrate on recanalization in the biodegradable graft model was examined. Sildenafil citrate is a type-5 phosphodiesterase inhibitor that has been shown to promote neovascularization in other systems [43]. Rats received a daily dose of 5 mg/kg of oral sildenafil citrate following reconstruction of the vas deferens with a biodegradable graft. At 16 weeks, the rats on sildenafil citrate had a significantly increased number of microcanals (29 vs. 4) though the average length of the canals was constant at 2 mm. This observation was confirmed by an increase in staining for CD31, an endothelial marker. An ongoing study involves combining both oral sildenafil citrate with increasing the local concentration of TGF-beta and platelet-derived growth factors via microspheres. Areas of future research into this field include examining different substrates of which the conduit itself is composed and embedding the growth factors directly into the conduit to maximize local concentration.

Expert Commentary

Grafting of the male reproductive tract is an exciting new area of tissue engineering which may allow natural conception for patients with significant lengths of obstructed vas deferens. While stents had a significant and important role in increasing patency and pregnancy rates in the pre-microsurgical era, their role in the modern era of microsurgical two-layered anastomosis remains to be defined. To date, if the vasal obstruction is amenable to a primary watertight, tension-free anastomosis, microsurgical non-stented techniques remain the gold standard. Cases where a tension-free anastomosis is not possible because of the physical length of the obstruction remain problematic, but further research into tissue engineering in the form of implantable conduits holds much promise.

Five-Year View

The potential role of implantable conduits in reconstruction of the male reproductive tract remains to be fully investigated. Currently, biodegradable conduits have been shown limited success in guiding regrowth of vasal tissue elements along the entire length of a 5-mm long segment though further research into supplementing naturally occurring growth factors in the hopes of maximizing regrowth is ongoing. As the obstructed segment of vas deferens that is bridged by bioengineered conduits lengthens, the barriers to success mount. One such barrier is that oxygen and other nutrients necessary for cell survival can diffuse approximately 2–3 mm with the need for angiogenesis. The 5-mm segment under current investigation approaches the length that could be bridged without angiogenesis. The use of sildenafil citrate to increase angiogenesis is one possible approach to minimize this problem. Other specific research problems that need to be addressed include maximizing local delivery of growth factors. While current research employs nanoparticles, another possibility is the impregnation of the conduit itself with growth factors. The specific design and engineering issues that this approach raises are under investigation.

Key Issues

- Microsurgical two-layered anastomosis to correct vasal obstruction remains the gold standard.
- The role of vasal stenting in the era of microsurgical two-layered anastomosis is limited.
- Biodegradable conduits to bridge segments of obstructed vas deferens where a primary microsurgical two-layered anastomosis is impossible remain investigational but hold significant long-term promise.

Acknowledgment We would like to thank Kris Greiner for her editorial assistance in preparing this chapter.

References

1. Barone MA, Hutchinson PL, Johnson CH, et al. Vasectomy in the United States, 2002. J Urol. 2006;176:232–6.
2. Magnani RJ, Haws JM, Morgan GT, et al. Vasectomy in the United States, 1991 and 1995. Am J Public Health. 1999;89:92–4.
3. Holman CD, Wisniewski ZS, Semmens JB, et al. Population-based outcomes after 28,246 in-hospital vasectomies and 1,902 vasovasostomies in Western Australia. BJU Int. 2000;86:1043–9.
4. Schiff J, Li PS, Goldstein M. Toward a sutureless vasovasostomy: use of biomaterials and surgical sealants in a rodent vasovasostomy model. J Urol. 2004;172:1192–5.
5. Castaldo G, Tomaiuolo R, Vanacore B, et al. Phenotypic discordance in three siblings affected by atypical cystic fibrosis with the F508del/D614G genotype. J Cyst Fibros. 2006;5:193–5.
6. Stricker H, Kunin J, Faerber G. Congenital prostatic cyst causing ejaculatory duct obstruction: management by transrectal cyst aspiration. J Urol. 1993;149:1141–3.
7. Engin G, Kadioglu A, Orhan I, et al. Transrectal US and endorectal MR imaging in partial and complete obstruction of the seminal duct system. A comparative study. Acta Radiol. 2000;41: 288–95.
8. Handelsman DJ, Conway AJ, Boylan LM, et al. Young's syndrome. Obstructive azoospermia and chronic sinopulmonary infections. N Engl J Med. 1984;310(1):3–9.
9. Thomas AH, Sabanegh Jr ES. Microsurgical treatment of male infertility. In: Lipshultz LI, Howards SS, Niederberger CS, editors. Infertility in the Male. 4th ed. New York: Cambridge University; 2009. p. 392–406. A very well written summary of current microsurgical surgical techniques.
10. Kolettis PN, Woo L, Sandlow JI. Outcomes of vasectomy reversal performed for men with the same female partners. Urology. 2003;61:1221–3.
11. Silber SJ. Microscopic vasectomy reversal. Fertil Steril. 1977;28:1191–202.
12. Vrijhof HJ, Delaere KP. Vasovasostomy results in 66 patients related to obstructive intervals and serum agglutinin titres. Urol Int. 1994;53:143–6.
13. Belker AM, Thomas Jr AJ, Fuchs EF, et al. "Results of 1,469 microsurgical vasectomy reversals by the Vasovasostomy Study Group. J Urol. 1991;145:505–11.
14. Vrijhof EJ, de Bruine A, Zwinderman A, et al. New nonabsorbable stent versus a microsurgical procedure for vasectomy reversal: evaluating tissue reactions at the anastomosis in rabbits. Fertil Steril. 2005;84:743–8.
15. Carbone Jr DJ, Shah A, Thomas Jr AJ, et al. Partial obstruction, not antisperm antibodies, causing infertility after vasovasostomy. J Urol. 1998;159:827–30.
16. Practice Committee of the American Society for Reproductive Medicine. Vasectomy reversal. Fertil Steril. 2008;90:S78–82.

17. Lipshultz LI, Rumohr JA, Bennett RC. Techniques for vasectomy reversal. Urol Clin North Am. 2009;36:375–82. The most recent definitive treatise on surgical techniques.
18. Kolettis PN. Restructuring reconstructive techniques—advances in reconstructive techniques. Urol Clin North Am. 2008;35:229–34.
19. Derrick Jr FC, Yarbrough W, D'Agostino J. Vasovasostomy: results of questionnaire of members of the American Urological Association. J Urol. 1973;110:556–7.
20. Kim HH, Goldstein M. History of vasectomy reversal. Urol Clin North Am. 2009;36:359–73. A concise and fascinating summary of the history of the vasectomy reversal.
21. Amelar RD, Dubin L. Vasectomy reversal. J Urol. 1979;121:547–50.
22. Dorsey JW. Surgical correction of post-vasectomy sterility. J Urol. 1973;110:554–5.
23. Montie JE, Stewart BH, Levin HS. Intravasal stents for vasovasostomy in canine subjects. Fertil Steril. 1973;24:877–83.
24. Fernandes M, Shah KN, Draper JW. Vasovasostomy: improved microsurgical technique. J Urol. 1968;100:763–6.
25. Rowland R, Nanninga JB, O'Connor VJ. Improved results in vasovasostomies using internal plain catgut stents. Urology. 1977;10:260–2.
26. Silber SJ. Microsurgery in clinical urology. Urology. 1975;6:150–3.
27. Owen ER. Microsurgical vasovasostomy: a reliable vasectomy reversal. Aust N Z J Surg. 1977;47:305–9.
28. Silber SJ, Galle J, Friend D. Microscopic vasovasostomy and spermatogenesis. J Urol. 1977;117:299–302.
29. Silber SJ. Vasectomy and vasectomy reversal. Fertil Steril. 1978;29:125–40.
30. Flam TA, Roth RA, Silverman ML, et al. Experimental study of hollow, absorbable polyglycolic acid tube as stent for vasovasostomy. Urology. 1989;33:490–4.
31. Rothman I, Berger RE, Cummings P, et al. Randomized clinical trial of an absorbable stent for vasectomy reversal. J Urol. 1997;157:1697–700.
32. Nudell DM, Conaghan J, Pedersen RA, et al. The mini-micro-epididymal sperm aspiration for sperm retrieval: a study of urological outcomes. Hum Reprod. 1998;13:1260–5.
33. Miller C, Shanks H, Witt A, et al. Oriented Schwann cell growth on micropatterned biodegradable polymer substrates. Biomaterials. 2001;22:1263–9.
34. Kamischke A, Nieschlag E. Analysis of medical treatment of male infertility. Hum Reprod. 1999;14 Suppl 1:1–23.
35. Romero-Maroto J, Escribano G, Egea L, et al. Transplant of a pediculate segment of vas deferens. Experimental study. Eur Urol. 1989;16:133–7.
36. Gilis J, Borovikov AM. Treatment of vas deferens large defects. Int Urol Nephrol. 1989;21:627–34.
37. Carringer M, Pedersen J, Schnurer LB. Experimental vas replacement by either vas or a vascular graft. Scan J Urol Neprhol. 1995;29:97–102.
38. Rutkowski GE, Miller CA, Jeftinija S, et al. Synergistic effects of micropatterned biodegradable conduits and Schwann cells on sciatic nerve regeneration. J Neural Eng. 2004;1:151–7.
39. Miller C, Jeftinija S, Mallapragada S. Synergistic effects of physical and chemical guidance cues on neurite alignment and outgrowth on biodegradable polymer substrates. Tissue Eng. 2002;8:367–78.
40. Labrecque M, Hays M, Chen-Mok M, et al. Frequency and patterns of early recanalization after vasectomy. BMC Urol. 2006;6:25.
41. Stahl BC, Ratliff TL, De Young BR, et al. Involvement of growth factors in the process of post-vasectomy micro-recanalization. J Urol. 2008;179:376–80.
42. Simons CM, De Young BR, Griffith TS, et al. Early microrecanalization of vas deferens following biodegradable graft implantation in bilaterally vasectomized rats. Asian J Urol. 2009;11:373–8.
43. Koneru S, Varma Penumathsa S, Thirunavukkarasu M, et al. Sildenafil-mediated neovascularization and protection against myocardial ischaemia reperfusion injury in rats: role of VEGF/angiopoietin-1. J Cell Mol Med. 2008;12:2651–64.

Chapter 12
Mini-Incision Vasectomy Reversal Using the No-Scalpel Vasectomy Instruments and Principles

Darby J. Cassidy, Keith Jarvi, Ethan D. Grober, and Kirk C. Lo

A wide variety of techniques have been described in the literature for vasectomy reversal, and as with most techniques, they continue to evolve in current surgical practice. We have developed a mini-incision technique at the University of Toronto for vasectomy reversal using the principles and instruments used for the no-scalpel vasectomy.

History

Like most surgical procedures, vasectomy reversal techniques are in constant evolution. The genesis of the techniques used for vasectomy reversal dates back to the work of Dr. Edward Martin at the University of Pennsylvania in the early 1900s. In 1902 Martin performed the first documented vasoepididymostomy for a man with obstructive azoospermia secondary to gonorrhea [1]. In 1909 he published a series of 11 azoospermic men who underwent vasoepididymostomies with a patency rate of 64% and pregnancy rate of 27%. Martin's publication and the demonstrated effectiveness of his vasoepididymostomy technique served to dispel the earlier and widely held belief that such anastomoses were hardly worth pursuing given their technical challenges and expected low success rates. Francis Hagner subsequently reproduced Martin's outcomes in his series of 33 patients with reported patency and pregnancy rates of 64 and 48% respectively, solidifying its role as an effective technique in the management of obstructive azoospermia [1].

D.J. Cassidy, MD (✉)
Department of Urology, University Hospital of Northern British Columbia,
Prince George, BC, Canada

K. Jarvi, MD • E.D. Grober • K.C. Lo, MD, CM
Division of Urology, Department of Surgery,
University of Toronto, Mount Sinai Hospital, Toronto, ON, Canada
e-mail: kjarvi@mtsinai.on.ca; klo@mtsinai.on.ca

S.J. Parekattil, A. Agarwal (eds.), *Male Infertility for the Clinician*,
© Springer Science+Business Media New York 2013

Quinby reported the first successful vasovasostomy in 1919 on a man who underwent vasectomy 8 years earlier [1]. O'Connor, Quinby's former assistant, subsequently published a series of 14 vasectomy reversals using Quinby's technique in 14 men with an overall patency rate of 64%, once again demonstrating vasovasostomy as an effective technique for vasectomy reversal [1].

As the interest in family planning and the role of women in the workplace evolved over the ensuing decades, the rates of vasectomy increased substantially as did the inevitable demand for vasectomy reversal that followed.

Vasectomy remains the most commonly performed urologic procedure in North America, with over 500,000 vasectomies performed annually in the United States alone [1–3]. In 1974, the no-scalpel vasectomy was introduced and provided surgeons with a technique that minimized discomfort and postprocedural morbidity without compromising patient outcomes [4–6]. Between 2 and 11% of vasectomized men will ultimately request a reversal of their vasectomy for a variety of reasons such as a new partner or death of a child [3]. As a result, vasectomy reversal is a very commonly requested procedure for the urologist, and the demand continues to grow.

Vasectomy Reversal Techniques

The original descriptions for vasectomy reversal were macrosurgical techniques with or without the use of loupe magnification. The early techniques used in the 1900s used thin silver wire for the vasal anastomosis, which ultimately evolved into the use of nonabsorbable 4-0 to 6-0 sutures during the 1970s [2]. The reported patency rates for these techniques ranged from 79 to 88% with pregnancy rates of 34–50%. These techniques were largely abandoned when the operating microscope became widely available in most centers.

Silber and Owen are both credited with the first description of a microsurgical vasovasostomy in humans in 1977, although several authors had previously described this technique using animal models [2]. These anastomoses were performed with an operating microscope using 16–25 times magnification and 9-0 nylon sutures in a one- or two-layer closure. In the two-layer technique, the initial three sutures are placed through the mucosa and the immediately adjacent muscular layer along the anterior wall. Once these were tied, the vas was then rotated to expose the posterior wall, allowing the placement and tying of the remaining three mucosal sutures. The 9-0 nylon is then used to separately place the second layer of six seromuscular sutures. The one-layer closure is done with 6–7 full thickness 9-0 nylon sutures.

Further evolution and refinements of the original techniques have been taken place over time. In the 1980s, the two-layer closure technique evolved to use 10-0 nylon for the mucosal anastomosis and 8 or 9-0 nylon for the seromuscular layer. Marc Goldstein invented and introduced the microspike vas approximator clamp and microdot suture placement technique which allowed for greater stabilization of the vasal ends and more precise placement of the 10-0 anastomotic sutures by following the preplaced microdots, especially when the vasal lumens are of disparate caliber [1, 7].

The current technique for vasovasostomy has been very well described by Larry Lipshultz and his group and is commonly used by today's microsurgeons [2]. With this technique, the testicles and spermatic cords are delivered via a single 4–6 cm midline or bilateral 4–6 cm paramedian scrotal incision(s). The vasectomy site is identified, and the healthy testicular and abdominal ends of the vas are mobilized using iris scissors and Jacobsen mosquitoes, with care taken to preserve as much perivasal adventitia and vasal blood supply as possible so as not to compromise the vasal ends; 5-0 absorbable stay sutures are placed superficially on both the testicular and abdominal vas 1–2 cm from the intended transection sites. The testicular vas is then transected sharply in a guillotine fashion with a fresh scalpel blade, and the expressed fluid is examined immediately with light microscopy at 100–400 times magnification to confirm patency by identifying the presence of sperm or sperm parts in the fluid. The abdominal vas is transected in an identical fashion and its patency confirmed with saline vasogram or methylene blue vasography with temporary insertion of a Foley catheter. Hemostasis is managed with bipolar electrocautery to minimize vasal injury. If the intraoperative findings are suitable for vasovasostomy (copious thin fluid and/or the presence of sperm or sperm parts and normal vasography), the two vasal ends are approximated and stabilized either by placement within a vas approximator clamp or microvascular clamp or by placing 1–2 adventitial holding stitches at the 6 o'clock position. The operating microscope is now brought into the field, and a two-layer anastomosis is begun. A double-armed 10-0 nylon mucosal suture is placed and tied at the 6 o'clock position. Three to five additional 10-0 mucosal sutures are placed around the circumference of the vasal lumen and tied. Interrupted single-armed 9-0 nylon sutures are placed in the seromuscular layer circumferentially to complete the second layer. A common modification to this technique eliminates the delivery of the testicle in an effort to minimize postoperative morbidity [7]. With this technique, a 4–6-cm incision is made in the upper scrotum angled toward the external inguinal ring along the path of the vas deferens on each side. This allows for the easy identification of the vasectomy site and mobilization of the testicular and abdominal vasal ends. The anastomosis is then performed in an identical fashion to the previous description.

The patency and pregnancy rates reported in the literature are widely variable and dependent on a number of preoperative, operative, and postoperative factors that may or may not have been controlled for. It is universally accepted that the microsurgical approach yields superior patency and pregnancy rates compared to macrosurgical anastomoses given the ability to more precisely place more delicate sutures [3]. Unpublished data also demonstrates that surgeons with microsurgery training experience superior outcomes with an average patency rate of 89% compared to 53% in inexperienced hands [3]. The Vasovasostomy Study Group reviewed the outcomes of 1,469 contemporary microsurgical vasovasostomies [3, 8]. They demonstrated a 97% patency rate and 76% pregnancy rate in men less than 3 years from their vasectomy. As the interval from vasectomy increases, the rates decline with a 71% patency rate and 30% pregnancy rate when 15 years or more from the vasectomy. The Vasovasostomy Study Group also determined that there was no statistically significant difference in patency or pregnancy rates between one-layer and two-layer anastomosis, with the decision based on surgeon preference and experience [1, 8].

The morbidity of vasovasostomy has been poorly examined with no published studies discussing the morbidity associated with the various techniques for vasectomy reversal. Postoperative pain, swelling, bruising, and activity limitation are all commonly seen after vasectomy reversal especially if the testicle and its investing tunica vaginalis are delivered. Most men are counseled to wear supportive briefs or scrotal supports for 2 weeks, to take 1–2 weeks off work, and to limit themselves to light physical exertion for 3–4 weeks.

We have already discussed many technical modifications that have been developed in an attempt to improve surgical outcomes, but none were specifically developed to help reduce the morbidity of the procedure.

Mini-Incision Vasectomy Reversal

In an effort to maintain the established effectiveness of microsurgical vasovasostomy and to reduce postoperative morbidity, Keith Jarvi and his group at the University of Toronto applied the established gold standard technique used for vasectomy (no-scalpel vasectomy) to vasovasostomy [4, 9]. The mini-incision and no-scalpel techniques for performing vasectomy are familiar to most practicing urologists and have been shown to reduce complication rates and decrease recovery times without compromising vasectomy outcomes, making these techniques attractive to urologists performing vasectomy reversals.

Technique of Mini-Incision Vasectomy Reversal

The instruments required for this technique are those used for no-scalpel vasectomy and the traditional vasectomy reversal. These include two no-scalpel ring vasectomy clamps, one no-scalpel sharpened snap clamp, multiple fresh 15-blade scalpels, two nontoothed Adson forceps, two to three jeweler's forceps, two microscopic tying forceps, one nonlocking microscopic needle driver, microscopic scissors, Wexel sponges, and the appropriate sutures.

In an identical fashion to the no-scalpel vasectomy, the vas deferens is palpated, manipulated, and stabilized through the scrotal skin in the mid to upper scrotum lateral to the median scrotal raphe using the three-finger technique previously described (Fig. 12.1). It is important to bring the vas deferens at least 1 cm lateral to the midline to be in the more pliable portion of the scrotal skin. The no-scalpel vasectomy ring

Fig. 12.1 The vas deferens is identified and secured using the three-finger technique

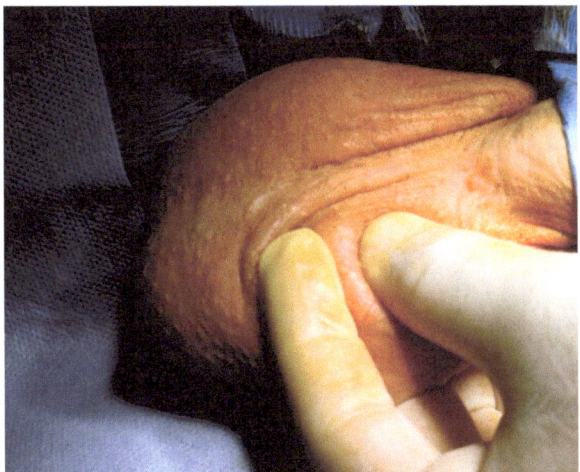

Fig. 12.2 Abdominal end of the vas deferens is grasped with a ring vasectomy clamp approximately 5 mm away from vasectomy defect and elevated

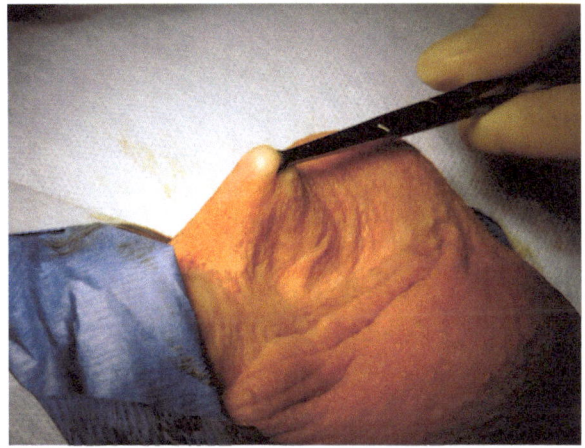

clamp is then used to grasp the vas deferens approximately 5 mm from the previous vasectomy site or directly onto the site of vasectomy occlusion if possible in an effort to minimize vasal injury (Fig. 12.2). Using the ring forceps, the abdominal vas is gently elevated to just below the scrotal skin and a 15-blade scalpel or no-scalpel sharpened snap is used to make a small subcentimeter skin incision directly over the vas (Fig. 12.3). This incision is then carried down through the skin and dartos muscle layer using the sharpened snap, being careful not to injure the underlying vas. Once the vas is exposed, the second ring clamp is used to regrasp the exposed vas within the incision and elevate it gently out of wound (Figs. 12.4 and 12.5). The vas is then carefully mobilized and a perivasal window is created with a combination of blunt and sharp dissection for a length of approximately 1 cm with care taken to preserve the vasculature within the perivasal adventitia and finally secured with a vessel loop (Figs. 12.6 and 12.7). At every step, meticulous hemostasis is essential, particularly

Fig. 12.3 Using no-scalpel vasectomy techniques, the skin and dartos muscle layers are opened directly over the vas deferens for a length of 8–10 mm

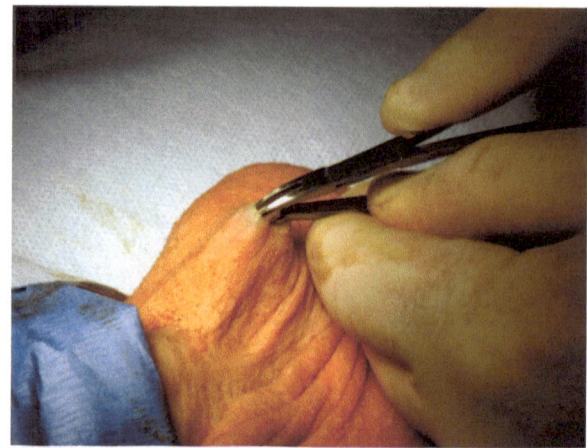

Fig. 12.4 A second no-scalpel vasectomy ring clamp is used to grasp the vas within the incision

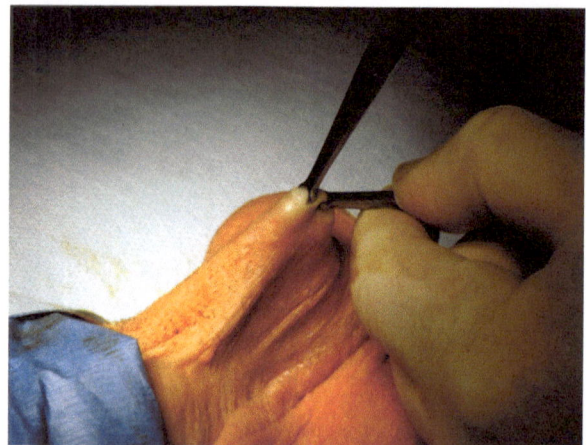

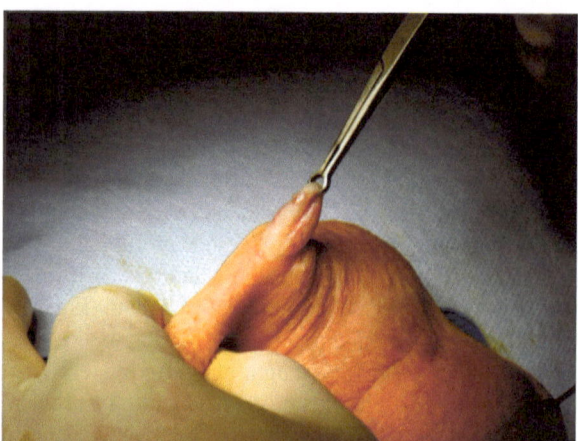

Fig. 12.5 The abdominal end of the vas is gently delivered out the incision

Fig. 12.6 A sharpened snap is used to create a small 1–1.5 cm perivasal window

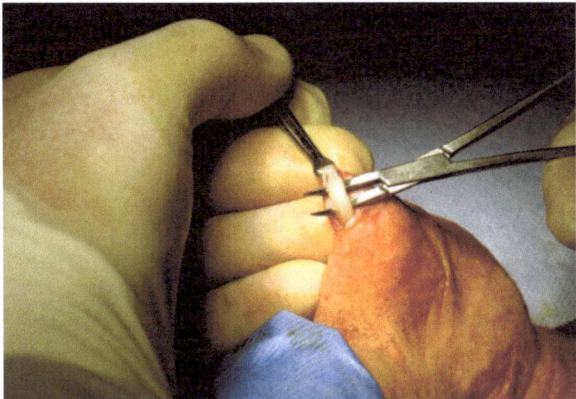

Fig. 12.7 The abdominal end of the vas is secured with vessel loops

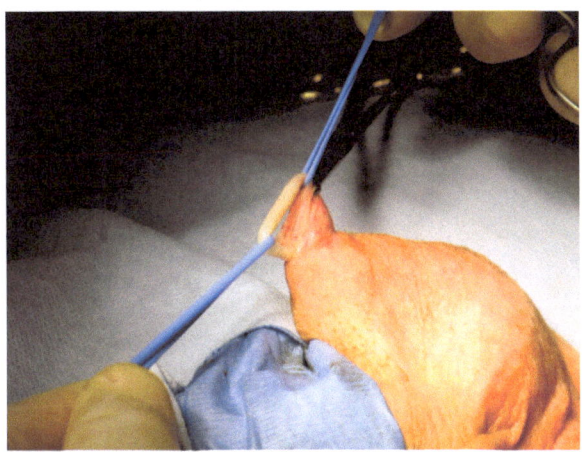

since the blood vessels in the dartos and subcutaneous layer may be difficult to control through the mini-incision after they retract into the scrotum. This is best achieved with the judicious use of microscopic bipolar electrocautery. With the abdominal end of the vas mobilized and secured, the testicular end of the vas is palpated through the incision beyond the identified vasectomy site and is regrasped with the ring forceps through the mini-incision in the scrotal skin and gently pulled out of the incision, mobilized, and secured in a manner identical to the abdominal vas (Fig. 12.8). Using this technique, a substantial portion of the vas can be delivered through the mini-incision given the inherent compliance of the scrotal skin (Fig. 12.9). Care must be taken during the mobilization of the testicular vas as the convoluted portion is often encountered and is very thin and easily injured. Stay sutures of 5-0 Biosyn or PDS are carefully placed through the superficial seromuscular layer of the vas approximately 5–10 mm away from the anticipated transection site on both the abdominal and testicular vas. These stay sutures, once tied, function to allow both control of the vasal ends to prevent retraction into the incision but also can be tied after the

Fig. 12.8 With the
abdominal end of the vas
secured, the testicular end of
the vas is delivered through
the same incision and
mobilized in an identical
fashion to the abdominal end
(note the vasectomy defect
between the clamps)

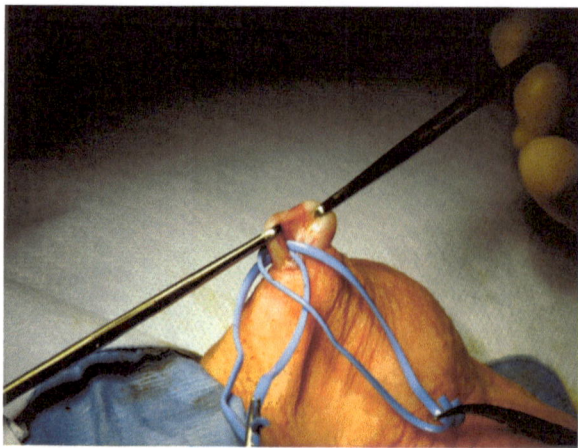

Fig. 12.9 Both vasal ends
easily delivered through the
mini-incision

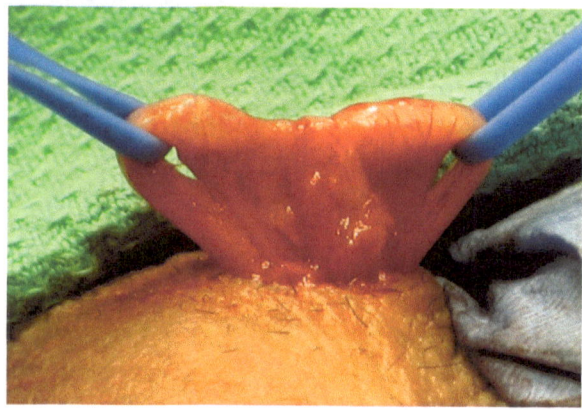

microsurgical anastomosis is complete to relieve tension on the repair. With both
vasal ends secured, each vas is then transected sharply using a fresh 15-blade scalpel
in a guillotine fashion stabilizing the vas over a nontoothed Adson forceps
(Fig. 12.10). A commercially available vas approximator clamp or small vascular
clamp is then used to control the vasal ends and bring them into close proximity to
each other just outside the incision. Finally, a solid, high-contrast backing is placed
beneath both the vasal ends and the vas approximator clamp to improve visualization
of the sutures and provide support during the microscopic anastomosis (Fig. 12.11).
The anastomosis is then performed under operating microscope magnification in a
standard fashion. We begin by placing 4 10-0 double-armed nylon sutures through
the mucosal and smooth muscle layer anteriorly in an inside out fashion on both vasa.
Once all four anterior sutures are placed, they are tied down using microscopic tying
forceps after cutting the needles off. The second anterior layer is then completed by
placing 3 9-0 single-armed nylon sutures between the tied 10-0 sutures incorporating
the seromuscular layers only. Once the 9-0 sutures are tied down, the vas

Fig. 12.10 Stay sutures of 5-0 Biosyn or PDS are placed superficially into the seromuscular layer of the vasal ends approximately 1 cm from the intended transection site, and the ends are then transected with a fresh 15 scalpel blade in a guillotine fashion

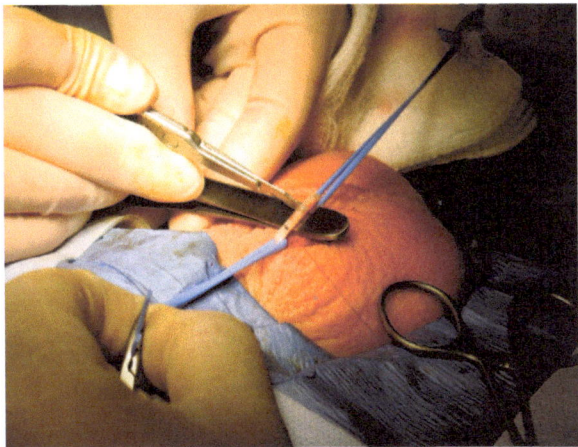

Fig. 12.11 The vasal ends are then secured in place in a vas approximating clamp and the plastic backboard in placed under the vasa and clamp

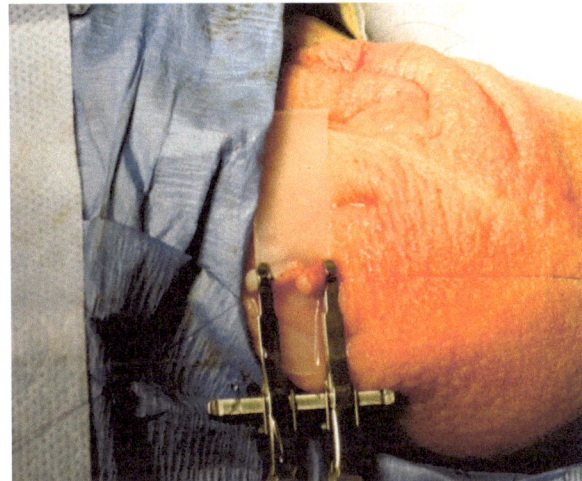

approximator is rotated to expose the posterior wall of the vasa. The patency of the two vasal lumens is easy to assess visually under magnification and can also be confirmed by gentle probing with a jeweler forceps. Two to three additional 10-0 nylon sutures are then placed through the posterior mucosal layer depending on luminal size disparity between the two ends. Once they are tied down, three additional 9-0 nylon seromuscular sutures are placed between the 10-0 sutures to complete the two-layer anastomosis. As previously mentioned, the 5-0 stay sutures can be tied loosely together to prevent tension on the anastomosis, or they can be removed at this point. The vas is then returned to the scrotum and the operating microscope removed from the operative field. Hemostasis of the skin edges and dartos muscle is managed with electrocautery. Typically, only one stitch is needed for closure, and in many cases, no stitch is needed at all. The opening in the skin is typically 8–10 mm in length (Fig. 12.12). Intraoperatively, a local incision block is performed using 5 cm^3 of

Fig. 12.12 Final incision length of <1 cm

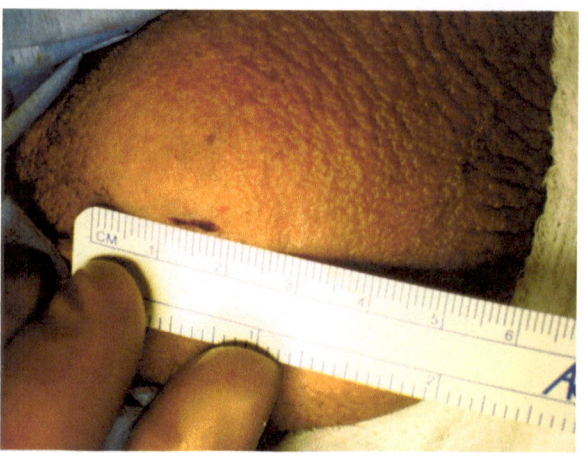

0.25% bupivacaine on each side at the conclusion of the case. All patients are discharged home the same day with a prescription for 30 tablets of narcotic analgesia and are counseled to use a scrotal support for 7 days, refrain from sexual intercourse for 2 weeks, and avoid strenuous exercise and heavy lifting for 3 weeks. Office follow-up is arranged for 4–6 weeks time, and semen analysis is arranged for 2 and 4 months post-op and then every 3 months until pregnancy is achieved.

For primary vasectomy reversal or redo vasectomy reversals, the mini-incision approach is technically feasible in the majority of men. Occasionally, scarring around the vas deferens or indistinct anatomy may preclude the use of the mini-incision technique and the larger, traditional surgical incision is then required.

Outcome of Mini-Incision Vasectomy Reversal

To date over 200 mini-incision vasectomy reversals have been performed by three different surgeons at the University of Toronto. Using a single surgeon's data, 164 consecutive vasectomy reversals from 2004 to 2010 were reviewed [9]. All patients were followed-up in the office or by telephone call 4 weeks after surgery. All postoperative complications were recorded, and pain scores were documented using a validated postvasectomy pain scale subsequently adapted to vasectomy reversals [10]. Patients were also asked to quantify the number of days required for return of work and resumption of daily activities after surgery. Semen analysis was also carried out at 2 and 4 months postoperatively and evaluated according to WHO 1992 criteria [11].

Of the 164 men, 139 underwent bilateral vasectomy reversal with 55% having a mini-incision technique. The patency rate for the mini-incision technique was 96% and was not statistically different from the patency rate of men who had undergone the traditional incision vasectomy reversal. Mean semen parameters also did not differ between the mini-incision technique and the traditional incision.

Fifty-three men completed the pain and recovery assessment including 20 men who underwent mini-incision vasectomy reversal. Reported pain severity in the

Fig. 12.13 Pain severity during the first 48 h following surgery was less among patients who received a bilateral MIVR compared to patients who received a traditional incision VR

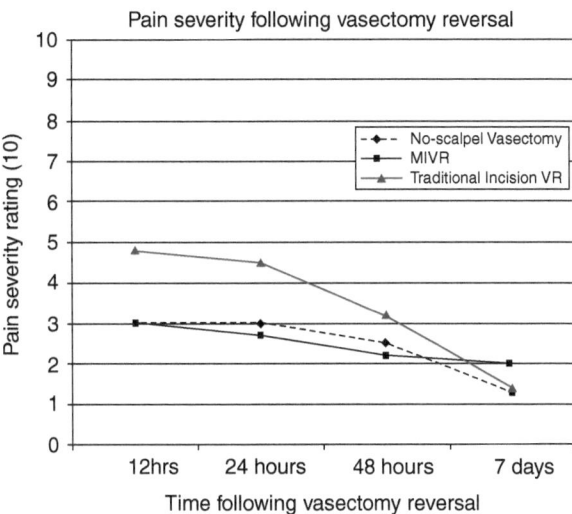

Pain severity following vasectomy reversal

mini-incision group was significantly less during the first 48 h postprocedure compared to men who underwent vasectomy reversal using the traditional incision, although at 1 week, there was no statistically significant difference in pain scores (Fig. 12.13).

Following the mini-incision vasectomy reversal patients returned to self-reported "normal everyday activities" 2 days earlier compared to men following traditional incision vasectomy reversal. Time to return to work however was not different between the two groups and averaged 5 days for both.

Key Issues

The mini-incision vasectomy reversal technique developed at the University of Toronto uses techniques and instruments familiar to most urologists. By taking advantage of the compliance of the scrotal wall, a substantial length of vas deferens can safely be delivered through a mini-incision for an efficient approach to vasectomy reversal. By avoiding a longer incision, delivery of the testicle and more extensive tissue dissection, one can significantly reduce postoperative pain and hasten return to daily activities without compromising patient outcomes as evidenced by our experience.

References

1. Kim H, Goldstein M. History of vasectomy reversal. Urol Clin North Am. 2009;36(3):359–73.
2. Lipshultz LI, Rumohr JA, Bennett RC. Techniques for vasectomy reversal. Urol Clin North Am. 2009;36(3):375–82.

3. Nagler HM, Jung H. Factors predicting successful microsurgical vasectomy reversal. Urol Clin North Am. 2009;36(3):383–90.
4. Jarvi K, Grober ED, Lo KC, et al. Mini-incision microsurgical vasectomy reversal using no-scalpel vasectomy techniques and instruments. Urology. 2008;72(4):913–5.
5. Li SQ, Goldstein M, Zhu J, Huber D. The no-scalpel vasectomy. J Urol. 1991;145(2):341–4.
6. Weiss RS, Li PS. No-needle jet anesthetic technique for no-scalpel vasectomy. J Urol. 2005;173(5):1677–80.
7. Goldstein M, Li PS, Matthews GJ. Microsurgical vasovasostomy: the microdot technique of precision suture placement. J Urol. 1998;159(1):188–90.
8. Belker AM, Thomas Jr AJ, Fuchs EF, et al. Results of 1,469 microsurgical vasectomy reversals by the Vasovasostomy Study Group. J Urol. 1991;145(3):505–11.
9. Grober E, Jarvi K, Lo K, Shin EJ. Mini-incision vasectomy reversal using no-scalpel vasectomy principles: efficacy and postoperative pain compared with traditional approaches to vasectomy reversal. Urology. 2011;77(3):602–6.
10. Aggarwal H, Chiou RK, Siref LE, Sloan SE. Comparative analysis of pain during anesthesia and no-scalpel vasectomy procedure among three different local anesthetic techniques. Urology. 2009;74(1):77–81.
11. World Health Organization. WHO Laboratory Manual for the examination of human semen and sperm-cervical mucus interaction. 4th ed. Cambridge, UK/New York: World Health Organization; 1999.

Chapter 13
Robotic Assisted Microsurgery for Male Infertility

Jamin V. Brahmbhatt and Sijo J. Parekattil

Since the use of the operating microscope for microsurgery in 1975 [1], there has been a steady increase in the use of such technology in the operative management of male infertility and chronic testicular or groin pain [1–11]. Added to the reports relating to greater patency rates and fertility rates of vasovasostomy performed with the operating microscope [12], the concepts of magnification have been successfully applied to vasoepididymostomy and varicocele ligation. More recently, microscopic spermatic cord neurolysis has demonstrated applicability to the treatment of groin and testicular discomfort [13, 14]. These techniques require varying degrees of microsurgical skills and an array of supporting technology, neither of which may be part of many urologists' personal or technical armamentarium. The melding of improved visualization with magnification to an ergonomic platform that can be operated remotely has a significant application to testicular and reproductive surgery. Robotic assistance during surgical procedures has been utilized in a wide array of surgical fields with the above mentioned benefits [15–19]. This chapter covers the latest developments in the robotic microsurgical platform, robotic microsurgical tools, and current evaluations of various robotic microsurgical applications for male infertility and patients with chronic testicular or groin pain.

J.V. Brahmbhatt, MD
Department of Urology, University of Tennessee Health Science Center,
Memphis, TN, USA
e-mail: jaminbrahmbhatt@gmail.com

S.J. Parekattil, MD (✉)
Director of Urology, Winter Haven Hospital, University of Florida,
200 Avenue F. N.E., Winter Haven, FL 33881, USA
e-mail: sijo.parekattil@winterhavenhospital.org

S.J. Parekattil, A. Agarwal (eds.), *Male Infertility for the Clinician*,
© Springer Science+Business Media New York 2013

Novel Equipment

With any new field, the development of novel tools or instruments that can enable surgeons to create new solutions for existing clinical needs is of paramount importance. Below are some new products that enhance the ability to perform robotic-assisted microsurgery.

New Robotic Surgical Platform

Intuitive Surgical (Sunnyvale, CA) now offers an enhanced four-arm da Vinci-type Si robotic system with high-definition digital visual magnification that allows for greater magnification than the standard robotic system (up to 10–15×). The enhanced magnification capability allows the surgeon to position the camera 6–7 cm away from the operative field to avoid any local tissue effects from the heat emitted from the camera lighting (this was a problem with the older system, where the camera had to be placed within 2–3 cm of the operative field for microsurgery). This new system (Fig. 13.1) allows greater range of motion and better microsurgical instrument handling. The additional fourth arm has improved range of motion and positioning capabilities to provide the microsurgeon with one additional tool during procedures. The robot is positioned from the right side of the patient for microsurgical cases as illustrated in Fig. 13.2.

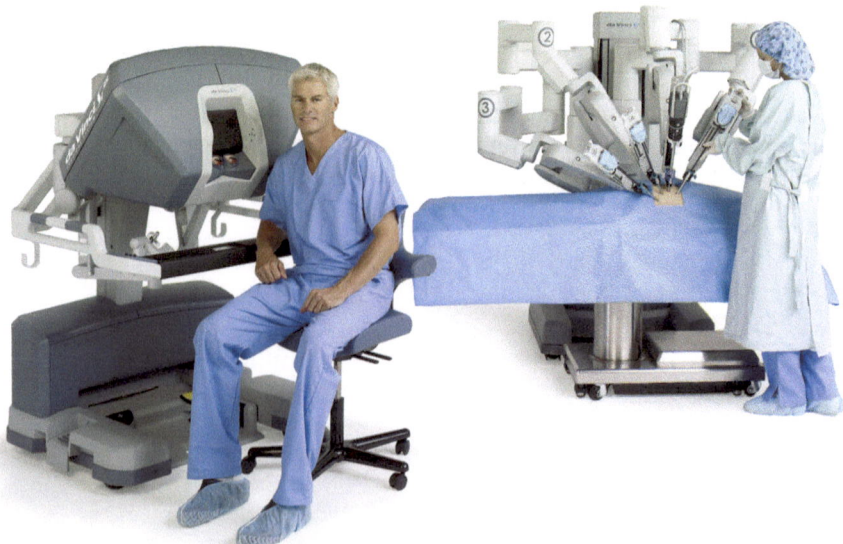

Fig. 13.1 daVinci Si Robotic platform (Courtesy of Intuitive Surgical © 2010)

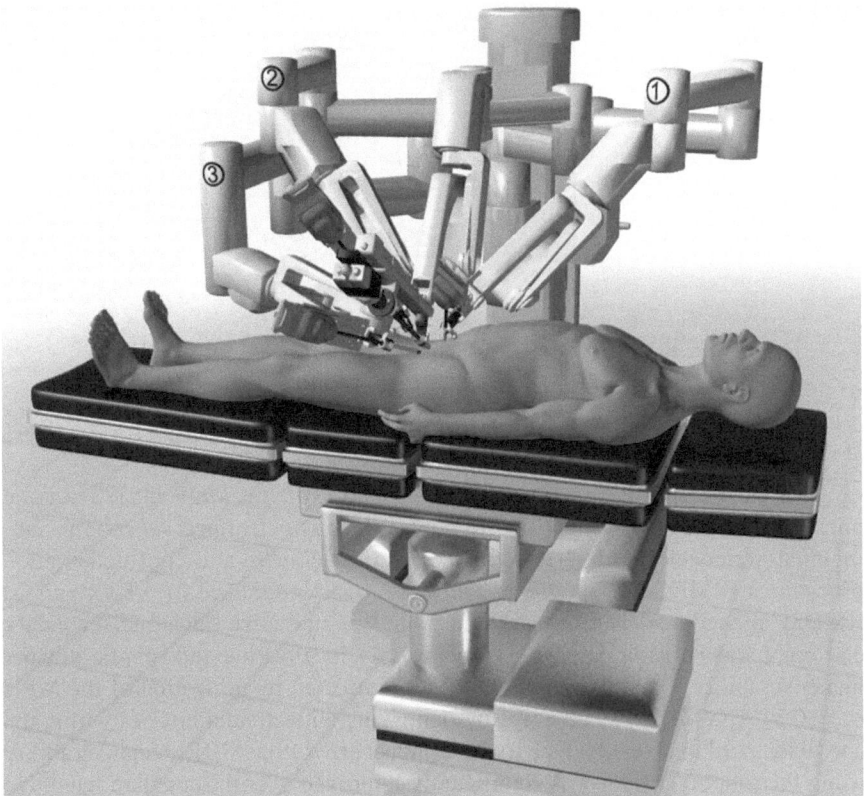

Fig. 13.2 Robotic platform positioning for microsurgical cases

Refined Robotic Doppler Flow Probe

Cocuzza et al. [20] have shown that the systematic use of intraoperative vascular Doppler ultrasound during microsurgical subinguinal varicocelectomy improves precise identification and preservation of testicular blood supply. During robotic microsurgical cases, the standard Doppler probe has to be held by a surgical assistant and cannot be manipulated readily with the robotic graspers. A new revised micro-Doppler flow probe (MDP) has been developed by Vascular Technology Inc. (Nashua, NH) that is designed specifically for use with the robotic platform (Fig. 13.3). This new probe allows for easy manipulation of the probe with the fourth arm and allows the surgeon to perform real-time Doppler monitoring of the testicular artery during cases such as robotic-assisted microscopic varicocelectomy (RAVx) and robotic-assisted microscopic denervation of the spermatic cord (RMDSC). This allows the surgeon to hear the testicular artery flow while dissecting out the veins and nerves with the other two robotic arms.

Fig. 13.3 Robotic micro-
Doppler probe

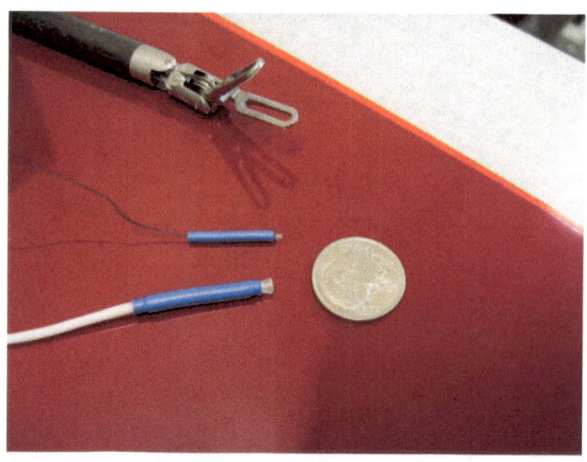

A recent prospective randomized control trial of the MDP in 273 robotic microsurgical cases from Jul 2009 to Sept 2010 was performed: 67 robotic sub-inguinal varicocelectomies (RVx) and 206 robotic spermatic cord denervation procedures (RMDSC). The use of the MDP was randomized to 5 RVx and 20 RMDSC procedures. The primary end point was operative time, and secondary end point was surgeon ease in testicular artery localization and robotic grasper maneuverability. Operative duration was not affected by utilization of the MPD ($p = 0.5$). The MDP was effective in identifying all testicular arteries within the spermatic cord in all cases. Due to the compact size of the MDP, maneuverability using the robotic grasper was significantly improved over the standard handheld Doppler probe. MDP allowed for full range of motion of the robotic arms allowing the surgeon to easily scan vessels from a wide range of angles. No complications from use of the MDP occurred. The new micro-Doppler probe for robotic microsurgical procedures appears to have performed effectively in this study.

Vascular Technology Inc. (Nashua, NH) has recently developed an even smaller microprobe that can detect flow through vessels at about 0.5-mm diameter (Fig. 13.3). This just expands further potential applications for this technology.

Enhanced Digital Visual Magnification

The miniaturization and development of advanced digital microscopic cameras (100–250×) allow even greater magnification than the standard robotic (10–15×) and microscopic (10–20×) magnification in use at this time. Our group is currently involved in clinical trials of a 100× digital camera (Digital Inc., China) that can be utilized via the TilePro™ da Vinci Si robotic system (Intuitive Surgical, Sunnyvale, CA) to allow the surgeon to toggle or use simultaneous 100× and 10–15× visualization. This provides the surgeon with unparalleled visual acuity for complex microsurgical procedures.

Karl Storz (El Segundo, CA) also offers a robotic arm platform to hold an optical mini-scope that offers 16–20× magnification that can then be used during the da Vinci robotic cases to provide an additional enhanced magnification view (routed through the da Vinci console).

New Saline-Enhanced Electrosurgical Micro Blade

Saline-enhanced electrosurgical resection (SEER) has been utilized for cauterization of vessels in a number of liver and renal applications. It is a form of electrosurgical cautery and resection that leads to minimal smoke and scar formation. A new robotic SEER micro blade is in development (Bovie Inc., Clearwater, FL) that may provide an option for ablation of veins during robotic-assisted subinguinal varicocelectomy.

Robotic Microsurgical Procedures

Robotic-Assisted Microscopic Vasectomy Reversal

A number of groups have developed robotic-assisted techniques to perform robotic-assisted microscopic vasectomy reversal (RAVV) in animal and ex vivo human models [21–25]. Some studies suggest that robotic-assisted reversal may have advantages over microsurgical reversal in terms of ease of performing the procedure and improved patency rates [23, 24]. A few groups have actually performed human robotic-assisted vasovasostomies using the initial da Vinci robotic system [26] (Intuitive Surgical, Sunnyvale, CA).

These efforts have been recently confirmed in human RAVV cases performed using the new da Vinci Si system [27, 28]. A recent prospective control study of robotic versus pure microsurgical vasovasostomy in 90 vasectomy reversal cases performed from Aug 2007 to Sept 2010 by a single fellowship trained microsurgeon was performed (this was an extension to a previously published study) [29]. The primary end point was operative duration. The secondary end point was total motile sperm count at 2, 5, 9, and 12 months postoperatively. Case breakdown was as such: 45 robotic-assisted cases and 45 pure microsurgical cases. Selection of approach (robotic vs. pure microscopic) was based on patient choice (robotic was more expensive than microscopic). Preoperative patient characteristics were similar in both groups. The same suture material and suturing technique (2 layer 10-0 and 9-0 nylon anastomosis) was used in both approaches.

Median clinical follow-up was 14 months (range 1–37 months). Median duration from vasectomy in the robotic group was 8 years (1–19) and in the microscopic group 6.5 years (1–19). Ninety-four percentage overall patency was achieved in the RAVV cases and 79% in MVV (>1 million sperm/high power field). Median operative duration was significantly decreased in RAVV at 90 min (60–180) compared to MVV at 120 min (60–180), $p = 0.004$. Mean postoperative total motile sperm counts were not significantly higher in RAVV versus MVV, but the rate of postoperative sperm count recovery was significantly greater in RAVV.

The use of robotic assistance in microsurgical vasovasostomy may have potential benefit over MVV with regard to decreasing operative duration and improving the rate of recovery of postoperative total motile sperm counts. Further evaluation and longer follow-up are needed to assess its clinical potential and the true cost–benefit ratio.

Robotic-Assisted Microscopic Varicocelectomy

Although reports of robotic-assisted laparoscopic intra-abdominal varicocelectomy have been published [30], there are a number of publications that suggest that microscopic subinguinal varicocelectomy(MVx) may provide superior outcomes compared to intra-abdominal varicocelectomy [31–34]. Shu, Wang et al. were the first to publish on robotic-assisted microsurgical subinguinal varicocelectomy (RAVx) [35]. They compared standard microsurgical to robotic-assisted varicocelectomy and found that the robotic approach provided advantages in terms of slightly decreasing operative duration and complete elimination of surgeon tremor.

To further explore these findings, we performed a prospective randomized control trial of MVx to RAVx in a canine varicocele model by a fellowship-trained microsurgeon. The surgeon performed cord dissection and ligation of three veins with 3-0 silk ties. Twelve canine varicocelectomies were randomized into two arms of six: MVV versus RAVx. Procedure duration, vessel injury, and knot failures were recorded. The RAVx mean duration (9.5 min) was significantly faster than MVV (12 min), $p = 0.04$. The duration for robot setup and microscope setup was not significantly different. There were no vessel injuries or knot failures in either group.

A review of our prospective clinical database of 97 RAVx cases from Jun 2008 to Sept 2010 (median follow-up 11 months: range 1–27) is as follows. The median duration per side was 30 min (10–80). Indications for the procedure were the presence of a grade two or three varicocele and the following conditions: 10 with azoospermia, 42 with oligoospermia, and 49 with testicular pain (with or without oligoospermia, and failed all other conservative treatment options). Three-month follow-up was available for 81 patients: 75% with oligoospermia had a significant improvement in sperm count or motility; one with azoospermia was converted to oligoospermia. For testicular pain, 92% had complete resolution of pain (targeted neurolysis of the spermatic cord had been performed in addition to varicocelectomy). One recurrence or persistence of a varicocele occurred (by physical and ultrasound exam), one patient developed a small postoperative hydrocele, and two patients had small postoperative scrotal hematomas (treated conservatively). The fourth robotic arm allowed the surgeon to control one additional instrument during the cases decreasing reliance on the microsurgical assistant. The fourth arm also enabled the surgeon to perform real-time intraoperative Doppler mapping of the testicular arteries while dissecting the veins with the other arms if needed.

Robotic-assisted microsurgical subinguinal varicocelectomy appears to be safe, feasible, and efficient. The preliminary human results appear promising. Further evaluation and comparative effectiveness studies are warranted.

Robotic-Assisted Microscopic Denervation of the Spermatic Cord

Recent studies by Levine et al. [13] and Oliveira et al. [14] have shown that microscopic denervation of the spermatic cord is an effective treatment option for men with chronic testicular pain. Our group has been developing a robotic-assisted microsurgical approach for the denervation of the spermatic cord (RMDSC) to assess if there may be any potential benefit over the standard microscopic technique.

A review of our initial 230 RMDSC cases from Oct 2008 to Sept 2010 was performed (median follow-up of 8 months). Selection criteria for patients were as such: chronic testicular pain (>6 months), failed standard pain management treatments, and negative urologic workup. A robotic-assisted subinguinal, inguinal, or intra-abdominal approach was utilized based on the location of pain. Pain was assessed utilizing a standardized validated tool (PIQ-6). The median operative duration was 20 min (7–150). The fourth robotic arm allowed the surgeon to control one additional instrument leading to less reliance on the microsurgical assistant.

Postoperatively, 77% (176) patients had complete resolution of pain and 8% (19) had a 50% decrease in pain. RMDSC was successful in eliminating testicular and or groin pain for a number of possible etiologies: postvasectomy pain syndrome (PVPS), postinguinal hernia pain, sports hernia or groin trauma pain, chronic epididymitis or idiopathic pain, varicocele pain, postrobotic prostatectomy groin or testicular pain, postnephrectomy or donor nephrectomy groin or testicular pain, postpelvic radiation or brachytherapy groin or testicular pain, and fibromyalgia groin pain. Figure 13.4 illustrates the outcomes in these various pain categories.

Single Port and Abdominal Robotic Microsurgical Neurolysis

Chronic groin pain can be debilitating for patients. Microsurgical subinguinal denervation of the spermatic cord (MDSC) is a treatment option for this pain. However, there are limited further options for patients who fail this treatment or who have phantom pain after orchiectomy. Our goal was to develop a single port and abdominal robotic microsurgical neurolysis technique to ligate the genitofemoral and inferior hypogastric nerve fibers within the abdomen above the internal inguinal ring.

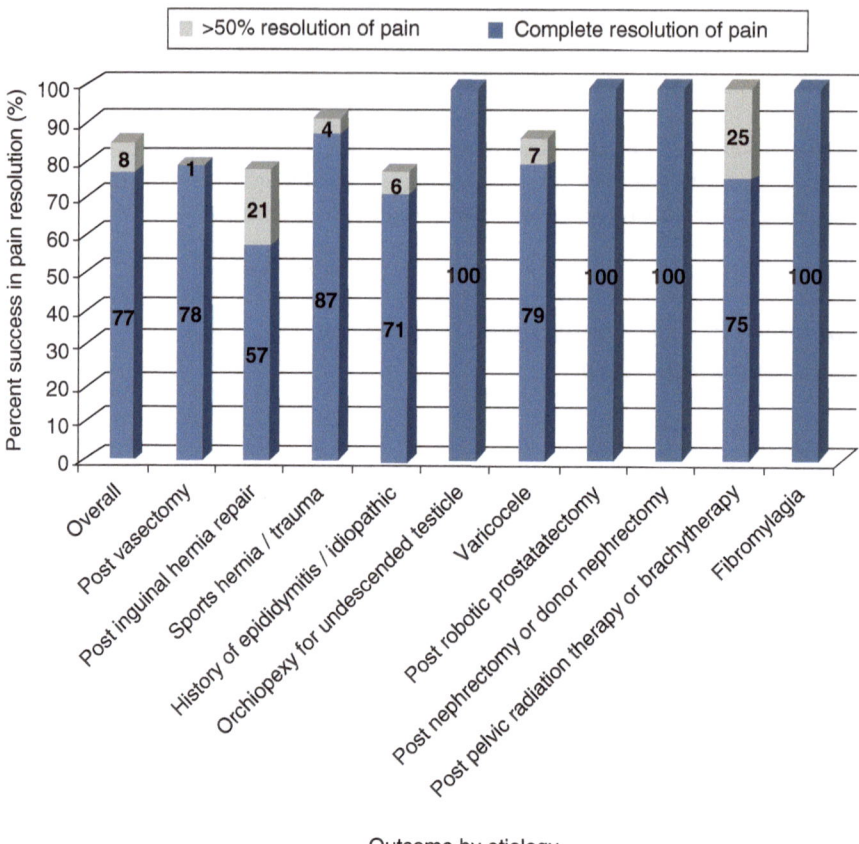

Outcome by etiology

Fig. 13.4 Pain elimination outcomes for robotic-assisted microsurgical denervation of the spermatic cord for various groin or testicular pain etiologies

We performed a prospective study of patients with chronic groin pain who had either failed previous MDSC or had phantom pain after orchiectomy. Primary end point was impact of pain on quality of life (PIQ-6 pain impact questionnaire from RAND) and secondary end point was operative robotic duration. PIQ-6 scores were collected pre-op and at 1, 3, 6, and 12 months post-op.

We completed 30 cases (five single port) from Jun 2009 to Sept 2010. Elimination of pain occurred in 60% (18 cases), and a greater than 50% reduction in pain occurred in an additional 13% (4 cases) within 1 month post-op. Two of the failures were patients that had pain elimination for 6 months, but then pain returned thereafter. Median OR duration was 10 min (5–30). There were three complications: one post-op scrotal hematoma that resolved with conservative measures, one patient had pain at one of the port sites, and one patient had pain that shifted from the groin to the leg. Single port and abdominal robotic microsurgical neurolysis appears to be an option for treatment in this difficult patient population. Further follow-up and evaluation is warranted.

Expert Commentary

The use of robotic assistance during microsurgical procedures is expanding. The application of this technology in other microsurgery fields apart from urology is also expanding, such as ophthalmology, hand surgery, and plastic and reconstructive microsurgery. The advantages of a stable microsurgical platform, ergonomic surgeon instrument controls, elimination of tremor, and magnified immersive 3D vision are all intuitively apparent. Further comparative effectiveness studies are ongoing and will be forthcoming on the true applicability of this new surgical platform. However, the preliminary results so far are quite impressive.

Five-Year View

The use of robotic assistance during microsurgical procedures is likely to expand in all areas of microsurgery. In order to provide a structured evidence-based platform to develop these procedures and protect patient safety, a dedicated society has been formed (Robotic-Assisted Microsurgical and Endoscopic Society: RAMSES—www. roboticmicrosurgeons.org). This society has developed a core curriculum for robotic microsurgical training that could be utilized in the fields of urology, hand surgery, plastic/reconstructive, ophthalmology, and vascular surgery. The goal of this group is to further the prudent and scientific use of such techniques. Such organizations may be able to influence the direction of instrument/equipment development by industry.

Key Issues

- Robotic assistance during microsurgery provides microsurgeons with many advantages: improved operative efficiency, elimination of tremor, scaling of motion, and enhanced imaging.
- Improved clinical outcomes appear likely with robotic assistance, and preliminary studies appear to support this concept.
- Novel treatment options for men with chronic testicular or groin pain, postvasectomy pain, sports hernia pain, postnephrectomy, donor nephrectomy, and phantom groin pain are now available with this technology.
- Structured evidence-based platforms for the scientific development of this technology are necessary to protect patient safety. Groups such as RAMSES may provide guidance.

Acknowledgments We would like to thank Dr. Johannes Vieweg, Dr. Li-Ming Su, Dr. Philip Li, Dr. Hany Atalah, Katy Lyall, David Regan, Dr. Rachana Suchdev, Intuitive Surgical and Vascular Technology Inc. for their continued support in the pursuit and refinement of robotic microsurgical techniques and tools.

References

1. Silber SJ. Microsurgery in clinical urology. Urology. 1975;6:150–3.
2. Marmar JL. Modified vasoepididymostomy with simultaneous double needle placement, tubu-lotomy and tubular invagination. J Urol. 2000;163:483–6.
3. Berger RE. Triangulation end-to-side vasoepididymostomy. J Urol. 1998;159:1951–3.
4. Chan PT, Li PS, Goldstein M. Microsurgical vasoepididymostomy: a prospective randomized study of 3 intussusception techniques in rats. J Urol. 2003;169:1924–9.
5. Fogdestam I, Fall M. Microsurgical end-to-end and end-to-side epididymovasostomy to cor-rect occlusive azoospermia. Scand J Plast Reconstr Surg. 1983;17:137–40.
6. Marmar JL, Kim Y. Subinguinal microsurgical varicocelectomy: a technical critique and sta-tistical analysis of semen and pregnancy data. J Urol. 1994;152:1127–32.
7. Owen ER. Microsurgical vasovasostomy: a reliable vasectomy reversal. Aust N Z J Surg. 1977;47:305–9.
8. Schlegel PN. Testicular sperm extraction: microdissection improves sperm yield with minimal tissue excision. Hum Reprod. 1999;14:131–5.
9. Schultheiss D, Denil J. History of the microscope and development of microsurgery: a revolu-tion for reproductive tract surgery. Andrologia. 2002;34:234–41.
10. Silber SJ. Microscopic vasoepididymostomy: specific microanastomosis to the epididymal tubule. Fertil Steril. 1978;30:565–71.
11. Thomas Jr AJ. Vasoepididymostomy. Urol Clin North Am. 1987;14:527–38.
12. Owen ER. Microsurgical vasovasostomy: a reliable vasectomy reversal. J Urol. 1977;47:305–9.
13. Levine LA. Microsurgical denervation of the spermatic cord. J Sex Med. 2008;5:526–9.
14. Oliveira RG, Camara C, Alves Jde M, et al. Microsurgical testicular denervation for the treat-ment of chronic testicular pain initial results. Clinics (Sao Paulo). 2009;64:393–6.
15. Bourla DH, Hubschman JP, Culjat M, et al. Feasibility study of intraocular robotic surgery with the da vinci surgical system. Retina. 2008;28:154–8.
16. Casale P. Robotic pediatric urology. Expert Rev Med Devices. 2008;5:59–64.
17. Colombo Jr JR, Santos B, Hafron J, et al. Robotic assisted radical prostatectomy: surgical techniques and outcomes. Int Braz J Urol. 2007;33:803–9.
18. Guru KA, Wilding GE, Piacente P, et al. Robot-assisted radical cystectomy versus open radical cystectomy: assessment of postoperative pain. Can J Urol. 2007;14:3753–6.
19. Rodriguez E, Chitwood Jr WR. Minimally invasive, robotic cardiac surgery. Ann Thorac Surg. 2008;85:357–8.
20. Cocuzza M, Pagani R, Coelho R, et al. The systematic use of intraoperative vascular doppler ultrasound during microsurgical subinguinal varicocelectomy improves precise identification and preservation of testicular blood supply. Fertil Steril. 2010;93(7):2396–9.
21. Kuang W, Shin PR, Matin S, Thomas Jr AJ. Initial evaluation of robotic technology for micro-surgical vasovasostomy. J Urol. 2004;171:300–3.
22. Kuang W, Shin PR, Oder M, Thomas Jr AJ. Robotic-assisted vasovasostomy: a two-layer technique in an animal model. Urology. 2005;65:811–4.
23. Schiff J, Li PS, Goldstein M. Robotic microsurgical vasovasostomy and vasoepididymostomy: a prospective randomized study in a rat model. J Urol. 2004;171:1720–5.
24. Schiff J, Li PS, Goldstein M. Robotic microsurgical vasovasostomy and vasoepididymostomy in rats. Int J Med Robot. 2005;1:122–6.
25. Schoor RA, Ross L, Niederberger C. Robotic assisted microsurgical vasal reconstruction in a model system. World J Urol. 2003;21:48–9.
26. Fleming C. Robot-assisted vasovasostomy. Urol Clin North Am. 2004;31:769–72.
27. Parekattil SJ, Moran ME. Robotic instrumentation: evolution and microsurgical applications. Indian J Urol. 2010;26:395–403.
28. Parekattil S, Cohen M, Vieweg J. Human robotic assisted bilateral vasoepididymostomy and vasovasostomy procedures: initial safety and efficacy trial. Proc SPIE. 2009;7161:71611L.

29. Parekattil S, Atalah H, Cohen M. Video technique for human robotic assisted microsurgical vasovasostomy. J Endourol. 2010;24:511–4.
30. Corcione F, Esposito C, Cuccurullo D, et al. Advantages and limits of robot-assisted laparoscopic surgery: preliminary experience. Surg Endosc. 2005;19:117–9.
31. Chen XF, Zhou LX, Liu YD, et al. comparative analysis of three different surgical approaches to varicocelectomy. Zhonghua Nan Ke Xue. 2009;15:413–6.
32. Cayan S, Shavakhabov S, Kadioglu A. Treatment of palpable varicocele in infertile men: a meta-analysis to define the best technique. J Androl. 2009;30:33–40.
33. Al-Said S, Al-Naimi A, Al-Ansari A, et al. Varicocelectomy for male infertility: a comparative study of open, laparoscopic and microsurgical approaches. J Urol. 2008;180:266–70.
34. Al-Kandari AM, Shabaan H, Ibrahim HM, et al. Comparison of outcomes of different varicocelectomy techniques: open inguinal, laparoscopic, and subinguinal microscopic varicocelectomy: a randomized clinical trial. Urology. 2007;69:417–20.
35. Shu T, Taghechian S, Wang R. Initial experience with robot-assisted varicocelectomy. Asian J Androl. 2008;10:146–8.

Chapter 14
Robot-Assisted Vasectomy Reversal

Peter Frank De Wil, Vincenzo Ficarra, George A. de Boccard, and Alexandre Mottrie

Since the early part of the twentieth century, vasectomy was used for eugenic, puni-tive, and therapeutic purposes. Nowadays, this procedure is widely used as a contra-ceptive tool, and it is calculated that about 50 million men have relied on vasectomy for family planning. More than in Europe, in the United States, vasectomy is employed as contraceptive method by nearly 11% of married couples [1]. Second indication for vasectomy is after transurethral resection of prostate or adenomec-tomy for benign prostatic hyperplasia (BPH) to prevent urogenital infections.

In the early years of past century, Dr. Edward Martin, surgeon at the University of Pennsylvania was the first to perform reversal procedures. He performed vasoepididy-mostomies in men who had obstruction secondary to epididymitis and not vasectomy.

This work is what led Jeequier to label Martin as the "father of andrology" [2].

The number of vasectomy reversals is rising because of the rising popularity of vasectomy combined with the continuing upward trend of divorce and remarriage,

P.F. De Wil, MD (✉)
Urological Department, Kliniek Sint Jan,
Kruidtuinlaan 32, 1000, Brussels, Belgium
e-mail: peter_dewil@hotmail.com

V. Ficarra, MD, PhD
Department of Oncological and Surgical Sciences,
Urology Clinic, University of Padua, Monoblocco Ospedaliero,
IV Floor, Via Giustiniani 2, 35100 Padua, Italy
e-mail: vincenzo.ficarra@unipd.it

G.A. de Boccard, MD
Clinique Generale Beaulieu, Robot-Assisted Laparoscopic Surgery Center,
20 Chemin Beau Soleil, 1206 Geneva, Switzerland
e-mail: boccard@iprolink.ch

A. Mottrie,
Department of Urology, O.L.V. Clinic Aalst, Aalst, Belgium
e-mail: a.mottrie@telenet.be

S.J. Parekattil, A. Agarwal (eds.), *Male Infertility for the Clinician*,
© Springer Science+Business Media New York 2013

especially in industrialized countries. In order to plan the more appropriate intervention to reach pregnancy, the chances of success in terms of patency of vas and/or pregnancy should be counseled based on the personal experience of the surgeon, patient's health history, age, results of physical examination, and reproductive potential of his partner. A potential alternative is sperm extraction for IVF or ICSI. In most men, vasectomy reversal is technically feasible, but success rates depend on a variety of factors determined by both male and female fertility factors [3].

Vasectomy reversal is a technically challenging procedure, and a number of microsurgical advances have enhanced outcomes (e.g., use of the operating microscope with optical magnification). A number of techniques where developed using microsurgical technique [4, 5], one-layer [6–8], microdot [9], stents [10], and oblique technique [11]. This chapter reviews the application of robotic-assisted microsurgery for vasectomy reversal.

Robotic Vasovasostomy

So why use robotic assistance for microsurgical vasectomy reversal? Robotic assistance provides a number of benefits for the microsurgeon: elimination of tremor, scaling of motion (1:5), and enhanced magnification—all in a fixed stable microsurgical platform. It obviates the need for specialized tissue support platforms and reduces the reliance of the microsurgeon on a skilled microsurgical assistant. These are all important advantages for technically challenging procedures.

From an economical point of view, only centers already equipped with a da Vinci robot should perform robotic vasovasostomy because the additional cost is only a few hundred euro/dollars [12]. Five studies have reported the results of robot-assisted vasectomy reversal in experimental animal models and in humans: Kuang et al. [13, 14], Schiff et al. [15], Parekattil et al. [16], and De Boccard et al. [17]. This chapter focuses on our technique.

Personal Surgical Technique

The personal surgical technique has been previously described in detail [18]. The surgical technique in preparing the vas deferens for vasovasostomy is identical to the microsurgical technique. A scrotal median raphe approach is utilized (incision about 5 cm in length). The previous vasectomy sites are identified, and the proximal and distal ends of the vas deferens are dissected free. The distal end of the vas (testicular side) is transected, and the fluid from this end is evaluated. The proximal vas end is flushed with 2 cm³ of saline to assess for patency. The two ends of the vas deferens are now loosely approximated using either a 4-0 or 7-0 absorbable suture to create a tension-free anastomosis.

Once the vas ends have been prepared, the robotic platform (da Vinci Si system, Intuitive Surgical, Sunnyvale, CA) is brought into the field. The robotic system is placed in between the legs of the patient as in a robotic prostatectomy placement. The first assistant remains on the left of the patient, and the primary surgeon moves from the right of the patient to the surgical console. A 0° lens is utilized and placed at an 80° angle to the patient. The right-side anastomosis is performed first, and the camera is positioned in such a manner that the camera can be moved to the left anastomosis at the same angle (by simply sliding it over to the left by a few centimeters). Black Diamond microforceps are utilized in arms 1 and 2. They are positioned at 45° to the camera lens. Arm 3 carries the Potts scissors and is positioned in front of the camera at 30° to the patient. The standard robotic trocars are placed for all arms even though the procedure in not being performed intracorporeally in order to stabilize the instruments.

The anastomosis is now completed utilizing 8-0 or 9-0 nylon interrupted sutures. Three posterior full-thickness (muscularis and mucosa) sutures are placed and then tied down to secure the posterior plate of the anastomosis. Five full-thickness sutures are placed anteriorly and then tied down to complete the anastomosis. Two or three additional sutures may be placed to secure the supporting muscularis. The use of the third arm with the Potts scissors improves the efficiency of the procedure and obviates the need for a skilled microsurgical assistant (a scrub nurse is sufficient). After completion of the anastomosis on both sides, the robot is now undocked and the scrotal incision is closed with a 4-0 absorbable suture in two layers.

Our experience in robotic-assisted microsurgical vasovasostomy includes 11 cases performed from January 2006 to December 2009 in Aalst, Belgium, and 14 cases performed in Geneva. We have only had one scrotal hematoma that was treated conservatively, and all cases were patent 6 months postsurgically. Our mean total sperm count was 48.6 million/ml after RAVV (robotic-assisted vasovasostomy) and 22.8 million/ml after MAVV (microsurgical-assisted vasovasostomy). The RAVV cases performed in Belgium where compared to 17 cases who underwent MAVV at that same institution, and so far, the pregnancy rates for RAVV vs. MAVV where 36–41%, respectively.

Expert Commentary

The advantages of the da Vinci system include improved visibility with a three-dimensional view, a comfortable and ergonomically superior position during surgery, and increased degrees of freedom of motion of instruments. Another important advantage is improved stability during suturing as a result of the motion reduction feature in the robot.

For all these reasons, the da Vinci surgical robotic system was applied in the fields of general, vascular, cardiac, pediatric, gynecologic, and urologic surgery in only a few years time. Recently, a number of reports have shown that the robot allows surgeons to significantly simplify the more complex reconstructive steps of the lapa-roscopic procedures. There has been an explosive increase in the number of urologic procedures being attempted using da Vinci assistance, and we believe that robotic technology represents the future of minimally invasive surgery, and applications for the robot will expand as more centers report their results. As reported by Fleming in 2004 [12], robot-assisted vasectomy reversal is an attractive alternative to both tradi-tional microsurgical vasovasostomy and vasoepididymostomy for several reasons:

- Greater ease and precision of suture placement are possible with elimination of the physiological tremor. While the magnification of the robotic camera (10–15×) is not as high as that of the operating microscope (up to 25×), enhanced control with motion reduction compensated for this difference. Data coming from the literature showed that the precision of suture placement resulted in a more rapid suture placement and watertight anastomosis. Moreover, the robotic technology minimizes the differences between placing sutures with the left or right hand, which further facilitates suturing. These concepts find clinical confir-mation in the percentages of patent anastomosis and in the percentages of the presence of sperm granuloma.
- The training period is probably shorter than traditional microscopic techniques and benefits achieved with the surgical robot were acquired with a short learning curve. The learning curve period was considered nonexistent for experienced microsurgeons and probably fewer cases are necessary to become competent also for robotic surgeons without specific microsurgical training. As reported by Fleming et al., a surgeon without expertise in microsurgical technique should participate in a rat microsurgery course and should have extensive lab animal microsurgery experience, performing at least five to eight cases [12]. Vice versa, experienced microsurgeons need to learn to use the robot approximatively 30 min in a "dry lab," practicing suturing with a piece of Gore-tex vascular graft and 9-0 nylon suture [12]. However, to be critical, no studies yet demonstrated the exact impact of learning curve for vasectomy reversal procedures.
- More surgeons with expertise in robotic surgery will be able to provide high-quality surgical care for their patients. Although data coming from literature are promising, the robot-assisted reversal vasectomy is still in its feasibility phase and most of the available studies were performed in experimental models. Our personal experience confirms the good results reported in Literature in terms of patent anastomoses rate and mean sperm count and pregnancy rate in compari-son with the current gold standard treatment represented by microsurgical-assisted techniques.

Potential drawbacks to use a robot for reversal of vasectomy are the suboptimal instrumentation available, not designed for microsurgery, and the lack of tactile feedback. Another critical issue could be represented by the costs of the procedure. However, it is clear that RAVV must be considered an optional procedure to per-form only in centers performing routinely robotic surgery. We believe that the con-tribution of the robotic surgery to the microsurgical technique has the potential for a more profound impact.

Five-Year View

Robot-assisted vasovasostomy is a promising and attractive alternative to the micro-surgical reversal vasectomy procedures. In the next years, this technique must reach a more acceptable level of evidence to justify its use. Only seven records are retrieved when we perform a Medline database search using as search terms *vasovasostomy* and *robot*. This shows this procedure is in its infancy or feasibility step. The wide diffusion in the United States and Europe of the da Vinci device allows us to believe that in the next years also the RAVV will be performed in an increasing number of cases and urologic centers. Further studies with adequate sample size and longer follow-up are needed to assess the clinical impact of the robotic surgery in the reversal vasectomy. Parallel, it would be useful that Intuitive Surgical Systems provides more dedicated instruments to further improve the clinical results.

Key Issues

- Conventional microscope-assisted reversal vasectomy (MAVV) (vasovasostomy and vasoepididymostomy) is a technically difficult procedure that is most successful in the hands of well-trained microsurgeons.
- Robot-assisted vasovasostomy (RAVV) is an attractive and promising procedure alternative to traditional microscopic techniques.
- Data of literature coming from few experimental studies performed in animal models and preliminary human clinical studies.
- In the last decade, the feasibility of robot-assisted vasovasostomy becomes more realistic.
- Preliminary results showed that RAVV is associated with low complications, high patent anastomosis rate, and good pregnancy rate in comparison with MAVV.
- The training period is probably shorter than traditional microscopic techniques, and benefits achieved with the surgical robot were acquired with a short learning curve.
- Further studies with adequate sample size and longer follow-up are needed to assess the clinical impact of the robotic surgery in the reversal vasectomy.

References

1. Sandlow JI, Nagler HM. Vasectomy and vasectomy reversal: important issues. Urol Clin North Am. 2009;36(3):xiii–xiv.
2. Jequier AM. Edward Martin (1859–1938). The founding father of modern clinical andrology. Int J Androl. 1991;14(1):1–10.
3. Belker AM, Thomas Jr AJ, Fuchs EF, et al. Results of 1469 microsurgical vasectomy reversals by the Vasovasostomy Study Group. J Urol. 1991;145:505.
4. Yarbro ES, Howards SS. Vasovasostomy. Urol Clin North Am. 1987;14(3):515–26.

5. Meacham RB, Niederberger CS. Use of a moderated international Internet information exchange in the study of male reproduction. Urology. 1996;48(1):3–6.
6. Thomas Jr AJ, Pontes JE, Buddhdev H, Pierce Jr JM. Vasovasostomy: evaluation of four surgical techniques. Fertil Steril. 1979;32(3):324–8.
7. Fuse H, Kimura H, Katayama T. Modified one-layer microsurgical vasovasostomy in vasectomized patiens. Int Urol Nephrol. 1995;27(4):451–6.
8. Fischer MA, Grantmyre JE. Comparison of modified one- and two-layer microsurgical vasovasostomy. BJU Int. 2000;85(9):1085–8.
9. Goldstein M, Li PS, Matthews GJ. Microsurgical vasovasostomy: the microdot technique of precision suture placement. J Urol. 1998;159(1):188–90.
10. Rothman I, Berger RE, Cummings P, et al. Randomized clinical trial of an absorbable stent for vasectomy reversal. J Urol. 1997;157(5):1697–700.
11. Hendry WF. Vasectomy and vasectomy reversal. Br J Urol. 1994;73(4):337–44.
12. Fleming C. Robot-assisted vasovasostomy. Urol Clin North Am. 2004;31:769–72.
13. Kuang W, Shin PR, Matin S, et al. Initial evaluation of robotic technology for microsurgical vasovasostomy. J Urol. 2004;171(1):300–3.
14. Kuang W, Shin PR, Oder M, et al. Robotic assisted vasovasostomy: a two-layer technique in an animal model. J Urol. 2005;65(4):811–4.
15. Schiff J, Li PS, Goldstein M. Robotic microsurgical vasovasostomy and vasoepididymostomy: a prospective randomized study in a rat model. J Urol. 2004;171:1720.
16. Parekattil SJ, Atalah HN, Cohen MS. Video technique for human robot-assisted microsurgical vasovasostomy. J Endourol. 2010;24(4):511–4.
17. De Boccard G-A. Robotic vasectomy reversal, video, posted YouTube. 25 Oct 2009. http://www.youtube.com/watch?v=4zHRyFHC7nE.
18. De Boccard G-A, Mottrie A. Robotic surgery in male infertility. In: Robotics in genitourinary surgery, vol. 7. New York: Springer; 2011. p. 617–23.

Further Reading

Boorjian S, Lipkin M, Goldstein M. The impact of obstructive interval and sperm granuloma on outcome of vasectomy reversal. J Urol. 2004;171:304–6.
Carbone Jr DJ, Shah A, Thomas Jr AJ, et al. Partial obstruction, not antisperm antibodies, causing infertility after vasovasostomy. J Urol. 1998;159:827–30.
Centers for Disease Control and Prevention. National summary and fertility clinic reports. www.cdc.gov/ART. Accessed 1 June 2011.
Chan PT, Goldstein M. Superior outcomes of microsurgical vasectomy reversal in men with the same female partners. Fertil Steril. 2004;81:1371–4.
Hinz S, Rais-Bahrami S, Kempkensteffen C, et al. Fertility rates following vasectomy reversal: importance of age of the female partner. Urol Int. 2008;81:416–20.
Kim HH, Goldstein M. History of vasectomy reversal. Urol Clin North Am. 2009;36:359–73.
Kolettis PN. Is physical examination useful in predicting epididymal obstruction? Urology. 2001;57:1138–40.
Meinertz H, Linnet L, Fogh-Andersen P, et al. Antisperm antibodies and fertility after vasovasostomy: a follow-up study of 216 men. Fertil Steril. 1990;64:315–8.
Parekattil SJ, Kuang W, Kolettis PN, et al. Multi-institutional validation of vasectomy reversal predictor. J Urol. 2006;175:247–9.
Potts JM, Pasqualotto FF, Nelson D, Thomas AJ, Agarwal A. Patient characteristics associated with vasectomy reversal. J Urol. 1999;161:1835–9.

Chapter 15
Robotic-Assisted Varicocelectomy

Tung Shu and Run Wang

A varicocele is defined as a meshwork of distended blood vessels in the scrotum. It is usually left-sided resulting from the dilatation of the spermatic veins or pampiniform plexus. It is currently the most common surgically correctable finding identified in men being evaluated for infertility and is observed in 8–16.2% of the normal male population and in 21–39% of infertile men [1, 2].

Several theories have been proposed to explain the observed pathophysiology of varicoceles. Semen quality uniformly declines in animals with induced varicoceles, even when there is only a left varicocele. The reduction in scrotal temperature after varicocele ligation supports a causative role of increased temperature on the infertility produced by varicocele. It has been hypothesized that varicoceles cause hypoxia, which might play a role in altering spermatogenesis in the varicocele patients [3]. A higher frequency of sperm cells with fragmented DNA has been reported in the ejaculate of subjects with varicocele, in comparison with fertile donors, a phenomenon that might be correlated with an increase in reactive oxygen species [4].

Numerous studies have reported the significant benefits on semen parameters with surgical treatment of varicocele [4–8]. Currently, there are several surgical approaches available for the treatment of varicocele [9–12], including the retroperitoneal approach, (high ligation via open, laparoscopic, retroperitoneoscopic, single-incision laparoscopic, or robotic-assisted), the inguinal approach (open), and the subinguinal approach (open microscopic). Of these approaches, the subinguinal microscopic

T. Shu, MD (✉)
Department of Urology, Baylor College of Medicine,
Center for Kidney Health at the Vanguard Urologic Institute,
6400 Fannin, Suite 2300, Houston, TX 77030, USA
e-mail: tung.shu@vanguardurology.com

R. Wang, MD, FACS
Department of Urology, University of Texas Medical School at Houston,
6431 Fannin Street, MSB 6.018, Houston, TX 77030, USA

MD Anderson Cancer Center, Houston, TX, USA
e-mail: run.wang@uth.tmc.edu, runwang@mdanderson.org

S.J. Parekattil, A. Agarwal (eds.), *Male Infertility for the Clinician*,
© Springer Science+Business Media New York 2013

approach offers the best outcomes, including shorter hospital stays, preservation of the testicular arteries and lymphatics, least number of postoperative complications, recurrence, and a higher number of pregnancies [2, 12]. The microscopic assistance, however, takes longer time to perform due to surgeons who are unaccustomed to use microinstruments, two-dimensional vision, and inability to see their own hands.

The da Vinci® Surgical System has helped surgeons overcome the limitations for both traditional open and conventional minimally invasive surgeries. With miniaturized wristed instruments, 3D camera, and computer technologies, the da Vinci® Surgical System filters and translates surgeon's hand movements seamlessly into precise micromovements of the da Vinci instruments. With added experience from using the da Vinci® Surgical System, dramatic improvements in tissue handling, time, and skill can be achieved [13, 14]. With preliminary experience, we have used the da Vinci® Surgical System to perform robotic-assisted subinguinal varicocelectomy in comparison to the standard microscopic approach for the treatment of varicocele [15].

Materials and Methods

Eight patients aged 29.1 ± 12.5 years underwent microscopic subinguinal varicocelectomies: seven patients with left-sided repair and one patient with bilateral repair. Eight patients aged 22.0 ± 8.0 years underwent robot-assisted varicocelectomies: seven patients with left-sided repair and one patient with bilateral repair.

All varicocelectomies were performed through inguinal incisions (Fig. 15.1a). The spermatic cord was exposed and delivered out of the wound with a Penrose drain placed underneath the cord structures (Fig. 15.1b). At this time, the da Vinci® Surgical System or operating microscope was brought in and placed above the surgical field (Fig. 15.1c). The testicular artery and vas deferens with vassal artery and small vassal veins were identified and isolated (Fig. 15.1d). Other veins within the cord were isolated (Fig. 15.1e) and ligated with 5-0 Vicryl sutures and divided (Fig. 15.1f). At the completion of the varicocelectomy, only the testicular artery, lymphatics, and vas deferens with its vessels remained.

Results

The average operative time for the microscopic subinguinal varicocelectomy was 73.9 ± 12.2 min, whereas the robotic-assisted approach took 71.1 ± 21.1 min. Average follow-up time for the patients in the microscopic group was 34.3 ± 6.4 months, whereas the robotic-assisted group was 10.9 ± 7.1 months (Table 15.1).

In our experience, there was no difficulty in identifying and isolating vessels and the vas deferens with the robotic-assisted approach. A short learning curve for tying with 5-0 sutures was required because of the lack of tactile sensation when using the

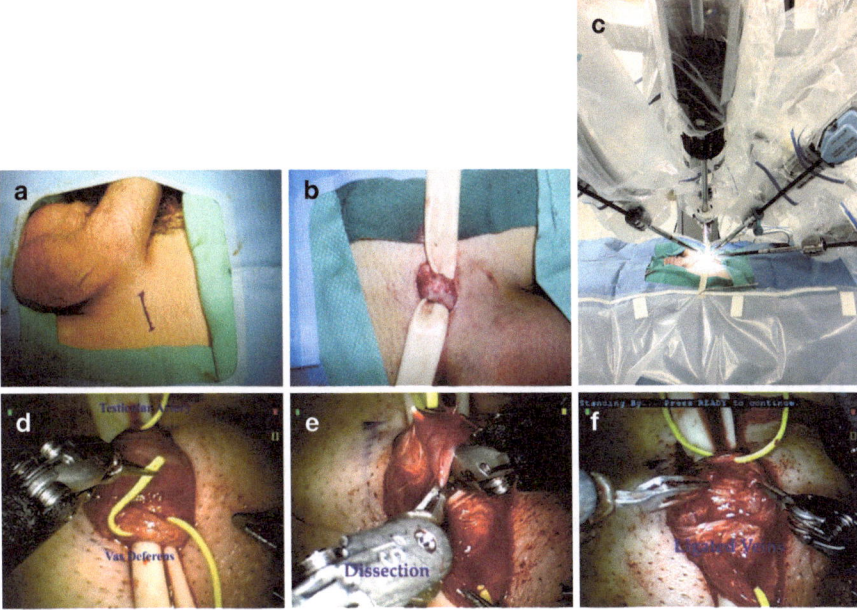

Fig. 15.1 (**a**) Subinguinal incision, (**b**) spermatic cord exposure, (**c**) da Vinci robot set up, (**d**) testicular artery and vas deferens isolation, (**e**) spermatic vein isolation, (**f**) spermatic vein ligated and divided

Table 15.1 Data of microscopic and robot-assisted varicocelectomies

	Age (years)	Average operative time (min)	Follow-up time (months)
Microscopic technique 8 patients, 9 varicocelectomies	29.1 ± 12.5	73.9 ± 12.2	34.3 ± 6.4
Robot-assisted technique 8 patients, 9 varicocelectomies	22.0 ± 8.0	71.1 ± 21.1	10.9 ± 7.1

da Vinci® Surgical System. Patients in both groups were able to resume daily activities on the day of surgery and full activities within 2 weeks. There was no intraoperative or postoperative complication. No recurrence of varicocele was observed in either group of patients.

Expert Commentary

In 2006, we perform the first robotic-assisted subinguinal varicocelectomy using the da Vinci® Surgical System [15]. From our continuing experience, we believe that the robotic-assisted varicocelectomy can be safely and effectively performed when compared to traditional microscopic approach. There was not a significant difference with regards to operative time; however, with increased experience with the da Vinci® Surgical System, the time should decrease. When compared to the microscopic approach, the tremor is completely eliminated with the robot. More importantly, the advantage of decreased intraoperative and postoperative complications experienced with microsurgical approach is maintained with the robotic approach.

We are currently studying the cost-effectiveness and efficacy with regard to the improvement of semen quality and pregnancy for patients with infertility with our described robotic-assisted subinguinal varicocelectomy.

Five-Year View

Given the advantages of decreased hand tremor, scaling of motion, and enhanced magnification, robotic assistance for microsurgical procedures appears to be a natural advantage for microsurgeons. This is yet to be proven, but as the technology improves and more surgeons adapt these techniques, this evidence is likely to be forthcoming.

Key Issues

- The subinguinal microscopic approach offers the best outcomes, including shorter hospital stays, preservation of the testicular arteries and lymphatics, least number of postoperative complications, recurrence, and a higher number of pregnancies [2, 12].
- Robotic assistance provides the microsurgeon with advantages in terms of decreased hand tremor, scaling of motion, and enhanced magnification.
- The average operative time for the microscopic subinguinal varicocelectomy was 73.9 ± 12.2 min, whereas the robotic-assisted approach took 71.1 ± 21.1 min.
- When compared to the microscopic approach, the tremor is completely eliminated with the robot. More importantly, the advantage of decreased intraoperative and postoperative complications experienced with microsurgical approach is maintained with the robotic approach.

References

1. Jarow JP. Effects of varicocele on male fertility. Hum Reprod Update. 2001;7:59–64.
2. Watanabe M, Nagai A, Kusumi N, Tusboi H, Nasu Y, Kumon H. Minimal invasiveness and effectivity of subinguinal microscopic varicocelectomy: a comparative study with retroperitoneal high and laparoscopic approaches. Int J Urol. 2005;12:892–8.

3. Pasqualotto FF, Sobreiro BP, Hallak J, Pasqualotto EB, Lucon AM. Induction of spermatogenesis in azoospermic men after varicocelectomy repair: an update. Fertil Steril. 2006;85:635–9.
4. Enciso M, Muriel L, Fernandez J, Goyanes V, Segrelles E, Marcos M, et al. Infertile men with varicocele show a high relative proportion of sperm cells with intense nuclear damage level, evidenced by the sperm chromatin dispersion test. J Androl. 2006;27:106–11.
5. Daitch J, Bedaiwy M, Pasqualatto E, Hendin B, Hallak J, Falcone T, et al. Varicocelectomy improves intrauterine insemination success rates in men with varicocele. J Urol. 2001;165:1510–3.
6. Lee JS, Park HJ, Seo JT. What is the indication of varicocelectomy in men with nonobstructive azoospermia? Urology. 2007;69:352–5.
7. Zucchi A, Mearini L, Mearini E, Fioretti F, Bini V, Poreno M. Varicocele and fertility: relationship between testicular volume and seminal parameters before and after treatment. J Androl. 2006;27:548–51.
8. Gat Y, Zukerman Z, Chakraborty J, Gornish M. Varicocele, hypoxia and male infertility. Fluid mechanics analysis of the impaired testicular venous drainage system. Hum Reprod. 2005;20:2614–9.
9. Palomo A. Radical cure of varicocele by a new technique: preliminary report. J Urol. 1949;152:1127–32.
10. Belloli G, D'Agostino S, Zen F, Loverno E. Fertility rates after successful correction of varicocele in adolescence and adulthood. Eur J Pediatr Surg. 1995;5:216–8.
11. Kaouk JH, Palmer JS. Single-port laparoscopic surgery: initial experience in children for varicocelectomy. BJU Int. 2008;102:97–9.
12. Al-Kandari AM, Shabaan H, Ibrahim HM, Elshebiny YH, Shokeir AA. Comparison of outcomes of different varicocelectomy techniques: open inguinal, laparoscopic, and subinguinal micro-scopic varicocelectomy: a randomized clinical trial. Urology. 2007;69:417–20.
13. Nguyen MM, Das S. The evolution or robotic urologic surgery. Urol Clin North Am. 2004;31:653–8.
14. Corcione F, Esposito C, Cuccurullo D, Settembre A, Miranda N, Amato F, et al. Advantages and limits of robot-assisted laparoscopic surgery: preliminary experience. Surg Endosc. 2005;19:117–9.
15. Shu T, Taghechian S, Wang R. Initial experience with robot-assisted varicocelectomy. Asian J Androl [serial online]. 2008;10(1):146–8.

Chapter 16
Ethical Considerations in Male Infertility

Marc S. Cohen and Ray E. Moseley

In recent years, the progression of medical science has led to what used to be extremely rare ethical problems on the cutting edge of urological management of male infertility to become a more routine part of urological practice. These ethical problems, even though they have become more common in urological practice, still cause significant issues for the physician. In this chapter we discuss four cases that illustrate the ethical problems associated with identification and framing of the ethical problem, analysis of the problem, and the resolution of the problem. The basic purpose of these case discussions is that it is much easier to avoid and/or satisfactorily resolve an ethical problem when it is recognized early before a crisis mode arises or before poor ethical decisions are made and have to be unraveled after the fact. These cases represent four possible scenarios but are by no means exhaustive of the possible ethical issues that may arise from the current urological practice.

Physicians are traditionally trained to find and fix problems. Ethical dilemmas are not so directly rectified. It is hoped that by posing the following case scenarios and suggesting the various ethical subtleties and concerns, physicians will begin to appreciate the spectrum of responses that each scenario contains. By appreciating these subtleties, it is hoped that physicians and nonphysicians will appreciate the complex tapestry that each poses and the value of considering these dilemmas and solutions before such events occur. What follows, therefore, is not a set of fixed answers for those particular cases as no single answer or combinations of responses exists. Rather, we hope this chapter will provide a framework for consideration of these and similar scenarios. As opposed to dealing with clinical pathology, there is

M.S. Cohen, MD (✉)
Department of Urology, Shands at the University of Florida,
1600 SW Archer Boulevard, Box 100247 HSC, Gainesville, FL 32610, USA
e-mail: cohenms@urology.ufl.edu, marc.cohen@urology.ufl.edu

R.E. Moseley, PhD
Department of Community Health and Family Medicine,
University of Florida Health Science Center,
Box 100237, Gainesville, FL 100234, USA

S.J. Parekattil, A. Agarwal (eds.), *Male Infertility for the Clinician*,
© Springer Science+Business Media New York 2013

no true "standard of care" other than to do the right thing, which may, depending on the situation, be a matter of conjecture and prospective. The physician must now consider not just a disease but the unique environment and circumstances superimposed on this disease. To the end, institutional policies may exist (or be created) to address issues that are controversial.

One of the particular and frequent recurring themes in these scenarios is the need to recognize and reflect not only on the disease and the patient but also the need to address the spectrum and mores of the family and society. In doing so, the focus of the physician must frequently shift from the effect of the disease on the patient to the effect on the family.

Case Studies

Case 1

A 11-year-old male patient recently diagnosed with leukemia is to be started on chemotherapy shortly. The parents are interested in fertility preservation for their child. At this point, there is no data on human spermatogonia being matured to produce mature sperm. There have been some animal studies that have done this in a lab setting (in vitro), which indicate that this might be possible. There are no established guidelines on the cryopreservation of testicular tissue and spermatogonia in prepubertal males for future fertility preservation. However, the technology is advancing at a pace such that this may be possible in the near future.

Analysis

The major ethical issue facing the urologist is "Should the urologist honor the wishes of the parents and cryopreserve this tissue in preparation for the possible future ability of the 11-year-old patient to use it to produce offspring?" If the answer is "yes" then there are several procedural/ethical issues that will arise. These include: What is the appropriate role of the 11-year-old patient in this decision? and Should "assent" by the patient be required before this procedure is undertaken.

In analyzing the first ethical issues, the urologist must first determine if this procedure is in the appropriate scope of medical practice. In other words, would the results of this procedure, i.e., cryopreservation, storage conditions and options, and the future medical use of this tissue have a reasonable chance of actually being able to be used to produce future offspring? This entails both a practice issue, since physicians should not ethically or professionally engage in medical procedures that offer no reasonable chance of success and an informed consent issue, since any appropriate informed consent should detail the chance of success for a procedure and help the decision makers evaluate the options. Many physicians and medical ethicists would argue that this type of procedure at this early stage of development should not be offered outside of an approved research trial or without the prerequisite scientific studies validating the safety and efficacy of this type of procedure in producing future offspring [1]. Another powerful argument to consider is that this will be a very expensive procedure with long-term storage costs and will be made by parents who are under significant stress of caring for their very ill child, who may be inappropriately swayed by guilt or manipulated by for profit cryopreservation businesses.

A more straightforward ethical issue is whether or not the patient should be asked, whether he agrees or "assents" to having the procedure, and whether this should be encouraged or required. Assent is the concept that persons with diminished capacity who may not fully understand all of the relevant information about a medical procedure should still be asked if they wish to participate in the medical procedure and should agree to participation. The determining factor is the level of capacity and understanding of the child. The literature on child assent (mostly involving the issue of assent to participate in medical research) suggests that a relatively mature 11-year-old should be asked for agreement [2]. This, however, would involve a relatively in-depth discussion to assess the child's capacity and agreement by the parents. What is clear is that as the child matures, assuming that the treatment for the leukemia is successful, he should at the minimum be informed of this cryopreserved tissue, and he should eventually become the decision maker over the use of this tissue, and when he reaches 18 will have the legal authority to decide what to do with the tissue.

There are additional ethical issues related to this case. These include: Whether this procedure is an appropriate allocation of medical resources?, Who owns this tissue?, and Whether it is ethically permissible to use the tissue in the event the patient dies from the leukemia? This second set of ethical issues are certainly not separate from health policy issues and legal issues, and they clearly are not just decisions that should be made by the individual physician on a case-by-case basis. The danger for the individual urologist facing this case would be, if he or she were to unduly influence the decision based on their own personal views, of whether this is an appropriate allocation of general medical resources. This would run the risk of violating the formal principle of justice of treating similar cases in a similar manner, since different urologists would have widely divergent views on this aspect and there is no clear professional or ethical policy that was enlightened by transparent and open debate.

Case 2

A 26-year-old man, recently engaged, has met brain death criteria and has now been pronounced dead after a severe MVA. His parents and fiancée want to cryopreserve his testicular tissue and sperm so that the fiancée can eventually have his children.

Analysis

The major ethical issue is "Whether the parents and/or the fiancée have the right to either make this decision to cryopreserve his testicular tissue and sperm, and/or to speak for their dead loved one, if they believe that this is what he would want?" In analyzing this issue, the urologist should consider a number of subquestions that should have bearing on the ethical resolution of this issue. For example, it would be nice to know what the recently deceased person thought about this issue. Admittedly, it is unlikely that a 26-year old would have given much thought to this issue; however, he may have expressed values and views which may be related and would give some insight on what he would want. For example, the range of things this deceased person may have believed or done could include previously expressed his wishes on this subject. Who knows for sure if he had seen a television show that discussed this very issue. He may have clearly expressed his desire to have children some day, or he may have expressed his wishes in writing given that more and more persons are writing Living Wills with specific wishes detailed. He may also have expressed the views that having a family and/or passing on his family name was extremely important to him.

The answers to these questions could certainly make us more confident (or less confident) that the deceased would actually want to have his tissue harvested and cryopreserved; however, this would not necessarily help in the resolution of this issue unless we hold the position that the dead have any rights at all, and if next of kin and loved ones have the moral authority to make these decisions. Traditionally, next of kin make burial decisions and help make sure that a dead person's estate is fairly distributed to survivors according to the deceased wishes. However, harvesting this type of tissue for this purpose seems pretty far afield from these traditional and established roles of family and loved ones.

There are also a number of possible scenarios that could follow from such a decision that involve both legal and ethical issues. Who does the sperm belong to—parents, fiancée, or both? Does the one who pays for the cryopreservation have any bearing on this? If the fiancée marries someone does she lose authority over the cryopreserved sperm? Do any children who are produced from this sperm have a claim on the estate of the "father"?

From the perspective of the urologist, this decision should require some careful thought and a lot of information for the decision makers. The general ethical principle involved in this type of case is that a person, and in this case a dead person, should generally not be used as a means to some end especially if the person does not or has not agreed to this use. In this case, the deceased person's sperm should not be used to produce a child that he may or may not have wanted to produce. It would seem at minimum that there should be some pretty good indications that the deceased person would have wanted this cryopreservation in this type of situation, before cryopreservation is undertaken.

This case illustrates a highly complex ethical decision superimposed on a highly time-sensitive issue. There are truly no right answers to the acute emotional issues it poses. What it does demonstrate is the need to seriously consider the "what if…"

issues, inevitably, of these unnerving acute episodes. Because of the inevitable nature of such events an institutional policy is a recommended suggestion. That being said, these policies tend to be a legal defense mechanism, founded in the environment of litigious society that without emotion gives the physician the protection from having to make a decision usually based on a family member's or romantic partner's opinion of the patient's unexpressed and undocumented thoughts of their own personal legacy. These policies are frequently a way for obvious (and perhaps legally appropriate) reasons "wash its hands" of responsibility.

Case 3

A 19-year-old White man with attention deficit disorder schedules an appointment to discuss elective vasectomy. The patient is a junior in college. He visits you on one occasion accompanied by his mother. At the time of the original visit where he was accompanied by his mother, the patient notes that he has no physical problems. The patient states that he is in love with his fiancée and they both have agreed that they do not want children as a couple. That patient's mother is upset by the idea of a vasectomy and hoping that you will convince the patient otherwise. The patient claims that he is "sure" that he does not want to have children under alternative circumstances. The visit by the patient and his fiancée reveals a very upset 18-year-old woman who has been intolerant to birth control pills and hormone implants. She is not willing to use condoms, foam, or diaphragm, because of concerns related to efficiency. The fiancée feels that vasectomy would offer better efficiency and would represent less of a surgical risk as compared to tubal ligation. The patient wishes to support his fiancée in this decision.

Analysis

This case illustrates the importance of communication that inevitably exists in fertility issues. As has been previously suggested, physician training is founded in identifying and fixing problems. When superimposed onto a hostile environment a patient or partner in distress may be seen as a stereotype of that environment; in other words, the patient may be seen as the problem, rather than an unfortunate victim. When so perceived and inappropriately managed, the outcomes can be disastrous.

Approaching such scenarios requires the physician to reorder his or her priorities. Rather than focusing on "finding the problem" a more useful approach in these types of cases may be as Stephen Covey ("Seven Habits of Highly Effective People") suggests, "Seek first to understand, then to be understood" [3]. As suggested by a number of patient-centered interview processes, it is important to acknowledge the emotional aspects of this volatile situation of the client and the physician and seek first to find meaning (if possible) for both. Fortunately, as compared to Case 2, the only time restraints superimposed here are self-imposed. There is time to address these issues if the physician chooses to do so. Recognizing and acknowledging the emotional aspects of these encounters can be equally important being able to recognize and call upon external support can be of the utmost importance (e.g., in this instance Planned Parenthood Organizations) can provide additional support.

Should the physician honor the patient's request for a vasectomy? Is this request "outside" of the range of reasonable medical alternatives for the patient's situation? A cornerstone of modern medical ethics is that adult competent patients generally, and except in very rare circumstances, have an unrestricted right to choose between medical procedures that are viable and appropriate medical alternatives for a legitimate medical need. This presumes that the patient receives information about the acceptable medical alternatives, understands those alternatives, and can make a free and uncoerced decision.

The first thing the physician must decide is whether the patient is requesting a medical procedure that is not just technically possible but that is also one of the appropriate medical alternatives for the patient's medical situation. Although most physicians would probably not recommend the requested intervention as the first choice, it does appear to be in the range of possible alternatives. The contraindications for the procedure all appear to be social concerns and not strictly medical concerns. Even though the patient is an adult he is only 19 years old, and persons of that age commonly change their minds about issues such as marriage and family. The significance of this concern is magnified since the results of the procedure are difficult if not impossible to reverse. For this reason alone, extra care and time should be taken with the patient to insure that this is the best alternative and that he carefully considers the alternatives and long-term consequences.

An additional feature of this case that adds to the ethical difficulty is that the patient seems to be making a choice of medical interventions based, not on a direct medical need, but mainly on the medical issues and personal preferences of his partner. For this reason, in some real sense both involved individuals are patients. Although the fiancée was present during one visit, it is not clear that this would constitute a through workup or exploration of her contraception concerns. This issue should be thoroughly explored by the physician (namely that his fiancée has received a through medical workup of her medical issues). For example, it is far from clear that this couple understands the data on the effectiveness of birth control pills when used correctly.

Additionally, in this case the physician should be concerned about whether the patient really understands the ramifications of choosing this medical procedure as a solution to his problem, and whether the patient is making a free and uncoerced decision. This patient is clearly under significant and conflicting pressure from both his mother and his fiancée, and this conflict alone should lead to the physician offering advice to not rush into this procedure. A valid informed consent requires not just that the appropriate information is given to the patient but also that the patient understands the information and that the patient's decision is not coerced [4].

So what can the physician do to be reassured that the patient really understands the requested procedure and that the patient is not being somehow forced into this decision? The first thing to note is that this is not an emergency situation, and that the patient should be given adequate time to thoroughly consider this decision. Secondly, the patient should be informed about how many people change their minds about desiring family and the chances of a successful vasectomy reversal in that event [5]. Also, the physician should probably discuss and consider recommending the possible cryopreservation of the patient's sperm.

Case 4

A 30-year-old "mentally challenged" man is brought to your office by his mother. The patient has been known to be sexually active and his mother, who is his legal guardian, has been concerned that this may result in an unwanted child. The patient has limited understanding secondary to his mental state; however, the patient does seem to understand that this would mean he would not be able to have children, but he voices no objections. You want to help the family, but have concerns regarding your ethical/legal positions regarding a request by the mother to perform a vasectomy.

Analysis

This case raises a number of significant ethical and legal concerns. Before any of the ethical and legal issues can even be framed and addressed additional medical information is required. Exactly what is the mental status of the 30-year-old patient? What is the nature of the "known sexual activity?" What are the risks of pregnancy and are there less restrictive and permanent ways to achieve birth control? The answer to these questions will frame the appropriate ethical questions and possible resolutions.

For this case, we will presume that this patient lives in a group facility for persons with a similar mental disability. We will also presume that this is a well-run and appropriate structured environment. However, even in the safest facility it is possible and even likely that sexual activity will occur between residents of this facility. It should be noted that, if the sexual activity is between staff or other nonresidents and the patient, it raises additional serious legal and ethical concerns that should be reported to the proper authorities. In a similar manner, if the patient lives alone or at home with his mother, this possible sexual activity raises the possibility of important safety and supervision concerns, which would need to be in turn explored by the physician or possibly referred to appropriate state agencies.

Before considering whether to proceed, with even considering a permanent surgical procedure, the relative risk of the patient having a child should be evaluated. If our presumed scenario is accurate, it would be relevant to know if the sexual activity and a possible resulting child was just a potential fear of the mother or if there was ongoing sexual activity. It should be noted that it is not uncommon for people with mental disability to be in long-term relationships with fellow facility residents. If, for example, this was the case, then it would be important to know if the patient's significant other could even become pregnant.

Should a parent be able to consent to sterilization of a mentally incompetent adult child? In most states, legal guardians for those who have mental disabilities have the legal authority to make these types of medical decisions [6]. However, it should be noted that these decisions are often controversial and some types of decisions have been challenged by disability rights advocates [7]. The important question for the physician involved in this type of case is, what is the potential for abuse? For example, is this procedure being for the convenience of the mother/guardian, or so that the facility does not need to so closely monitor the activities of residents? As opposed to what is in the best interest of the resident, or simply because of some misguided social Darwinian bias? We would suggest that any physician who is asked to participate in this type of permanent medical procedure should seek guidance and support by consulting with a second physician, and considering requesting judicial or ethics committee review. As an additional safeguard, we would suggest that the physician make every effort if possible to seek assent from the patient prior to any medical procedure.

Expert Commentary

We have tried to illustrate through the use of four clinical scenarios some of the ethical dilemmas that may arise as part of the day-to-day interactions involving male patients with infertility-/fertility-related issues. These cases, by necessity are meant to be thought productive but not all inclusive. The basic, key steps to approaching these problems are as follows in Sect. 16.4.

Five-Year View

As stated in the beginning of this chapter, what used to be rare has become commonplace and routine. This text itself is a testament to the rapid advancement in our understanding of male infertility and the exponential technological changes that have taken place to meet the challenges posed; it is intuitive that these advances are only the beginning. As these technologies continue to "push the envelope" over the ensuing 5 years, it is also understood that the ethical dilemmas will continue to increase.

Key Issues

General Steps to Resolving Ethical Problems

1. Identify the ethical problem both in terms of the decisions to be made and the conflicting values present in the case.

2. *Critically* analyze the reasons for and against the various possible courses of action, paying special attention not to overstate or understate the reasons.
3. Clearly state the resolution or the range of acceptable options, both in terms of the decision to be made and of the prevailing supporting values.

Potential Mistakes to Avoid

1. Using value-laden language in both the description of the ethical problem and the analysis, thus introducing unacknowledged bias.
2. Not adequately taking into account long-term consequences when analyzing the various courses of actions.
3. Failure to verify facts or to recognize crucial lack of factual information, thus making unsupported assumptions.

References

1. Neal MS, Nagel K, Duckworth J, Bissessar H, Fischer MA, Portwine C, Tozer R, Barr RD. Effectiveness of sperm banking in adolescents and young adults with cancer: a regional experience. Cancer. 2007;110:1125–30.
2. Miller VA, Drotar D, Kodish E. Children's competence for assent and consent: a review of empirical findings. Ethics Behav. 2004;14:255–96.
3. Covey Stephen R. The seven habits of highly effective people: powerful lessons in personal change. New York: Simon and Schuster Inc.; 1990. p. 237.
4. Goldstein MM. Health information technology and the idea of informed consent. J Law Med Ethics. 2010;38:27–36.
5. Howard G. Who asks for vasectomy reversal and why? Br Med J (Clin Res Ed). 1982;285:490–3.
6. Lachance D. In re Grady: the mentally retarded individual's right to choose sterilization. Am J Law Med. 1981;6:559–91.
7. Zuba-Ruggieri R. Making links, making connections: internet resources for self-advocates and people with developmental disabilities. Intellect Dev Disabil. 2007;45:209–16.

Chapter 17
Management of Fertility in Male Cancer Patients

Daniel H. Williams IV

Cancer survival rates have improved dramatically over the last couple of decades due to advances in diagnostic techniques and therapies [1–3]. Roughly 15% of cases of newly diagnosed cancer in men are in those younger than 55 years of age, and about one quarter of them are younger than age 20 [4]. Consequently, the population of young cancer survivors has grown, and the focus of cancer treatments has shifted from one of survival alone to that of survival *and* quality of life after treatment.

For many men and their families, the maintenance and preservation of fertility during and after treatment is important [5–11]. However, antineoplastic agents, radiation, and surgical therapies can all pose significant threats to a man's fertility potential, as can the presence of cancer itself. Male infertility due to cancer treatments may be temporary or permanent and can range from mild to severe. Because it is difficult—if not impossible—to predict the exact impact of cancer therapy on an individual man's ability to father a biological child, sperm cryopreservation *prior* to therapy remains the cornerstone of fertility preservation in this patient population [12–20]. Unfortunately, in many cases, sperm cryopreservation remains underutilized [6–9]. When sperm has not been banked prior to treatment and when men are azoospermic by their cancer treatment, surgical sperm retrieval in conjunction with advanced reproductive technologies (ART) is offered.

D.H. Williams IV, MD
Department of Urology, University of Wisconsin Hospital and Clinics,
1685 Highland Avenue, Madison, WI 53719, USA
e-mail: williams@urology.wisc.edu

S.J. Parekattil, A. Agarwal (eds.), *Male Infertility for the Clinician*,
© Springer Science+Business Media New York 2013

Effects of Cancer on Male Fertility

The causes of poor semen quality in patients with cancer are not well understood, and multiple factors are likely involved. Some of these factors include preexisting defects in germ cells, local tumor effects, endocrine disturbances, and autoimmune and systemic effects of cancer [21–24].

A number of studies report that cancer adversely affects semen quality. However, published results of large studies are conflicting. Some suggest that cancer adversely affects semen quality [14, 25, 26], while others have found no differences between semen analyses of men with and without cancer [27]. Additionally, some studies suggest that the type of malignancy impacts semen quality [14, 28–30] whereas others do not [31, 32].

Ragni et al. reported that 11.6% of men who wished to cryopreserve sperm at their institution were azoospermic [28]. This ranged from 3.9% of men with non-Hodgkin's lymphoma to 15.3% of men with testicular tumors. Lass et al. reported that 10.5% of untreated men were azoospermic including 9.6% with testicular tumors, 13.3% with leukemia or lymphoma, and 3.7% of men with other malignancies [14]. Colpi et al. reported normal semen parameters according to WHO criteria in only 40% of men with lymphoma, 37% with testicular cancer, and 37% with other tumors [26]. Men with Hodgkin's disease usually present with poor semen parameters [33, 34]. Likewise, Lass et al. reported that 50% of men with cancer who cryopreserved at their institution had fewer than ten million motile sperm per ejaculate [14]. Finally, men with testicular cancer had semen parameters that were inferior to those of normal controls [25, 30]. In contrast, Rofeim and Gilbert compared semen parameters of 214 men with a variety of cancers to 22 men without cancer and found no significant differences between the groups [27].

Some studies suggest that the type of malignancy impacts semen quality. A large study of 776 men with cancer demonstrated that sperm density was significantly reduced in men with testicular cancer but that sperm quality did not vary significantly among men with other malignancies [28]. Similarly, a study of 314 patients with cancer found that men with testicular cancer had the lowest pretreatment sperm concentrations compared to those with other malignant neoplasms [29]. A number of studies have found that men with testicular tumors had significantly lower sperm quality compared to those with hematological or other malignancies [14, 25, 30, 33, 35]. Sperm DNA integrity has also been shown to be worse in men with cancer prior to treatment compared to fertile controls [36].

However, there is also evidence to suggest that the type of malignancy does not impact semen quality. Meseguer et al. reviewed semen parameters of 184 men who banked sperm before cancer treatment and found no significant differences in total sperm counts among men with different malignancies [32]. Likewise, Chung et al. found that sperm counts and motility did not differ by type of cancer in 97 patients who froze sperm before the initiation of cancer therapy [31].

Effects of Chemotherapy on Male Fertility

Chemotherapy negatively affects spermatogenesis, either transiently or permanently [37–39]. These drugs directly damage proliferating cells, so early differentiating sperm cells are exquisitely sensitive to these agents. However, even the relatively quiescent sperm precursors can be damaged due to cumulative effects of multiple doses of chemotherapy [40]. Later-stage germ cells, namely spermatocytes and spermatids, are less sensitive to chemotherapy since they are not dividing, and this accounts for the finding of some sperm immediately following chemotherapy with a slow decline in counts over the ensuing months. Leydig cell function appears to be less effected by chemotherapy.

Improved chemotherapy regimens have resulted in lower rates of infertility; however, azoospermia after treatment continues to be a concern [41]. When men are rendered completely azoospermic after treatment, some report that only 20–50% of these men will have some recovery of spermatogenesis [42], while others report up to 80% recovery depending on the type of cancer and chemotherapeutic regimen [39].

Alkylating agents including cisplatin are widely used for testicular cancer and have a high risk of azoospermia, particularly when coupled with ifosfamide, and the risk of permanent azoospermia seems to be dose and agent dependent [26, 39, 43, 44]. Likewise, most regimens for Hodgkin's disease also put men at high risk for azoospermia [45]. The impact of newer chemotherapeutic agents like taxanes and monoclonal antibodies remains unknown [46]. Age at treatment may play a role in recovery of spermatogenesis; however, this remains unclear [47].

Efforts have been made to explore strategies that may offer protection to the germinal epithelium during cancer therapy. One such approach has been the use of luteinizing hormone-releasing hormone analogs during gonadotoxic therapies have been examined in men. While these medications held promise in some animal studies, they did not significantly protect against spermatogenic failure in humans [48, 49].

Effects of Radiation on Male Fertility

Radiation therapy negatively affects spermatogenesis, either transiently or permanently by directly inducing DNA damage [38, 50]. A number of variables can affect the deleterious effect of radiation therapy on gonadal function, including total dose, source of radiation, gonadal protection, scatter radiation, and individual susceptibility [26, 51]. Gonadal shielding should be routinely employed; however, small amounts of scatter radiation are inevitable. As little as 0.15 Gy can result in impaired sperm production [52, 53]. Doses over 0.5 Gy typically result in reversible azoospermia [38]. Semen parameters often reach their nadir 4–6 months after treatment. Doses over 2.5 Gy place men at risk for prolonged or permanent azoospermia [38, 51]. Leydig cell function is affected when doses reach >15 Gy [26, 39]. Regimens for malignancies such as testicular leukemia and for total body irradiation prior to bone marrow transplants usually result in irreversible damage to the spermatogonia and permanent sterility [44]. Newer radiotherapy strategies may result in less gonadal toxicity but results are pending.

Effects of Surgery on Male Fertility

Surgical procedures such as retroperitoneal lymph node dissection in men with testicular cancer can cause infertility as a result of ejaculatory dysfunction due to damage of the pelvic plexus [54]. Both anejaculation and retrograde may result. Modified RPLND templates have been shown to reduce the risk of ejaculatory dysfunction in these men [8, 55, 56].

While more prevalent in older men, prostate cancer may affect younger men of reproductive age. Additionally, many men are waiting until later in life to father children or begin second families. In removing an important male reproductive organ, radical prostatectomy renders these men sterile. Likewise, bilateral orchiectomy and cystectomy can put men at risk for reproductive failure. Low-anterior or abdominoperineal approaches to gastrointestinal malignancies may also put men at risk for ejaculatory failure [57].

Recovery of Spermatogenesis Following Cancer Treatment

Gonadotoxicity and testicular dysfunction are well-known side effects of cancer therapies since chemotherapy, radiotherapy, and surgery can all affect fertility potential [15, 41, 52, 58, 59]. Many men are rendered azoospermic following treatment. Spermatogenesis often returns in these men; however, the timing of the return (ranging from months to years) and the sperm quality when it returns are variable [29, 60–62]. Approximately 15–30% of childhood cancer survivors are permanently sterile following therapy [63].

A number of factors may influence the recovery of spermatogenesis following cancer therapy. In addition to the treatment regimen, the individual's pretreatment fertility potential and the influence of the cancer itself on the man's overall health can both impact posttreatment fertility [51, 64]. While the data are somewhat conflicting, certain malignancies, including testicular cancer and Hodgkin's disease, seem to influence pretreatment fecundity [14, 30].

Among testis cancer survivors, most were successful in achieving pregnancies, ranging from 71 to 82%, although successful paternity took many years in some cases and depended on the intensity of the chemo- or radiation therapy [65–67]. Men with low stage seminoma rarely become azoospermic after orchiectomy and radiation [68, 69]. High-dose testicular radiation for testicular intraepithelial neoplasia usually results in infertility [70].

Survivors of Hodgkin's lymphoma typically experience azoospermia after treatment. Depending on the chemotherapy and radiotherapy regimens, many patients recover some degree of spermatogenesis, but this may take up to 5–10 years [34, 71–73]. Non-Hodgkin's lymphoma regimens seem to be less gonadotoxic than those used to treat Hodgkin's disease [39]. Life-saving bone marrow transplantation strategies can also impair fertility, with azoospermia rates ranging from 10 to 70% depending on the agents, doses, and body irradiation templates employed [74, 75].

Men with genitourinary malignancies make up a unique subset of patients with cancer since their treatment directly and structurally impacts the male reproductive tract. Although few men undergoing prostate cancer treatment cite fertility as a concern, the prevalence of prostate cancer in young men is growing [76]. In a large review of over 14,000 men undergoing radical prostatectomy, 476 were 45 years of age or younger at the time of surgery [77]. For these men and their families, fertility needs may not yet have been met. If sperm are not cryopreserved preoperatively, testicular and/or epididymal sperm extraction, in conjunction with in vitro fertilization (IVF) and intracytoplasmic sperm injection (ICSI), is the only chance to father offspring. Regarding radiotherapy for prostate cancer, external beam therapy seems to have a greater negative impact on spermatogenesis than does brachytherapy [78, 79]. Like prostate cancer, fertility potential for most men with bladder cancer is not a significant concern due to age at diagnosis; however, young men may also develop urothelial carcinoma and elect to undergo various therapies. Smaller studies of men undergoing intravesical chemotherapy showed greater changes in semen parameters in men treated with BCG as opposed to mitomycin C [80]. A study of prostate-sparing cystectomy reported sperm in post-ejaculate urine samples [81]. Fertility following treatment of thyroid cancer with radioactive iodine is excellent; however, the treatment of pediatric sarcomas and rectal cancers results in a high rate of testicular dysfunction [82–84].

Risk of Malignancy in the Offspring of Men with Cancer

Two main concerns have been raised regarding risk of cancer in the children of cancer patients: does having cancer increase the risk of passing on this risk to one's offspring, and do cancer therapies portend any mutagenic risk? In particular, in the era of assisted reproductive technologies (ART) such as IVF/ICSI, is there any greater risk than in the past?

Prior to IVF/ICSI, studies did not demonstrate any increased risk of malignancy in the offspring of cancer survivors except in cases of known heritable diseases [85–87]. However, immediately following chemotherapy, there is a risk of sperm chromosomal abnormalities and aneuploidy which seems to lessen over time [88–92]. Chromosome analyses of testicular cancer patients after chemotherapy demonstrated no significant difference in the frequency of chromosomal abnormalities before and after therapy [93].

Semen Collection for Male Cancer Patients

Semen for sperm cryopreservation is generally obtained by masturbation. For many men, this may be an embarrassing or uncomfortable process. It is critical that men understand how to collect semen and that they be offered a private and relaxing environment to do so. Alternatively, men may collect a semen sample at home or another location than the clinic, providing that they keep the specimen at body temperature and return it to the lab within approximately 45 min to an hour after collection. Lubricants should be avoided as they can contaminate the specimens. The entire specimen should be collected, particularly in light of the fact that more sperm are present at the beginning of the ejaculate than at the end [94]. Wide-mouth specimen containers should be tested by each laboratory to ensure that they are compatible with semen collection and are not harmful to sperm.

Some men have difficulty providing semen specimens with masturbation. An alternative is to collect the sample with a condom. However, the condom must be approved by the laboratory as commercially available condoms generally contain spermicides that will kill sperm. This method typically results in fewer sperm being collected but may be necessary for some men. Additionally, anxiety, religious beliefs, pain, medications, and other factors may make semen collection challenging.

The adolescent male population is one in which extremely careful counseling and tactful, age-appropriate instructions are necessary, as these patients are at risk for emotional distress from this process. Parents should be included in discussions, although separate sessions with the adolescent are oftentimes useful. Unfortunately, no guidelines exist for the best approach to semen cryopreservation in the adolescent male, but individual institutional strategies are available [44].

At the time of diagnosis, many cancer patients are inpatients, and it may be at this time that many are first offered sperm cryopreservation. The logistics of collecting a specimen in this setting can be challenging, given the disruptions and interruptions that can occur in an inpatient room or bathroom. Additionally, some men are quite ill and debilitated by their cancer at the time of presentation and are unable to produce a sample. In these cases, surgical sperm retrieval can be offered.

Semen analyses are performed on all samples prior to cryopreservation. Semen parameters should be documented in accordance with the WHO guidelines [94]. Sometimes multiple collections are recommended depending on the number of motile sperm seen, the time since the last ejaculation, and individual variability.

Sperm Cryopreservation

The freezing of spermatozoa was first described as early as the eighteenth century, but modern techniques made cryopreservation practical and feasible in the mid-1900s with the development of sperm cryoprotectants. Today, common uses of sperm cryopreservation include banking sperm prior to vasectomy, at the time of vasectomy reversal for backup, prior to men engaging in potentially life-threatening activities (e.g., military deployment), and—pertinent to this review—prior to gonadotoxic, life-saving cancer treatments.

When semen is cryopreserved, a small aliquot of it is frozen separately, thawed, and reanalyzed after the initial freeze. This "test thaw" allows the postthaw survival to be determined as it can vary among individuals and even among different ejaculates from the same person [44]. Postthaw sperm motility is a good representation of the entire ejaculate and gives a reliable estimate of the total motile sperm count for that sample in the future [95].

While paternity with cryopreserved sperm clearly is possible, the freeze–thaw process may either negatively affect sperm quality and/or enhance any underlying sperm defects [96, 97]. Currently, sperm are kept in vials with cryoprotective agents like glycerol in combination with test yolk buffer, and these vials can be stored indefinitely in liquid nitrogen. Future techniques of dry storage may afford less damage to sperm [98].

The number of specimens that should be cryopreserved will differ for each patient. Determining factors include age, number of previous children, and semen quality. Abstinence of at least 48 h will typically maximize the yield of sperm per sample [94]. Even with time constraints and pressing health issues, men should be encouraged to consider sperm banking. Particularly in the era of ART, it is now possible to cryopreserve samples with low sperm counts that in the past were considered inadequate for freezing [13]. Poor semen quality has not been shown to affect fertilization or pregnancy rates after cryopreservation and IVF–ICSI, as long as live sperm can be recovered [99].

It has been my practice to encourage patients to initiate and complete sperm cryopreservation *before* starting any cancer therapy that affects the reproductive system. For example, in the setting of radical orchiectomy for testicular cancer, it is easier for a patient to ejaculate without a fresh inguinal incision; also, if that patient is found to have azoospermia, arrangements can be made to perform surgical sperm retrieval under the same anesthetic. If chemotherapy or radiation treatment has already been initiated, cryopreservation of semen is still possible during treatment, at least until the patient becomes azoospermic [42]. It should be noted that the effects of these gonadotoxic agents on sperm are largely unknown. Animal studies demonstrate a high incidence of mutagenic effects in offspring from matings that take place during immediately following treatment of the male with chemotherapy or radiation [100]. Increased frequency of sperm aneuploidy has also been reported after the initiation of chemotherapy and may persist up to 18 months or longer [89]. While the clinical impact of such effects in humans is unknown, sperm cryopreservation should ideally be performed before initiation of chemotherapy or radiotherapy. Otherwise, men are advised to wait 12–18 months after the completion of therapy before pursuing fertility treatments [101].

Attitudes About Sperm Banking

Over half of cancer patients desire future fertility, including over three quarters of those without children at the time of their cancer diagnosis [11, 102]. Currently, sperm banking is the only pretreatment strategy for male cancer patients to preserve their future fertility [103]. However, less than a quarter of cancer patients bank sperm, and the most common reason for not doing so is lack of information [102]. Only two-thirds of men awaiting cancer therapy are aware of sperm banking [104]. Schover et al. also showed that over 90% of responding oncologists felt that sperm banking should be offered to all men before treatment, but almost half failed to do so [105]. Reasons for this included time, high costs, and lack of convenient facilities. Only 10% claimed that they offered sperm banking to all eligible men despite evidence suggesting at least 50% of young men with cancer are interested in doing so [106].

Reebals et al. addressed oncology nurse practice issues in determining whether newly diagnosed adolescent male patients are offered the option of sperm banking before undergoing chemotherapy treatment. They distributed questionnaires to nurses and nurse practitioners who care for adolescent male cancer patients at the time of diagnosis, during chemotherapy, and during follow-up care. Over 95% of respondents agreed that all male patients undergoing cancer treatment should be offered sperm banking. Oncologists and nurse practitioners were seen as appropriate professionals to discuss this option. The authors concluded that lack of knowledge regarding sperm banking limited nurses' willingness to discuss this topic, and education regarding cryopreservation could improve knowledge and practice patterns [107].

Saito et al. reported a positive psychological effect in 80% of interviewed cancer patients who banked sperm. They found that in particular, if sperm was banked on the patient's own initiative, that doing so offered encouragement during therapy [11].

Obstacles to Sperm Banking

There are a variety of reasons why a patient may choose not to cryopreserve semen prior to starting cancer treatments, including modesty of both the patient and healthcare provider, privacy, discomfort, cost, urgency to begin treatment, and access to sperm banking facilities. Schover et al. found that the most common reason patients did not bank sperm was because of the lack of information [102].

In 1995, Koeppel reported over 50,000 new cases of cancer in men under the age of 35 and realized that with rising survival rates and the harmful effects of treatment on fertility potential that semen cryopreservation should be offered to these patients [108]. The author acknowledged the controversies regarding the practicality and usage of sperm banking including the challenges faced by health-care professionals in discussing such sensitive issues with patients. Oncology nurses were identified as key members of the treatment teams who could discuss infertility and sperm banking with patients at the most opportune time, before initiation of chemotherapy. It was recognized that improved knowledge would reinforce the importance of offering sperm banking to circumvent treatment-induced infertility.

Finding a sperm bank for a patient should not be a barrier in discussing the option. Information about sperm banks is readily available online. Most banks will have mail kits available that allow patients to collect sample at home and ship them to the sperm bank. This approach allows for privacy and convenience for the patient.

Cost has been identified as an obstacle for patients. Schover et al. demonstrated that both physicians and patients are under the impression that sperm cryopreservation is too costly [105]. Although cost varies by facility, it is estimated that initial processing fees are approximately $350 with monthly storage fees ranging from $10 to $50 per month. Insurance coverage is variable, but some will cover a portion of the cost, particularly in the setting of cancer treatment. National agencies such as the American Cancer Society may also have financial aid programs. Many sperm banks also offer payment plans based on need and income.

Canada and Schover acknowledged the limited time oncologists have with each patient and suggested that training oncology nurses, social workers, and nurse practitioners to discuss infertility with new cancer patients is a reasonable approach to this barrier [109]. Educational materials including patient education sheets and interactive computer programs for patients and their families are useful. Educating health-care providers via lectures, grand rounds, and in-service presentations is encouraged.

Developing an efficient, seamless system to provide this service to cancer patients during such an emotional time is also critical. Phone numbers and protocols should be readily available on inpatient wards and in outpatient clinics. Semen collection rooms should be readily accessible to patients.

Although semen collection is recommended prior to starting treatment, the urgency to start therapy sometimes trumps the ability to provide a sample for cryopreservation. In these cases, collection is possible after starting therapy; however, the impact of chemotherapeutic and radiotherapy regimens on the risk of genetic defects in the offspring remains unknown. Patients and their families must be counseled as such. Some authors report that samples collected within 10–14 days of starting treatment may still be safe to use for future ART, based on sperm transit times through the reproductive tract [110].

Lastly, there may be legal considerations surrounding sperm banking that need to be addressed. As summarized by Leonard et al., the law surrounding cryopreservation of semen is still uncertain [44]. It remains unclear if semen is categorized as property, person, or a unique material that is neither person nor property. Additionally, the disposition of cryopreserved specimens in the event of a dispute remains unclear [111]. Consent forms and contracts are important supporting documents for sperm banking, and they should address to whom the sperm belongs, what will happen in the event of death, and how payments for these services will be handled. Confounding factors may include cases of minors or in instances where there is potential for secondary gains (e.g., inheritance).

Semen Cryopreservation in Adolescent Male Cancer Patients

While adult male cancer patients may be more willing to accept the notion of sperm banking to preserve future fertility, adolescents may be intimidated and embarrassed by the concept. Their fertility wishes may not be realized for many years, and the long-term psychosocial impact of infertility on survivors of childhood cancer remains largely unknown [112]. In addition, opinions vary regarding the most appropriate age for discussing sperm banking and who should be responsible for addressing this issue.

The exact age at which sperm production first begins is unknown and probably varies based on individual factors. Enlargement of the testes represents a transition from Tanner stage I to II, and it is around and after this time that spermatogenesis likely begins, even prior to the adolescent growth spurt [113, 114]. Nevertheless, adolescent males with cancer, ranging from age 14 to 17 years, have been found to be good candidates for sperm banking [115, 116].

Ginsberg et al. examined the feasibility of offering sperm banking to young male cancer patients and determined the beliefs and decision-making processes of these patients and their parents. Of the 68 patients in their study who collected semen samples, 50 of them completed the study. They found that 80% of the patients made the decision to bank sperm with their parents and that all of the patients who banked sperm felt that they were making the right decision to do so. Patients and parents alike wanted information about semen cryopreservation. The authors concluded that because semen quality was dramatically reduced, even by one course of gonado-toxic therapy, sperm banking should be offered to all eligible patients prior to therapy. Parents played an important role in the decision to bank sperm [117].

Klosky et al. assessed sperm cryopreservation among males newly diagnosed with cancer aged 13 years and older. Oncologists assigned infertility risk to patients and reported whether their patients engaged in sperm cryopreservation. Less than 30% of their patients banked sperm. The authors found that the decision to cryopreserve semen was associated with a number of factors including a diagnosis of central nervous system malignancy or non-central nervous system solid tumor diagnosis, higher socioeconomic status, and not being a member of an Evangelical religious group. They concluded that sperm banking was underutilized by adolescent males and that newer strategies were needed to increase the number of these patients who participated in this fertility-preserving activity [118].

Emotional maturity is another important concept when discussing sperm banking in adolescent males. Boys who are not physically mature may still be able to collect sperm. Conversely, a physically mature adolescent may not be emotionally or sexually mature to perform a semen collection by masturbation.

Surgical Sperm Retrieval

A low—but still clinically significant—percentage of men with cancer who present for sperm banking will be azoospermic or will be unable to collect a semen sample. In such cases, surgical sperm retrieval techniques may be offered. Oftentimes, these procedures require a concerted and coordinated effort between the urologist and the fertility laboratory. Time pressures are typically present as these patients generally need to begin urgent therapy. The various approaches are discussed below, and they may be able to be scheduled concomitantly with any oncologically related procedures such as vascular access, lymph node sampling, or bone marrow biopsies.

Testicular sperm extraction (TESE) refers to an incisional testicular biopsy performed to obtain sperm for cryopreservation. Sperm obtained with this approach may only be used for ART [119]. For these men, it is difficult to predict success rates for sperm retrieval, although roughly half of azoospermic men with testicular cancer or malignant lymphomas will have sperm found on TESE [120, 121]. Additionally, men with testicular cancer undergoing radical orchiectomy may have microdissection TESE performed on the removed testicle [122, 123]. These men may also be scheduled for a simultaneous sperm retrieval procedure under anesthesia on the contralateral testicle.

For male cancer survivors who are azoospermic and who did not cryopreserve sperm prior to their cancer therapy, testicular sperm retrieval techniques in conjunction with ART can be offered [63, 124]. Microdissection TESE affords retrieval rates of approximately 50% in men with postchemotherapy azoospermia [125–127].

Microsurgical epididymal sperm aspiration is a procedure used to obtain sperm from the epididymides in the setting of obstructive azoospermia. An example where this approach would be indicated in a cancer patient with azoospermia is following a radical prostatectomy which from a reproductive perspective is similar to postvasectomy patient. In this patient population, testicular function is usually preserved, and cryopreserved sperm have been shown to be suitable for ART [128, 129].

Some patients with cancer have undergone surgical procedures that affect their ejaculatory function. Retroperitoneal lymph node dissections for testicular cancer and low-anterior and abdominoperineal resections for gastrointestinal malignancies can put men at risk for ejaculatory failure, despite improvements in surgical techniques. When medical treatment fails to improve emission and ejaculation, then electroejaculation (EEJ) may be offered. EEJ has been shown to be an effective way to retrieve sperm for ART [130, 131]. Sperm quality tends to be impaired in these patients, and pregnancy rates are better when these sperm are used for IVF/ICSI rather than intrauterine insemination [131–133]. EEJ should be used with caution in the setting of thrombocytopenia or leukopenia given the potential risks of bleeding or infection.

Outcomes of Using Cryopreserved Sperm for ART

While it is generally accepted that cancer and cancer therapies adversely affect a man's reproductive potential, the outcomes of ART up until recently have only been addressed in case reports and small studies. This is due, in part, to the advances in ICSI which has revolutionized the treatment of male infertility due to the need for only a few sperm either in the ejaculate or testicular tissue. Cryopreserved sperm may be used for intrauterine insemination (IUI) and/or IVF with ICSI. How to best use frozen sperm for ART depends on the quantity and quality of the sperm, how well the sperm survive the freeze–thaw process, the presence of any female factors, and patient/couple preference.

Sanger et al. reviewed the literature from an era prior to widespread use of ICSI. Fifty-four deliveries resulting from cryopreserved semen of male cancer survivors from fertility clinics and another 61 deliveries resulting from the use of cryopreserved semen from male cancer survivors were reported from sperm banks [13].

Naysmith et al. assessed the effect of cancer treatments on the natural and assisted reproductive potentials of men. Semen samples were analyzed before and after cancer therapy. Twenty-seven percent of the men had abnormal semen parameters before treatment. Following treatment, 68% of the samples were abnormal. Twenty-three percent of men developed azoospermia after treatment. Pretreatment sperm cryopreservation improved the fertility potential of 55% of their patients. The authors commented that improving awareness and education of patients and providers on the impact of cancer and cancer treatments on fertility is essential. They also stressed that with the advent of ICSI, all men with cancer should be offered pretreatment sperm cryopreservation as even men with very low sperm concentrations the chance of conception is very reasonable [15].

Tryde-Schmidt et al. reported their experience with couples referred for ART because of male-factor infertility due to cancer and cancer treatment. Most of their patients had testicular cancer and lymphomas. Ninety percent of the men had adjuvant treatment with chemo- and/or radiation therapy. Perhaps, most impressively, semen was cryopreserved in 82% of their men prior to treatment. Following cancer therapy, 43% of the men had motile spermatozoa in the ejaculate, while 57% were azoospermic. Both fresh and cryopreserved sperm were used, and the clinical pregnancy rates per cycle were 14.8% after IUI, 38.6% after ICSI, and 25% after ICSI–frozen embryo transfer, with corresponding delivery rates of 11.1, 30.5, and 21%. Cryopreserved semen was used in 58% of the pregnancies. Of note, the delivery rate per cycle was similar after use of fresh or cryopreserved sperm. The authors concluded that male cancer survivors have a good chance of fathering a child by using either fresh ejaculated sperm or cryopreserved sperm and that ICSI be used as a first choice, given the better success rates with ICSI as well as the need for overall higher total motile sperm counts for IUI which are not always available postthaw [134].

These reports of successful pregnancies with cryopreserved sperm in male cancer survivors are supported by numerous other studies [3, 14, 32, 135–139].

Van Casteren et al. reported their experience with ART using cryopreserved semen of cancer patients. Five hundred and fifty-seven male cancer patients banked 749 semen samples. Out of the total group of 557 men who cryopreserved semen, 218 (39%) returned for semen analysis after cancer treatment. Motile sperm were found in 155 (71.1%) of these 218 men. Twenty of these 218 men reported a spontaneous pregnancy. While only 42 of the cancer survivors (9.6%) ultimately requested the use of their banked semen, these men would have been unable to father their own child if their sperm had not been banked prior to therapy. Half of these men were successful in having live births using IVF/ICSI [140].

Conceptually, there could be differences in ICSI success rates when using fresh versus cryopreserved sperm; however, current studies indicate no difference in pregnancy outcomes between the two [141–143].

A few studies have looked at the utilization of cryopreserved sperm by male cancer survivors. In one study of 258 men, only 18 returned for treatment [16]. Ginsburg et al. found that at their fertility center, 19 male cancer survivors underwent a total of 35 IVF cycles, and 11 of these cycles used cryopreserved semen [138]. In a larger study, Magelssen et al. looked at posttreatment paternity in 1,388 testicular cancer survivors. Four hundred and twenty-two of these men had cryopreserved semen *after* orchiectomy. Overall, only 29 men (7%) used their cryopreserved semen for ART, while 67 men (17%) fathered at least one child with fresh semen [64, 106].

Lastly, according to a study by Saito et al., if male cancer survivors had return of spermatogenesis following treatment, none would choose to use their cryopreserved sperm. Even if the cryopreserved sperm was not used, as in most cases, a positive psychological effect of having banked sperm was achieved [11].

Five-Year View and Key Issues

An exciting new direction for fertility preservation in men with cancer is implementing stem cell technologies for germ cell transplantation and testicular grafting. Spermatogonial stem cells may be used in the future for preservation of testicular tissue and fertility preservation in men and boys prior to treatment, as these cells are capable of self-renewal, proliferation, and repopulation of the seminiferous tubules [101].

Schlatt et al. [144] recently reviewed the physiology of spermatogonial stem cells in rodent and primate testes and concluded that while germ cell transplantation has become an important research tool in rodents and other animal models [145–152], the clinical application in humans remains experimental. Regarding testicular grafting as another exciting strategy for fertility preservation in males prior to gonadotoxic therapy, both autologous and xenologous transfer of immature tissue revealed a high regenerative potential of immature testicular tissue and generation of sperm in rodents and primates. Like germ cell transplantation, however, further research is needed before an application in humans can be considered safe and efficient. Despite current limitations in regard to generation of sperm from cryopreserved male germ line cells and tissues, and since future improvements of germ cell transplantation and grafting approaches are likely, retrieval and cryopreservation of testicular tissue prior to therapy should be offered to young men with cancer who are at high risk of fertility loss, as this could be their only option to maintain their fertility potential after treatment [153, 154]. Additionally, prepubertal testicular tissue from boys facing gonadotoxic treatment may be cryopreserved under special conditions. Doing so may offer fertility preservation for young patients in the future [155].

A potential concern about using spermatogonial stem cells and testicular grafts is the theoretical risk of restoring cancer cells back into the recipient. This effect has been demonstrated in leukemic rat models [156]. But efforts have been made to reduce this risk using telomerase in culture [157]. The use of embryonic stem cell technology to treat infertile men is also under investigation; however, significantly more translational research is needed, before these technologies are applied to the treatment of human male infertility [158].

Summary

Improvements in cancer treatments have resulted in more men living into their reproductive years, and fertility is an important measure of quality of life in this patient population. However, *all* cancer therapies—chemotherapy, radiation, and surgery—are potential threats to a man's reproductive potential. The type of treatment(s) and individual susceptibilities to the deleterious effects of these treatments make it next to impossible to predict whether or not a man will recover spermatogenesis after therapy and what his sperms' potential is to safely fertilize an egg. Stem cell transplantation technologies may hold promise in the future but are unavailable for use in humans at this time. Advances in ART now provide more men with opportunities to become biological fathers, even in the setting of poor semen parameters. Thus, sperm cryopreservation *prior* to initiating life-saving cancer treatment offers men and their families hope and the best chances to father biologically related children in the future. It is a safe and effective means of preserving a man's fertility and should be offered to all men with cancer before treatment. Posttreatment male infertility also may be treated with ART and advances in surgical sperm retrieval. Barriers to sperm banking still exist, but the sensitive nature of many of these can be overcome by patient and provider education, as well as deliberate, coordinated strategies at comprehensive cancer care centers to make fertility preservation for male cancer patients a priority during pretreatment planning.

References

1. Mcvie JG. Cancer treatment: the last 25 years. Cancer Treat Rev. 1999;25:323–31.
2. Lass A, Akagbosu F, Brinsden P. Sperm banking and assisted reproduction treatment for couples following cancer treatment of the male partner. Hum Reprod Update. 2001;7:370–7.
3. Agarwal A, Ranganathan P, Kattal N, Pasqualotto F, Hallak J, Khayal S, et al. Fertility after cancer: a prospective review of assisted reproductive outcome with banked semen specimens. Fertil Steril. 2004;81:342–8.
4. Steliarova-Foucher E, Stiller C, Kaatsch P, Berrino F, Coebergh JW, Lacour B, et al. Geographical patterns and time trends of cancer incidence and survival among children and

adolescents in Europe since the 1970s (the ACCISproject): an epidemiological study. Lancet. 2004;364:2097–105.

5. Gritz ER, Wellisch DK, Wang HJ, Siau J, Landsverk JA, Cosgrove MD. Long-term effects of testicular cancer on sexual functioning in married couples. Cancer. 1989;64:1560–7.

6. Rieker PP, Fitzgerald EM, Kalish LA, Richie JP, Lederman GS, Edbril SD, et al. Psychosocial factors, curative therapies, and behavioral outcomes. A comparison of testis cancer survivors and a control group of healthy men. Cancer. 1989;64: 2399–407.

7. Rieker PP, Fitzgerald EM, Kalish LA. Adaptive behavioral responses to potential infertility among survivors of testis cancer. J Clin Oncol. 1990;8:347–55.

8. Hartmann JT, Albrecht C, Schmoll HJ, Kuczyk MA, Kollmannsberger C, Bokemeyer C. Long-term effects on sexual function and fertility after treatment of testicular cancer. Br J Cancer. 1999;80:801–7.

9. Schover LR, Rybicki LA, Martin BA, Bringelsen KA. Having children after cancer. A pilot survey of survivors' attitudes and experiences. Cancer. 1999;86:697–709.

10. Mackie E, Hill J, Kondryn H, Mcnally R. Adult psychosocial outcomes in long-term survivors of acute lymphoblastic leukaemia and Wilms' tumour: a controlled study. Lancet. 2000;355: 1310–4.

11. Saito K, Suzuki K, Iwasaki A, Yumura Y, Kubota Y. Sperm cryopreservation before cancer chemotherapy helps in the emotional battle against cancer. Cancer. 2005;104:521–4.

12. Fossa SD, Aass N, Molne K. Is routine pre-treatment cryopreservation of semen worthwhile in the management of patients with testicular cancer? Br J Urol. 1989;64:524–9.

13. Sanger WG, Olson JH, Sherman JK. Semen cryobanking for men with cancer—criteria change. Fertil Steril. 1992;58:1024–7.

14. Lass A, Akagbosu F, Abusheikha N, Hassouneh M, Blayney M, Avery S, et al. A programme of semen cryopreservation for patients with malignant disease in a tertiary infertility centre: lessons from 8 years' experience. Hum Reprod. 1998;13:3256–61.

15. Naysmith TE, Blake DA, Harvey VJ, Johnson NP. Do men undergoing sterilizing cancer treatments have a fertile future? Hum Reprod. 1998;13:3250–5.

16. Audrins P, Holden CA, Mclachlan RI, Kovacs GT. Semen storage for special purposes at Monash IVF from 1977 to 1997. Fertil Steril. 1999;72:179–81.

17. Agarwal A. Semen banking in patients with cancer: 20-year experience. Int J Androl. 2000;23 Suppl 2:16–9.

18. Kelleher S, Wishart SM, Liu PY, Turner L, Di Pierro I, Conway AJ, et al. Long-term outcomes of elective human sperm cryostorage. Hum Reprod. 2001;16:2632–9.

19. Bahadur G, Ling KL, Hart R, Ralph D, Riley V, Wafa R, et al. Semen production in adolescent cancer patients. Hum Reprod. 2002;17:2654–6.

20. Saito K, Suzuki K, Noguchi K, Ogawa T, Takeda M, Hosaka M, et al. Semen cryopreservation for patients with malignant or non-malignant disease: our experience for 10 years. Nippon Hinyokika Gakkai Zasshi. 2003;94:513–20.

21. Petersen PM, Skakkebaek NE, Rorth M, Giwercman A. Semen quality and reproductive hormones before and after orchiectomy in men with testicular cancer. J Urol. 1999;161:822–6.

22. Petersen PM, Skakkebaek NE, Vistisen K, Rorth M, Giwercman A. Semen quality and reproductive hormones before orchiectomy in men with testicular cancer. J Clin Oncol. 1999;17: 941–7.

23. Rueffer U, Breuer K, Josting A, Lathan B, Sieber M, Manzke O, et al. Male gonadal dysfunction in patients with Hodgkin's disease prior to treatment. Ann Oncol. 2001;12:1307–11.

24. Agarwal A, Allamaneni SS. Disruption of spermatogenesis by the cancer disease process. J Natl Cancer Inst Monogr. 2005;34: 9–12.

25. Hallak J, Kolettis PN, Sekhon VS, Thomas Jr AJ, Agarwal A. Sperm cryopreservation in patients with testicular cancer. Urology. 1999;54:894–9.

26. Colpi GM, Contalbi GF, Nerva F, Sagone P, Piediferro G. Testicular function following chemoradiotherapy. Eur J Obstet Gynecol Reprod Biol. 2004;113 Suppl 1:S2–6.

27. Rofeim O, Gilbert BR. Normal semen parameters in cancer patients presenting for cryopreservation before gonadotoxic therapy. Fertil Steril. 2004;82:505–6.

28. Ragni G, Somigliana E, Restelli L, Salvi R, Arnoldi M, Paffoni A. Sperm banking and rate of assisted reproduction treatment: insights from a 15-year cryopreservation program for male cancer patients. Cancer. 2003;97:1624–9.
29. Bahadur G, Ozturk O, Muneer A, Wafa R, Ashraf A, Jaman N, et al. Semen quality before and after gonadotoxic treatment. Hum Reprod. 2005;20:774–81.
30. Williams DHT, Karpman E, Sander JC, Spiess PE, Pisters LL, Lipshultz LI. Pretreatment semen parameters in men with cancer. J Urol. 2009;181:736–40.
31. Chung K, Irani J, Knee G, Efymow B, Blasco L, Patrizio P. Sperm cryopreservation for male patients with cancer: an epidemiological analysis at the University of Pennsylvania. Eur J Obstet Gynecol Reprod Biol. 2004;113 Suppl 1:S7–11.
32. Meseguer M, Molina N, Garcia-Velasco JA, Remohi J, Pellicer A, Garrido N. Sperm cryopreservation in oncological patients: a 14-year follow-up study. Fertil Steril. 2006;85: 640–5.
33. Hendry WF, Stedronska J, Jones CR, Blackmore CA, Barrett A, Peckham MJ. Semen analysis in testicular cancer and Hodgkin's disease: pre- and post-treatment findings and implications for cryopreservation. Br J Urol. 1983;55:769–73.
34. Viviani S, Bonfante V, Santoro A, Zanini M, Devizzi L, Di Russo AD, et al. Long-term results of an intensive regimen: VEBEP plus involved-field radiotherapy in advanced Hodgkin's disease. Cancer J Sci Am. 1999;5:275–82.
35. Berthelsen JG, Skakkebaek NE. Gonadal function in men with testis cancer. Fertil Steril. 1983;39:68–75.
36. Stahl O, Eberhard J, Cavallin-Stahl E, Jepson K, Friberg B, Tingsmark C, et al. Sperm DNA integrity in cancer patients: the effect of disease and treatment. Int J Androl. 2009;32: 695–703.
37. Spitz S. The histological effects of nitrogen mustards on human tumors and tissues. Cancer. 1948;1:383–98.
38. Apperley JF, Reddy N. Mechanism and management of treatment-related gonadal failure in recipients of high dose chemoradiotherapy. Blood Rev. 1995;9:93–116.
39. Howell SJ, Shalet SM. Spermatogenesis after cancer treatment: damage and recovery. J Natl Cancer Inst Monogr. 2005;34:12–7.
40. Schrader M, Muller M, Straub B, Miller K. The impact of chemotherapy on male fertility: a survey of the biologic basis and clinical aspects. Reprod Toxicol. 2001;15:611–7.
41. Meirow D, Schenker JG. Cancer and male infertility. Hum Reprod. 1995;10:2017–22.
42. Carson SA, Gentry WL, Smith AL, Buster JE. Feasibility of semen collection and cryopreservation during chemotherapy. Hum Reprod. 1991;6:992–4.
43. Pont J, Albrecht W. Fertility after chemotherapy for testicular germ cell cancer. Fertil Steril. 1997;68:1–5.
44. Leonard M, Hammelef K, Smith GD. Fertility considerations, counseling, and semen cryopreservation for males prior to the initiation of cancer therapy. Clin J Oncol Nurs. 2004;8: 127–31, 145.
45. Viviani S, Santoro A, Ragni G, Bonfante V, Bestetti O, Bonadonna G. Gonadal toxicity after combination chemotherapy for Hodgkin's disease. Comparative results of MOPP vs ABVD. Eur J Cancer Clin Oncol. 1985;21:601–5.
46. Lee SJ, Schover LR, Partridge AH, Patrizio P, Wallace WH, Hagerty K, et al. American Society of Clinical Oncology recommendations on fertility preservation in cancer patients. J Clin Oncol. 2006;24:2917–31.
47. Kenney LB, Laufer MR, Grant FD, Grier H, Diller L. High risk of infertility and long term gonadal damage in males treated with high dose cyclophosphamide for sarcoma during childhood. Cancer. 2001;91:613–21.
48. Kreuser ED, Klingmuller D, Thiel E. The role of LHRH-analogues in protecting gonadal functions during chemotherapy and irradiation. Eur Urol. 1993;23:157–63. discussion 163–4.
49. Cespedes RD, Peretsman SJ, Thompson Jr IM, Jackson C. Protection of the germinal epithelium in the rat from the cytotoxic effects of chemotherapy by a luteinizing hormone-releasing hormone agonist and antiandrogen therapy. Urology. 1995;46: 688–91.

50. Lushbaugh CC, Casarett GW. The effects of gonadal irradiation in clinical radiation therapy: a review. Cancer. 1976;37:1111–25.
51. Trottmann M, Becker AJ, Stadler T, Straub J, Soljanik I, Schlenker B, et al. Semen quality in men with malignant diseases before and after therapy and the role of cryopreservation. Eur Urol. 2007;52: 355–67.
52. Speiser B, Rubin P, Casarett G. Aspermia following lower truncal irradiation in Hodgkin's disease. Cancer. 1973;32:692–8.
53. Leiper AD, Grant DB, Chessells JM. Gonadal function after testicular radiation for acute lymphoblastic leukaemia. Arch Dis Child. 1986;61:53–6.
54. Fossa SD, Ous S, Abyholm T, Norman N, Loeb M. Post-treatment fertility in patients with testicular cancer. II. Influence of cis-platin-based combination chemotherapy and of retroperitoneal surgery on hormone and sperm cell production. Br J Urol. 1985;57:210–4.
55. Donohue JP. Evolution of retroperitoneal lymphadenectomy (RPLND) in the management of non-seminomatous testicular cancer (NSGCT). Urol Oncol. 2003;21:129–32.
56. Large MC, Sheinfeld J, Eggener SE. Retroperitoneal lymph node dissection: reassessment of modified templates. BJU Int. 2009;104: 1369–75.
57. Jones OM, Stevenson AR, Stitz RW, Lumley JW. Preservation of sexual and bladder function after laparoscopic rectal surgery. Colorectal Dis. 2009;11:489–95.
58. Jacobsen KD, Olsen DR, Fossa K, Fossa SD. External beam abdominal radiotherapy in patients with seminoma stage I: field type, testicular dose, and spermatogenesis. Int J Radiat Oncol Biol Phys. 1997;38:95–102.
59. Giwercman A, Petersen PM. Cancer and male infertility. Baillieres Best Pract Res Clin Endocrinol Metab. 2000;14:453–71.
60. Huyghe E, Matsuda T, Daudin M, Chevreau C, Bachaud JM, Plante P, et al. Fertility after testicular cancer treatments: results of a large multicenter study. Cancer. 2004;100:732–7.
61. Gandini L, Sgro P, Lombardo F, Paoli D, Culasso F, Toselli L, et al. Effect of chemo- or radiotherapy on sperm parameters of testicular cancer patients. Hum Reprod. 2006;21:2882–9.
62. Spermon JR, Ramos L, Wetzels AM, Sweep CG, Braat DD, Kiemeney LA, et al. Sperm integrity pre- and post-chemotherapy in men with testicular germ cell cancer. Hum Reprod. 2006;21: 1781–6.
63. Tournaye H, Liu J, Nagy PZ, Camus M, Goossens A, Silber S, et al. Correlation between testicular histology and outcome after intracytoplasmic sperm injection using testicular spermatozoa. Hum Reprod. 1996;11:127–32.
64. Magelssen H, Brydoy M, Fossa SD. The effects of cancer and cancer treatments on male reproductive function. Nat Clin Pract Urol. 2006;3:312–22.
65. Lampe H, Horwich A, Norman A, Nicholls J, Dearnaley DP. Fertility after chemotherapy for testicular germ cell cancers. J Clin Oncol. 1997;15:239–45.
66. Brydoy M, Fossa SD, Klepp O, Bremnes RM, Wist EA, Wentzel-Larsen T, et al. Paternity following treatment for testicular cancer. J Natl Cancer Inst. 2005;97:1580–8.
67. Huddart RA, Norman A, Moynihan C, Horwich A, Parker C, Nicholls E, et al. Fertility, gonadal and sexual function in survivors of testicular cancer. Br J Cancer. 2005;93: 200–7.
68. Joos H, Sedlmayer F, Gomahr A, Rahim HB, Frick J, Kogelnik HD, et al. Endocrine profiles after radiotherapy in stage I seminoma: impact of two different radiation treatment modalities. Radiother Oncol. 1997;43:159–62.
69. Nalesnik JG, Sabanegh Jr ES, Eng TY, Buchholz TA. Fertility in men after treatment for stage 1 and 2A seminoma. Am J Clin Oncol. 2004;27:584–8.
70. Classen J, Dieckmann K, Bamberg M, Souchon R, Kliesch S, Kuehn M, et al. Radiotherapy with 16 Gy may fail to eradicate testicular intraepithelial neoplasia: preliminary communication of a dose-reduction trial of the German Testicular Cancer Study Group. Br J Cancer. 2003;88:828–31.
71. Da Cunha MF, Meistrich ML, Fuller LM, Cundiff JH, Hagemeister FB, Velasquez WS, et al. Recovery of spermatogenesis after treatment for Hodgkin's disease: limiting dose of MOPP chemotherapy. J Clin Oncol. 1984;2:571–7.

72. Marmor D, Duyck F. Male reproductive potential after MOPP therapy for Hodgkin's disease: a long-term survey. Andrologia. 1995;27:99–106.
73. Tal R, Botchan A, Hauser R, Yogev L, Paz G, Yavetz H. Follow-up of sperm concentration and motility in patients with lymphoma. Hum Reprod. 2000;15:1985–8.
74. Jacob A, Barker H, Goodman A, Holmes J. Recovery of spermatogenesis following bone marrow transplantation. Bone Marrow Transplant. 1998;22:277–9.
75. Anserini P, Chiodi S, Spinelli S, Costa M, Conte N, Copello F, et al. Semen analysis following allogeneic bone marrow transplantation. Additional data for evidence-based counselling. Bone Marrow Transplant. 2002;30:447–51.
76. Boyd BG, Mccallum SW, Lewis RW, Terris MK. Assessment of patient concern and adequacy of informed consent regarding infertility resulting from prostate cancer treatment. Urology. 2006;68:840–4.
77. Magheli A, Rais-Bahrami S, Humphreys EB, Peck HJ, Trock BJ, Gonzalgo ML. Impact of patient age on biochemical recurrence rates following radical prostatectomy. J Urol. 2007;178:1933–7. discussion 1937-1938.
78. Daniell HW, Tam EW. Testicular atrophy in therapeutic orchiectomy specimens from men with prostate carcinoma: association with prior prostate bed radiation and older age. Cancer. 1998;83:1174–9.
79. Mydlo JH, Lebed B. Does brachytherapy of the prostate affect sperm quality and/or fertility in younger men? Scand J Urol Nephrol. 2004;38:221–4.
80. Raviv G, Pinthus JH, Shefi S, Mor Y, Kaufman-Francis K, Levron J, et al. Effects of intravesical chemotherapy and immunotherapy on semen analysis. Urology. 2005;65:765–7.
81. Colombo R, Bertini R, Salonia A, Da Pozzo LF, Montorsi F, Brausi M, et al. Nerve and seminal sparing radical cystectomy with orthotopic urinary diversion for select patients with superficial bladder cancer: an innovative surgical approach. J Urol. 2001;165:51–5. discussion 55.
82. Hyer S, Vini L, O'connell M, Pratt B, Harmer C. Testicular dose and fertility in men following I(131) therapy for thyroid cancer. Clin Endocrinol (Oxf). 2002;56:755–8.
83. Longhi A, Macchiagodena M, Vitali G, Bacci G. Fertility in male patients treated with neoadjuvant chemotherapy for osteosarcoma. J Pediatr Hematol Oncol. 2003;25:292–6.
84. Mansky P, Arai A, Stratton P, Bernstein D, Long L, Reynolds J, et al. Treatment late effects in long-term survivors of pediatric sarcoma. Pediatr Blood Cancer. 2007;48:192–9.
85. Hawkins MM, Draper GJ, Smith RA. Cancer among 1,348 offspring of survivors of childhood cancer. Int J Cancer. 1989;43:975–8.
86. Winther JF, Boice Jr JD, Mulvihill JJ, Stovall M, Frederiksen K, Tawn EJ, et al. Chromosomal abnormalities among offspring of childhood-cancer survivors in Denmark: a population-based study. Am J Hum Genet. 2004;74:1282–5.
87. Sankila R, Olsen JH, Anderson H, Garwicz S, Glattre E, Hertz H, et al. Risk of cancer among offspring of childhood-cancer survivors. Association of the Nordic Cancer Registries and the Nordic Society of Paediatric Haematology and Oncology. N Engl J Med. 1998;338:1339–44.
88. Robbins WA, Meistrich ML, Moore D, Hagemeister FB, Weier HU, Cassel MJ, et al. Chemotherapy induces transient sex chromosomal and autosomal aneuploidy in human sperm. Nat Genet. 1997;16:74–8.
89. De Mas P, Daudin M, Vincent MC, Bourrouillou G, Calvas P, Mieusset R, et al. Increased aneuploidy in spermatozoa from testicular tumour patients after chemotherapy with cisplatin, etoposide and bleomycin. Hum Reprod. 2001;16:1204–8.
90. Frias S, Van Hummelen P, Meistrich ML, Lowe XR, Hagemeister FB, Shelby MD, et al. NOVP chemotherapy for Hodgkin's disease transiently induces sperm aneuploidies associated with the major clinical aneuploidy syndromes involving chromosomes X, Y, 18, and 21. Cancer Res. 2003;63:44–51.
91. Thomas C, Cans C, Pelletier R, De Robertis C, Hazzouri M, Sele B, et al. No long-term increase in sperm aneuploidy rates after anticancer therapy: sperm fluorescence in situ hybridization analysis in 26 patients treated for testicular cancer or lymphoma. Clin Cancer Res. 2004;10:6535–43.
92. Wyrobek AJ, Schmid TE, Marchetti F. Relative susceptibilities of male germ cells to genetic defects induced by cancer chemotherapies. J Natl Cancer Inst Monogr. 2005;34:31–5.

93. Martin R. Human sperm chromosome complements in chemotherapy patients and infertile men. Chromosoma. 1998;107: 523–7.

94. World Health Organisation. WHO laboratory manual for the examination of human semen and sperm-cervical mucus interaction. 4th ed. Cambridge: Cambridge University Press; 1999.

95. Padron OF, Sharma RK, Thomas Jr AJ, Agarwal A. Effects of cancer on spermatozoa quality after cryopreservation: a 12-year experience. Fertil Steril. 1997;67:326–31.

96. Bolten M, Weissbach L, Kaden R. Cryopreserved human sperm deposits: usability after decades of storage. Urologe A. 2005;44: 904–8.

97. Gandini L, Lombardo F, Lenzi A, Spano M, Dondero F. Cryopreservation and sperm DNA integrity. Cell Tissue Bank. 2006; 7:91–8.

98. Meyers SA. Dry storage of sperm: applications in primates and domestic animals. Reprod Fertil Dev. 2006;18:1–5.

99. Kuczynski W, Dhont M, Grygoruk C, Grochowski D, Wolczynski S, Szamatowicz M. The outcome of intracytoplasmic injection of fresh and cryopreserved ejaculated spermatozoa—a prospective randomized study. Hum Reprod. 2001;16:2109–13.

100. Meistrich ML. Potential genetic risks of using semen collected during chemotherapy. Hum Reprod. 1993;8:8–10.

101. Shin D, Lo KC, Lipshultz LI. Treatment options for the infertile male with cancer. J Natl Cancer Inst Monogr. 2005;34:48–50.

102. Schover LR, Brey K, Lichtin A, Lipshultz LI, Jeha S. Knowledge and experience regarding cancer, infertility, and sperm banking in younger male survivors. J Clin Oncol. 2002;20:1880–9.

103. Dohle GR, Colpi GM, Hargreave TB, Papp GK, Jungwirth A, Weidner W. Eau guidelines on male infertility. Eur Urol. 2005;48:703–11.

104. Edge B, Holmes D, Makin G. Sperm banking in adolescent cancer patients. Arch Dis Child. 2006;91:149–52.

105. Schover LR, Brey K, Lichtin A, Lipshultz LI, Jeha S. Oncologists' attitudes and practices regarding banking sperm before cancer treatment. J Clin Oncol. 2002;20:1890–7.

106. Magelssen H, Haugen TB, Von During V, Melve KK, Sandstad B, Fossa SD. Twenty years experience with semen cryopreservation in testicular cancer patients: who needs it? Eur Urol. 2005;48:779–85.

107. Reebals JF, Brown R, Buckner EB. Nurse practice issues regarding sperm banking in adolescent male cancer patients. J Pediatr Oncol Nurs. 2006;23:182–8.

108. Koeppel KM. Sperm banking and patients with cancer. Issues concerning patients and healthcare professionals. Cancer Nurs. 1995;18:306–12.

109. Canada AL, Schover LR. Research promoting better patient education on reproductive health after cancer. J Natl Cancer Inst Monogr. 2005;34:98–100.

110. Chatterjee R, Haines GA, Perera DM, Goldstone A, Morris ID. Testicular and sperm DNA damage after treatment with fludarabine for chronic lymphocytic leukaemia. Hum Reprod. 2000;15:762–6.

111. Schuster TG, Hickner-Cruz K, Ohl DA, Goldman E, Smith GD. Legal considerations for cryopreservation of sperm and embryos. Fertil Steril. 2003;80:61–6.

112. Zebrack BJ, Zeltzer LK. Quality of life issues and cancer survivorship. Curr Probl Cancer. 2003;27:198–211.

113. Hirsch M, Lunenfeld B, Modan M, Ovadia J, Shemesh J. Spermarche—the age of onset of sperm emission. J Adolesc Health Care. 1985;6:35–9.

114. Nielsen CT, Skakkebaek NE, Richardson DW, Darling JA, Hunter WM, Jorgensen M, et al. Onset of the release of spermatozoa (spermarche) in boys in relation to age, testicular growth, pubic hair, and height. J Clin Endocrinol Metab. 1986;62:532–5.

115. Kliesch S, Behre HM, Jurgens H, Nieschlag E. Cryopreservation of semen from adolescent patients with malignancies. Med Pediatr Oncol. 1996;26:20–7.

116. Bahadur G, Ling KL, Hart R, Ralph D, Wafa R, Ashraf A, et al. Semen quality and cryopreservation in adolescent cancer patients. Hum Reprod. 2002;17:3157–61.

117. Ginsberg JP, Ogle SK, Tuchman LK, Carlson CA, Reilly MM, Hobbie WL, et al. Sperm banking for adolescent and young adult cancer patients: sperm quality, patient, and parent perspectives. Pediatr Blood Cancer. 2008;50:594–8.

118. Klosky JL, Randolph ME, Navid F, Gamble HL, Spunt SL, Metzger ML, et al. Sperm cryo-preservation practices among adolescent cancer patients at risk for infertility. Pediatr Hematol Oncol. 2009;26:252–60.
119. Vanderzwalmen P, Zech H, Birkenfeld A, Yemini M, Bertin G, Lejeune B, et al. Intracytoplasmic injection of spermatids retrieved from testicular tissue: influence of testicular pathology, type of selected spermatids and oocyte activation. Hum Reprod. 1997;12: 1203–13.
120. Kim ED, Gilbaugh 3rd JH, Patel VR, Turek PJ, Lipshultz LI. Testis biopsies frequently demonstrate sperm in men with azoospermia and significantly elevated follicle-stimulating hormone levels. J Urol. 1997;157:144–6.
121. Schrader M, Muller M, Sofikitis N, Straub B, Krause H, Miller K. "Onco-tese": testicular sperm extraction in azoospermic cancer patients before chemotherapy-new guidelines? Urology. 2003;61: 421–5.
122. Baniel J, Sella A. Sperm extraction at orchiectomy for testis cancer. Fertil Steril. 2001; 75:260–2.
123. Binsaleh S, Sircar K, Chan PT. Feasibility of simultaneous testicular microdissection for sperm retrieval and ipsilateral testicular tumor resection in azoospermic men. J Androl. 2004;25:867–71.
124. Devroey P, Liu J, Nagy Z, Goossens A, Tournaye H, Camus M, et al. Pregnancies after testicular sperm extraction and intracytoplasmic sperm injection in non-obstructive azoospermia. Hum Reprod. 1995;10:1457–60.
125. Chan PT, Palermo GD, Veeck LL, Rosenwaks Z, Schlegel PN. Testicular sperm extraction combined with intracytoplasmic sperm injection in the treatment of men with persistent azoospermia postchemotherapy. Cancer. 2001;92:1632–7.
126. Damani MN, Master V, Meng MV, Burgess C, Turek P, Oates RD. Postchemotherapy ejaculatory azoospermia: fatherhood with sperm from testis tissue with intracytoplasmic sperm injection. J Clin Oncol. 2002;20:930–6.
127. Meseguer M, Garrido N, Remohi J, Pellicer A, Simon C, Martinez-Jabaloyas JM, et al. Testicular sperm extraction (TESE) and ICSI in patients with permanent azoospermia after chemotherapy. Hum Reprod. 2003;18:1281–5.
128. Oates RD, Lobel SM, Harris DH, Pang S, Burgess CM, Carson RS. Efficacy of intracytoplasmic sperm injection using intentionally cryopreserved epididymal spermatozoa. Hum Reprod. 1996;11:133–8.
129. Janzen N, Goldstein M, Schlegel PN, Palermo GD, Rosenwaks Z, Hariprashad J. Use of electively cryopreserved microsurgically aspirated epididymal sperm with IVF and intracytoplasmic sperm injection for obstructive azoospermia. Fertil Steril. 2000;74:696–701.
130. Ohl DA, Denil J, Bennett CJ, Randolph JF, Menge AC, Mccabe M. Electroejaculation following retroperitoneal lymphadenectomy. J Urol. 1991;145:980–3.
131. Ohl DA, Wolf LJ, Menge AC, Christman GM, Hurd WW, Ansbacher R, et al. Electroejaculation and assisted reproductive technologies in the treatment of anejaculatory infertility. Fertil Steril. 2001;76:1249–55.
132. Chung PH, Verkauf BS, Mola R, Skinner L, Eichberg RD, Maroulis GB. Correlation between semen parameters of electroejaculates and achieving pregnancy by intrauterine insemination. Fertil Steril. 1997;67:129–32.
133. Schatte EC, Orejuela FJ, Lipshultz LI, Kim ED, Lamb DJ. Treatment of infertility due to anejaculation in the male with electroejaculation and intracytoplasmic sperm injection. J Urol. 2000;163:1717–20.
134. Schmidt KL, Larsen E, Bangsboll S, Meinertz H, Carlsen E, Andersen AN. Assisted reproduction in male cancer survivors: fertility treatment and outcome in 67 couples. Hum Reprod. 2004;19:2806–10.
135. Khalifa E, Oehninger S, Acosta AA, Morshedi M, Veeck L, Bryzyski RG, et al. Successful fertilization and pregnancy outcome in in-vitro fertilization using cryopreserved/thawed spermatozoa from patients with malignant diseases. Hum Reprod. 1992;7:105–8.
136. Palermo G, Joris H, Devroey P, Van Steirteghem AC. Pregnancies after intracytoplasmic injection of single spermatozoon into an oocyte. Lancet. 1992;340:17–8.

137. Rosenlund B, Sjoblom P, Tornblom M, Hultling C, Hillensjo T. In-vitro fertilization and intracytoplasmic sperm injection in the treatment of infertility after testicular cancer. Hum Reprod. 1998;13:414–8.
138. Ginsburg ES, Yanushpolsky EH, Jackson KV. In vitro fertilization for cancer patients and survivors. Fertil Steril. 2001;75:705–10.
139. Zorn B, Virant-Klun I, Stanovnik M, Drobnic S, Meden-Vrtovec H. Intracytoplasmic sperm injection by testicular sperm in patients with aspermia or azoospermia after cancer treatment. Int J Androl. 2006;29:521–7.
140. Van Casteren NJ, Van Santbrink EJ, Van Inzen W, Romijn JC, Dohle GR. Use rate and assisted reproduction technologies outcome of cryopreserved semen from 629 cancer patients. Fertil Steril. 2008;90:2245–50.
141. Ulug U, Bener F, Karagenc L, Ciray N, Bahceci M. Outcomes in couples undergoing ICSI: comparison between fresh and frozen-thawed surgically retrieved spermatozoa. Int J Androl. 2005;28:343–9.
142. Wald M, Ross LS, Prins GS, Cieslak-Janzen J, Wolf G, Niederberger CS. Analysis of outcomes of cryopreserved surgically retrieved sperm for IVF/ICSI. J Androl. 2006;27:60–5.
143. Borges Jr E, Rossi LM, Locambo De Freitas CV, Guilherme P, Bonetti TC, Iaconelli A, et al. Fertilization and pregnancy outcome after intracytoplasmic injection with fresh or cryopreserved ejaculated spermatozoa. Fertil Steril. 2007;87:316–20.
144. Schlatt S, Ehmcke J, Jahnukainen K. Testicular stem cells for fertility preservation: preclinical studies on male germ cell transplantation and testicular grafting. Pediatr Blood Cancer. 2009;53: 274–80.
145. Brinster RL, Avarbock MR. Germline transmission of donor haplotype following spermatogonial transplantation. Proc Natl Acad Sci USA. 1994;91:11303–7.
146. Dobrinski I. Germ cell transplantation. Semin Reprod Med. 2005;23:257–65.
147. Dobrinski I. Germ cell transplantation and testis tissue xenografting in domestic animals. Anim Reprod Sci. 2005;89:137–45.
148. Avarbock MR, Brinster CJ, Brinster RL. Reconstitution of spermatogenesis from frozen spermatogonial stem cells. Nat Med. 1996;2:693–6.
149. Izadyar F, Matthijs-Rijsenbilt JJ, Den Ouden K, Creemers LB, Woelders H, De Rooij DG. Development of a cryopreservation protocol for type a spermatogonia. J Androl. 2002;23: 537–45.
150. Nagano M, Patrizio P, Brinster RL. Long-term survival of human spermatogonial stem cells in mouse testes. Fertil Steril. 2002;78:1225–33.
151. Honaramooz A, Behboodi E, Megee SO, Overton SA, Galantino-Homer H, Echelard Y, et al. Fertility and germline transmission of donor haplotype following germ cell transplantation in immunocompetent goats. Biol Reprod. 2003;69: 1260–4.
152. Zhang X, Ebata KT, Nagano MC. Genetic analysis of the clonal origin of regenerating mouse spermatogenesis following transplantation. Biol Reprod. 2003;69:1872–8.
153. Goossens E, Tournaye H. Testicular stem cells. Semin Reprod Med. 2006;24:370–8.
154. Jahnukainen K, Ehmcke J, Schlatt S. Testicular xenografts: a novel approach to study cytotoxic damage in juvenile primate testis. Cancer Res. 2006;66:3813–8.
155. Keros V, Hultenby K, Borgstrom B, Fridstrom M, Jahnukainen K, Hovatta O. Methods of cryopreservation of testicular tissue with viable spermatogonia in pre-pubertal boys undergoing gonadotoxic cancer treatment. Hum Reprod. 2007;22:1384–95.
156. Jahnukainen K, Hou M, Petersen C, Setchell B, Soder O. Intratesticular transplantation of testicular cells from leukemic rats causes transmission of leukemia. Cancer Res. 2001;61: 706–10.
157. Feng LX, Chen Y, Dettin L, Pera RA, Herr JC, Goldberg E, et al. Generation and in vitro differentiation of a spermatogonial cell line. Science. 2002;297:392–5.
158. Toyooka Y, Tsunekawa N, Akasu R, Noce T. Embryonic stem cells can form germ cells in vitro. Proc Natl Acad Sci USA. 2003;100:11457–62.

Chapter 18
Novel Approaches in the Management of Klinefelter's Syndrome

Fnu Deepinder

Klinefelter syndrome [1] is the most common form of hypogonadism in men and is the leading genetic cause of male infertility. It also represents the most prevalent chromosomal aneuploidy in human beings [2, 3]. It is characterized by the presence of an extra X chromosome in a phenotypic male. The most abundant karyotype is 47, XXY, although other patterns including mosaicism (47, XY/47, XXY) and higher grade chromosomal aneuploidies containing supranumerous X chromosomes (48, XXXY, 49, XXXXY) are not uncommon. The latter phenotypes are more severely affected in terms of physical and mental development than men with classic 47, XXY karyotypes [4]. The genetic cause is either meiotic nondisjunction leading to failure of separation of the chromosome pair during first or second division of gametogenesis or from mitotic nondisjunction in the developing zygote. Increasing maternal age has been reported to raise the risk of Klinefelter syndrome [5].

The estimated prevalence of Klinefelter syndrome in men is 1:500 or 0.1–0.2% of the general population [2, 3]. However, extremely large discrepancies have been reported between prenatal and postnatal prevalence suggesting high rates of under diagnosis. A large Danish national registry study observed only 25% of the expected patients diagnosed after birth, and less than 10% of the expected diagnoses were made before puberty [6]. Some of the major reasons for this underdiagnosis are thought to be the variable phenotype of Klinefelter syndrome and low awareness of the disease among medical professionals. Recognition of clinical features is hence important for early detection of this syndrome.

F. Deepinder
Department of Endocrinology, Diabetes and Metabolism,
Cedars Sinai Medical Center, 8700 Beverly Boulevard, B-131,
Los Angeles, CA 90048, USA
e-mail: fnu.deepinder@cshs.org

S.J. Parekattil, A. Agarwal (eds.), *Male Infertility for the Clinician*,
© Springer Science+Business Media New York 2013

Diagnosis

A suspected diagnosis is based on a combination of typical clinical findings and laboratory investigations. Clinical signs and symptoms vary by age.

Prenatal

Although uncommon, fetus can be prenatally diagnosed to have 47, XXY karyotype by routine amniocentesis in high risk pregnancies especially in the presence of advanced maternal age. If confirmed, professional genetic counseling should be offered to the parents regarding the prognosis of the baby.

At Birth

Klinefelter syndrome is associated with several major and minor congenital abnormalities at birth including cleft palate, inguinal hernia, testis retention, clinodactyly, hypospadias, and microphallus [7]. Although these are not specific, it should prompt chromosomal evaluations to detect sex-chromosome aneuploidy, and if such screening is suggestive of Klinefelter syndrome, confirmatory karyotyping tests should follow [8].

School Age

Male children in this age group present with learning disability, language delay, and behavioral problems that often lead to chromosomal evaluation thus leading to the diagnosis of Klinefelter syndrome.

Adolescence

Adolescent boys present with delayed or incomplete pubertal development. These children may have varying signs and symptoms of androgen deficiency including eunuchoid body habitus with long legs, sparse body hair, gynecomastia, small phallus, and small firm testes [9].

Adults

Adults are often recognized through evaluation of decreasing libido, potency, and infertility. The development of secondary sexual characteristics such as beard growth, muscle bulk, and secondary body hair is either reduced or delayed. In addition, these men have several long-term consequences of hypogonadism including osteoporosis, glucose intolerance, and metabolic syndrome [8]. The incidence of breast cancer, mediastinal germ cell tumors, and non-Hodgkin lymphomas has also been found to be grossly elevated in these men [10].

A quick and reliable screening test for Klinefelter syndrome is Barr-body analysis. If suggestive, Klinefelter syndrome can be confirmed by chromosomal analysis in the lymphocytes. In certain cases such as chromosomal mosaicism, testicular biopsy is needed which generally reveals hyalinization and fibrosis of seminiferous tubules, absence of spermatogenesis, and relative hyperplasia of the Leydig cells [11].

All men with Klinefelter syndrome should have a full hormonal workup including testosterone, luteinizing hormone (LH), follicle-stimulating hormone (FSH), estradiol, prolactin, cortisol, sex hormone-binding globulins (SHBG), inhibin-B, thyroid function tests, and insulin-like growth factor-1 (IGF-1). These patients have normal levels of FSH, LH, and testosterone during prepubertal period; however, the serum testosterone declines after puberty and the levels of LH and FSH rise in most cases. The serum concentration of SHBG is also high causing further decline in free testosterone levels. The estrogen levels are usually higher than in normal men. The inhibin-B which is a marker of Sertoli cell function has demonstrated to be a better marker of spermatogenesis than FSH. The levels of inhibin-B decrease significantly after puberty in boys with Klinefelter syndrome reflecting loss of Sertoli cells [12]. At least three semen samples should be collected and analyzed, which usually reveal azoospermia. Cortisol levels should also be routinely measured to rule out any coexisting adrenal insufficiency [13].

In addition to the reproductive workup, it is important to monitor fasting blood glucose and lipids as these men have increased risk of diabetes and metabolic syndrome [8]. They also have increased risk of deep vein thrombosis and pulmonary embolism thus necessitating routine hematocrit checks to detect increased viscosity [14]. In addition, bone densitometry by dual-energy X-ray absorptiometry (DEXA) scan should be performed at 2- to 3-year intervals due to increased risk of osteoporosis, and their vitamin D status should be monitored. It is also suggested to do echocardiogram as a large proportion of these patients have been found to have mitral valve prolapse and their cardiovascular mortality is high [15].

Treatment

Treatment and care of Klinefelter males is a multidisciplinary approach and depends upon the patient's age.

Children

The most important problems associated with this syndrome in early childhood are delayed speech and learning disabilities. Parents should be counseled to anticipate communication problems in their child so as to avoid negative interactions. In addition, referral to speech therapist should be considered as soon the child shows signs of delayed speech. Language therapy is often required for these children in order to develop skills to better understand and deliver complex language [9].

Adolescents

At puberty, most patients with Klinefelter syndrome experience decline in testosterone and rise in LH and FSH. Testosterone treatment should be initiated in these boys around the age 12 years if their gonadotropin levels are elevated, even if their testosterone levels are in the lower limit of normal range [8]. Androgen replacement promotes development of secondary sexual characteristics, normalization of body proportions, prevention of gynecomastia, and improvement in energy, mood, and concentration among these adolescents [16, 17]. This aids in the development of normal male self-image and helps them build relationships with other people of same or opposite sex. The goal of testosterone therapy should be normalization of LH and testosterone levels in the age-appropriate mid-normal range [8].

Adult Males

Treatment in adult men with Klinefelter syndrome can be broadly classified into two categories.

Androgen Replacement

The patients who are not interested in fertility should be on lifelong testosterone-replacement therapy in order to prevent long-term manifestation of androgen deficiency such as osteoporosis, obesity, diabetes, and metabolic syndrome. In addition, androgen therapy improves mood, behavior, and self esteem and reduces fatigue and irritability [17]. Transdermal testosterone in either 5–10 mg/day patch or 5–10 g/day 1% gel is the preferred form of testosterone replacement as they lead to better steady state levels of serum testosterone than the injectable forms like testosterone cypionate or testosterone enanthate at doses of 50–400 mg intramuscular every 2–4 weeks. Other available testosterone preparations include buccal testosterone and subdermal implants. All patients on androgen replacement should have routine prostate examinations and measurement of PSA and hematocrit levels every 6 months.

Fertility

Until last decade, men with Klinefelter syndrome were considered sterile. However, recent literature suggests that Klinefelter syndrome males are born with spermatogonia which undergo massive apoptosis during early puberty [18, 19]. Spermatozoa have been found in the testes of these men, and in a minority of patients, viable sperm can also be seen in the ejaculate. With the advent of testicular sperm extraction (TESE) and intracytoplasmic sperm injection (ICSI), now it is possible to reproduce even when the spermatozoa are not present in the ejaculate but only in the testes.

Testicular sperm retrieval rates by microsurgical techniques in Klinefelter syndrome patients have been reported to be as high as 40–70% [20, 21]. Various studies have evaluated the parameters predicting sperm recovery in these men with varying results. While a small study by Madgar et al. reported that testicular volume, testosterone concentration, and the hCG test predicted sperm recovery in Klinefelter men [22], a recent study by Ramasamy et al. found no predictive value of serum FSH, LH, and testicular volume for sperm recovery [23].

Although optimal hormonal therapy prior to sperm retrieval has not been established so far, it is a common practice to stop testosterone replacement prior to any intervention due to possible deleterious effects of exogenous testosterone in suppressing spermatogenesis. Aromatase inhibitor such as anastrozole is used for 6 months prior to sperm extraction in order to decrease intratesticular estradiol and increase testosterone [13, 24]. In addition, few centers use human chorionic gonadotropin (hCG) and/or clomiphene citrate to stimulate endogenous testosterone production and spermatogenesis. However, hCG should be used along with aromatase inhibitors to prevent concomitant rise in estrogen levels [13]. Men with hypogonadism who respond to medical therapy with a resultant testosterone levels of greater than 250 ng/dL have been found to have a better chance of sperm retrieval than men who did not [23]. It is unclear if the rise in endogenous testosterone improves spermatogenesis or normalization of serum testosterone levels with medical therapy just occurs in men with greater potential for spermatogenesis without a cause and effect relationship [23].

Staessen et al. reported 20% live birth rate among 20 couples who underwent ICSI due to underlying Klinefelter syndrome in male partners [25]. Concerns are raised about any increased risk of chromosomal aberrations among offspring of Klinefelter syndrome patients born with assisted reproduction. A number of studies have reported an increased overall risk of both sex-chromosome and autosomal aneuploidies [26, 27]. However, most infants born have normal karyotype which is likely due to a high proportion of chromosomally normal spermatozoa in these men [28]. Nevertheless, couples should be counseled before undergoing any assisted reproductive procedure for all possible genetic risks. Furthermore, preimplantation genetic diagnostic techniques like embryo biopsy can be used as a tool for embryo selection by identifying good quality embryos prior to implantation [12].

Future Prospects

Klinefelter syndrome leads to infertility in eventually most of the men. Hence, children and adolescent boys with Klinefelter syndrome may be offered fertility preservation before they present with infertility. As of today, sperm cryopreservation is the only effective method of fertility preservation in men whereas fertility preservation options in prepubertal males are still experimental. Semen banking can be offered to those postpubertal boys with Klinefelter syndrome in whom spermatozoa can be retrieved from the ejaculate. Otherwise, microsurgical testicular biopsy can be utilized for sperm recovery. The optimal timing for testicular biopsy is the time of spermarche, i.e., production of spermatozoa so that motile sperm can be retrieved. Various techniques including scrotal ultrasound and magnetic resonance spectroscopy have been used in some centers to determine optimal timing for testicular biopsy in these adolescents [13].

The absence of spermatozoa and spermatids in testes of prepubertal boys prevents them from benefitting from the technique of sperm freezing. However, the spermatogonial stem cells are often present in prepubertal testicular tissue of patients with Klinefelter syndrome [18, 19] and can be isolated and successfully cryopreserved with almost 70% cells surviving freezing and thawing as demonstrated in animal experiments [29]. Although at present, it is impossible to generate haploid male gametes from diploid germ cells with the existing in vitro approaches, these stem cells can be either retransplanted autologously into the testes at a later time when fertility is desired or transplanted into the animals. The techniques are known as spermatogonial stem cell auto- and xenotransplantation, respectively [30–32]. There are concerns though with the later procedure that animal infectious agents like retroviruses may be introduced in human germ line when these cells are used to procure conception [33]. Some of the other challenges encountered with this technology include the ischemic damage to the transplanted testicular tissue, in vitro enrichment of stem cell spermatogonia, and noninvasive transfer of germ cell suspensions into the rete testis. Hence, in spite of latest developments suggesting bright prospects for fertility preservation, the technique needs to be developed for isolation, storage, and reinfusion of spermatogonial stem cells in humans and creating an in vitro culture system that supports full spermatogenesis.

Another investigational technique involves removal of testicular tissue from boys with Klinefelter syndrome and cryopreserving the tissue if spermatogonia are found. The cryopreserved testicular tissue can be transplanted to an ectopic site such as under the skin at a time when fertility is desired, known as ectopic autografting of testicular tissue, or into animals, called ectopic xenografting of testicular tissue. The grafted testicular tissue revascularizes in the ectopic site producing complete spermatogenesis [34, 35]. Sperm retrieval from grafted tissue can then be used to generate healthy offspring with assisted fertilization techniques. Grafting has been successfully demonstrated in animals including mice, hamsters, goats, calves, and monkeys [36–38].

Although recent advances in medicine have brightened the prospects of preserving paternity in males suffering from Klinefelter syndrome, at present, only sperm cryopreservation is considered accepted standard clinical practice. Cryopreservation of testicular tissue and spermatogonial stem cell transplantation should only be offered as a part of an approved research protocol after thorough counseling of patients and/or their family members as there are still many unresolved issues related to these technologies.

Five-Year View and Key Issues

Klinefelter syndrome is the most common sex-chromosome aberration in men but remains underdiagnosed. There is no published randomized, placebo-controlled trial on the effects of testosterone-replacement therapy in patients with Klinefelter syndrome. Such studies should be performed to evaluate the efficacy of testosterone replacement as compared to placebo and determine the appropriate doses and formulations that restore normal testosterone levels in men with Klinefelter syndrome.

Over the last decade, with advancements in assisted reproductive techniques and successful delivery of healthy children from men with Klinefelter syndrome, intense research has started to investigate optimal methods of hormonal manipulations, preservation of fertility in adolescents, and development of universal early screening programs. In some states, screening programs for Klinefelter syndrome are already in place, which might increase the number of such patients seen by endocrinologists and urologists in the near future. Development of randomized clinical trials comparing different forms of interventions in men and children with Klinefelter syndrome will hopefully provide the evidence that is essential to allow optimization of treatment in these patients.

References

1. Klinefelter HF, Reifenstein EC, Albright F. Syndrome characterized by gynecomastia, aspermatogenesis without Leydigism, increased, excretion of follicle stimulating hormone. J Clin Endocrinol Metab. 1942;2:615–27.
2. Philip J, Lundsteen C, Owen D, Hirschhom K. The frequency of chromosome aberrations in tall men with special reference to 47, XYY and 47, XXY. Am J Hum Genet. 1976;28:404–11.
3. Perwein E. Incidence of Klinefelter's syndrome. In: Bandmann HJ, Breit R, editors. Klinefeleter's syndrome. Berlin: Springer; 1984. p. 8–11.
4. Samango-Sprouse C. Mental development in polysomy X Klinefelter syndrome (47, XXY; 48, XXXY): effects of incomplete X inactivation. Semin Reprod Med. 2001;19:193–202.
5. Hook EB. Rates of chromosome abnormalities at different maternal ages. Obstet Gynecol. 1981;58:282–5.

6. Bojesen A, Juul S, Hojbjerg Gravholt C. Prenatal and postnatal prevalence of Klinefelter syndrome: a national registry study. J Clin Endocrinol Metab. 2003;88:622–6.
7. Robinson A, Lubs HA, Nielsen J, Sørensen K. Summary of clinical findings: profiles of children with 47, XXY, 47, XXX and 47, XYY karyotypes. Birth Defects Orig Artic Ser. 1979;15(1):261–6.
8. Bojesen A, Gravholt CH. Klinefelter syndrome in clinical practice. Nat Clin Pract Urol. 2007;4(4):192–204.
9. Visootsak J, Aylstock M, Graham Jr JM. Klinefelter syndrome and its variants: an update and review for the primary pediatrician. Clin Pediatr (Phila). 2001;40(12):639–51.
10. Aguirre D, Nieto K, Lazos M, Peña YR, Palma I, Kofman-Alfaro S, Queipo G. Extragonadal germ cell tumors are often associated with Klinefelter syndrome. Hum Pathol. 2006;37(4): 477–80.
11. Kamischke A, Baumgardt A, Horst J, Nieschlag E. Clinical and diagnostic features of patients with suspected Klinefelter syndrome. J Androl. 2003;24(1):41–8.
12. Lanfranco F, Kamischke A, Zitzmann M, Nieschlag E. Klinefelter's syndrome. Lancet. 2004;364(9430):273–83.
13. Paduch DA, Fine RG, Bolyakov A, Kiper J. New concepts in Klinefelter syndrome. Curr Opin Urol. 2008;18(6):621–7.
14. Campbell WA, Price WH. Venous thromboembolic disease in Klinefelter's syndrome. Clin Genet. 1981;19(4):275–80.
15. Fricke GR, Mattern HJ, Schweikert HU, Schwanitz G. Klinefelter's syndrome and mitral valve prolapse. An echocardiographic study in twenty-two patients. Biomed Pharmacother. 1984; 38(2):88–97.
16. Myhre SA, Ruvalcaba RH, Johnson HR, Thuline HC, Kelley VC. The effects of testosterone treatment in Klinefelter's syndrome. J Pediatr. 1970;76(2):267–76.
17. Nielsen J, Pelsen B, Sørensen K. Follow-up of 30 Klinefelter males treated with testosterone. Clin Genet. 1988;33(4):262–9.
18. Lin YM, Huang WJ, Lin JS, Kuo PL. Progressive depletion of germ cells in a man with nonmosaic Klinefelter's syndrome: optimal time for sperm recovery. Urology. 2004; 63(2):380–1.
19. Wikström AM, Raivio T, Hadziselimovic F, Wikström S, Tuuri T, Dunkel L. Klinefelter syndrome in adolescence: onset of puberty is associated with accelerated germ cell depletion. J Clin Endocrinol Metab. 2004;89(5):2263–70.
20. Schiff JD, Palermo GD, Veeck LL, Goldstein M, Rosenwaks Z, Schlegel PN. Success of testicular sperm extraction [corrected] and intracytoplasmic sperm injection in men with Klinefelter syndrome. J Clin Endocrinol Metab. 2005;90(11):6263–7.
21. Friedler S, Raziel A, Strassburger D, Schachter M, Bern O, Ron-El R. Outcome of ICSI using fresh and cryopreserved-thawed testicular spermatozoa in patients with non-mosaic Klinefelter's syndrome. Hum Reprod. 2001;16(12):2616–20.
22. Madgar I, Dor J, Weissenberg R, Raviv G, Menashe Y, Levron J. Prognostic value of the clinical and laboratory evaluation in patients with nonmosaic Klinefelter syndrome who are receiving assisted reproductive therapy. Fertil Steril. 2002;77(6):1167–9.
23. Ramasamy R, Ricci JA, Palermo GD, Gosden LV, Rosenwaks Z, Schlegel PN. Successful fertility treatment for Klinefelter's syndrome. J Urol. 2009;182(3):1108–13.
24. Raman JD, Schlegel PN. Aromatase inhibitors for male infertility. J Urol. 2002;167(2 Pt 1): 624–9.
25. Staessen C, Tournaye H, Van Assche E, Michiels A, Van Landuyt L, Devroey P, Liebaers I, Van Steirteghem A. PGD in 47, XXY Klinefelter's syndrome patients. Hum Reprod Update. 2003;9(4):319–30.
26. Hennebicq S, Pelletier R, Bergues U, Rousseaux S. Risk of trisomy 21 in offspring of patients with Klinefelter's syndrome. Lancet. 2001;357(9274):2104–5.
27. Morel F, Bernicot I, Herry A, Le Bris MJ, Amice V, De Braekeleer M. An increased incidence of autosomal aneuploidies in spermatozoa from a patient with Klinefelter's syndrome. Fertil Steril. 2003;79 Suppl 3:1644–6.

28. Levron J, Aviram-Goldring A, Madgar I, Raviv G, Barkai G, Dor J. Sperm chromosome analysis and outcome of IVF in patients with non-mosaic Klinefelter's syndrome. Fertil Steril. 2000;74(5):925–9.
29. Izadyar F, Matthijs-Rijsenbilt JJ, den Ouden K, Creemers LB, Woelders H, de Rooij DG. Development of a cryopreservation protocol for type A spermatogonia. J Androl. 2002; 23(4):537–45.
30. Orwig KE, Schlatt S. Cryopreservation and transplantation of spermatogonia and testicular tissue for preservation of male fertility. J Natl Cancer Inst Monogr. 2005;34:51–6.
31. Nagano M, Patrizio P, Brinster RL. Long-term survival of human spermatogonial stem cells in mouse testes. Fertil Steril. 2002;78(6): 1225–33.
32. Sofikitis N. Transplantation of human spermatogonia into the seminiferous tubules (STs) of animal testicles results in the completion of the human meiosis and the generation of human motile spermatozoa. Fertil Steril. 1999;72 suppl 1:S83–4.
33. Patience C, Takeuchi Y, Weiss RA. Infection of human cells by an endogenous retrovirus of pigs. Nat Med. 1997;3(3):282–6.
34. Brinster RL, Zimmermann JW. Spermatogenesis following male germ-cell transplantation. Proc Natl Acad Sci USA. 1994;91(24): 11298–302.
35. Ogawa T. Spermatogonial transplantation technique in spermatogenesis research. Int J Androl. 2000;23 Suppl 2:57–9.
36. Honaramooz A, Snedaker A, Boiani M, Scholer H, Dobrinski I, Schlatt S. Sperm from neonatal mammalian testes grafted in mice. Nature. 2002;418(6899):778–81.
37. Schlatt S, Kim SS, Gosden R. Spermatogenesis and steroidogenesis in mouse, hamster and monkey testicular tissue after cryopreservation and heterotopic grafting to castrated hosts. Reproduction. 2002;124(3):339–46.
38. Oatley JM, de Avila DM, Reeves JJ, McLean DJ. Spermatogenesis and germ cell transgene expression in xenografted bovine testicular tissue. Biol Reprod. 2004;71(2):494–501.

Chapter 19
Micro-testicular Sperm Extraction (MicroTESE)

Doron Sol Stember and Peter Schlegel

The condition of nonobstructive azoospermia (NOA) defines men with testicular failure who have severely deficient sperm production with no sperm in the ejaculate. NOA is the underlying diagnosis in approximately 10% of men seeking fertility evaluation. On testicular biopsy, these patients demonstrate hypospermatogenesis, maturation arrest, or Sertoli cell-only pattern (germinal cell aplasia). NOA may be related to genetic causes, as in Klinefelter Syndrome (KS) and XX-male syndrome, or may be acquired, as in testicular failure secondary to cryptorchidism or systemic chemotherapy administration. As recently as two decade ago, techniques were not available to assist patients with NOA conceive offspring and their options were limited to donor spermatazoa or child adoption.

A remarkable series of four distinct advancements have dramatically advanced the field in recent years, and today it is possible even for men with Sertoli cell-only pattern to initiate pregnancy with medical assistance. The first factor was the clinical recognition that successful fertilization is not dependent on epididymal transit. This concept allows for the direct retrieval of seminiferous tubules harboring sperm from the testes. Multiple techniques have been developed for this purpose and will be discussed herein.

The second critical factor was the development of intracytoplasmic sperm injection (ICSI), a technique that involves in vitro injection of a single sperm into an oocyte. ICSI removes many natural barriers to fertilization, theoretically requires

D.S. Stember, MD (✉)
Division of Urology, Department of Surgery,
Memorial Sloan-Kettering Cancer Center, 1275 York Avenue,
435, New York, NY 10065, USA
e-mail: stemberd@mskcc.org

P. Schlegel, MD
Department of Urology, Weill Cornell Medical College,
New York-Presbyterian/Weill Cornell Hospital,
525 East 6th Street, Starr 900, New York, NY 10065, USA
e-mail: pnschleg@med.cornell.edu

S.J. Parekattil, A. Agarwal (eds.), *Male Infertility for the Clinician,*
© Springer Science+Business Media New York 2013

only a single sperm, and can be successful even with nonmotile sperm. Surgical sperm retrieval by testicular extraction followed by ICSI was first described as a treatment for obstructive azoospermia in 1993 [1].

The third factor was the recognition, and histologic demonstration, that heterogeneity of seminiferous tubules exists in testis biopsy specimens. Patients with Sertoli cell-only as a predominant testicular histologic pattern, for example, often have microscopic foci of spermatogenesis. The indications for testicular sperm extraction (TESE) were thus expanded as it became apparent that viable spermatozoa could be obtained from men with sperm production so poor that no sperm or no viable sperm in the ejaculate, as with NOA [2, 3].

The fourth major factor has been the introduction of a sperm extraction technique that takes advantage of the opportunity to identify even microscopic sites of recognition of sperm production. Use of an operating microscope during TESE enables selective extraction of tubules that may harbor active spermatogenesis, even in a testicle otherwise overwhelmingly composed of nonproductive tubules. Under microscopic vision, normal-appearing tubules that are more likely to contain sperm can be selectively removed, while abnormal and sclerotic tubules are avoided. Microscopic vessels can also be avoided or coagulated, thereby significantly reducing the risk of post-procedure hematoma or devascularization of remaining testicular tissue.

In this chapter, we focus on considerations and techniques related to microscopic testicular sperm extraction (microdissection TESE). Microdissection TESE, a technique developed at New York-Presbyterian Hospital–Weill Cornell Medical Center, yields superior sperm retrieval rates and requires a minimal amount of testicular tissue compared with other methods of sperm extraction.

Microdissection Testicular Sperm Extraction

Nonobstructive Azoospermia

The formal diagnosis of NOA requires a histological diagnosis, but a preoperative biopsy is not required for microdissection TESE. A clinical diagnosis of NOA may be established with reasonable certainty on the combined basis of history, azoospermia on semen analysis, small testes, flat/empty epididymides, and elevated serum FSH levels. Definitive confirmation of the diagnosis can then be made by histologic analysis of tissue extracted at the time of the sperm retrieval procedure.

Multiple strategies to retrieve testicular tissue in patients with NOA have been developed. Successfully retrieved sperm may be cryopreserved for future use or, if timed to coincide with oocyte retrieval, can be immediately used for ICSI. Each technique has associated advantages and disadvantages. A variety of these sperm retrieval techniques can also be utilized by patients with obstructive azoospermia as an alternative to surgical reconstruction.

Conventional TESE

This procedure involves standard single or multiple testicular biopsies are performed in an open fashion under local or general anesthesia. A scrotal incision is made and the tunica albuginea is opened. Samples of testicular parenchyma are excised and subsequently evaluated for the presence of sperm by an embryologist. Conventional TESE may take less time than microdissection TESE and also has the advantage of not requiring microsurgical training.

However, in contrast to microdissection TESE, blind open tunical incision has a greater risk of interrupting the vascular supply and devascularizing testicular tissue. Loss of functional tissue is particularly problematic in NOA patients who tend to have limited volume and function of testicular tissue in the first place. The testicular blood vessels course under the tunica albuginea before penetrating the testicular parenchyma can be visualized and avoided by using an operating microscope.

Open or conventional TESE is also a relatively inefficient process, since a large proportion of tubules removed in patients with NOA are sclerotic. Multiple blind biopsies are obtained since there is no way to intraoperatively identify normal-appearing tubules. Open TESE does not allow for thorough dissection of all areas of the testis, because to do so would essentially remove all testicular tissue. Even though relatively large amounts of tissue may be removed in open TESE, the possibility of missing foci of spermatogenesis deep within the testes is high compared with microdissection TESE.

Fine Needle Aspiration/Testicular Mapping

Testicular fine needle aspiration (FNAB) is a cytologic technique that does not directly evaluate seminiferous tubule architecture, in contrast to standard biopsies, conventional or microdissection TESE. With a diagnosis of NOA made by other means, however, FNAB is generally considered the least involved procedure for acquiring sperm. It is usually performed under local anesthesia in the office setting, requires little time, is well tolerated by patients, and does not require advanced training on the practitioner's part. It is performed by inserting a 23-19-gage butterfly needle directly into the testis and aspirating contents into plastic tubing that is connected to the needle. Multiple needle punctures are usually directed into various parts of the testis.

A report of patients who underwent FNAB with 2–3 tissue samples from each testis demonstrated spermatozoa recovered in 47% of patients with NOA [4]. An earlier report of FNAB in which up to 15 samples were taken from each testis (with the patients under general anesthesia) had a 60% sperm retrieval rate in men with testicular failure, although most patients had too few sperm retrieved to inject all partner's eggs [5]. Other studies, however, have found that FNAB yields a much lower rate of sperm retrieval than TESE [6, 7]. The scarcity of high-quality literature regarding FNAB, the lack of careful follow-up of patients for potential complications, as well as a wide disparity of specific techniques used, makes critical evaluation of the technique difficult.

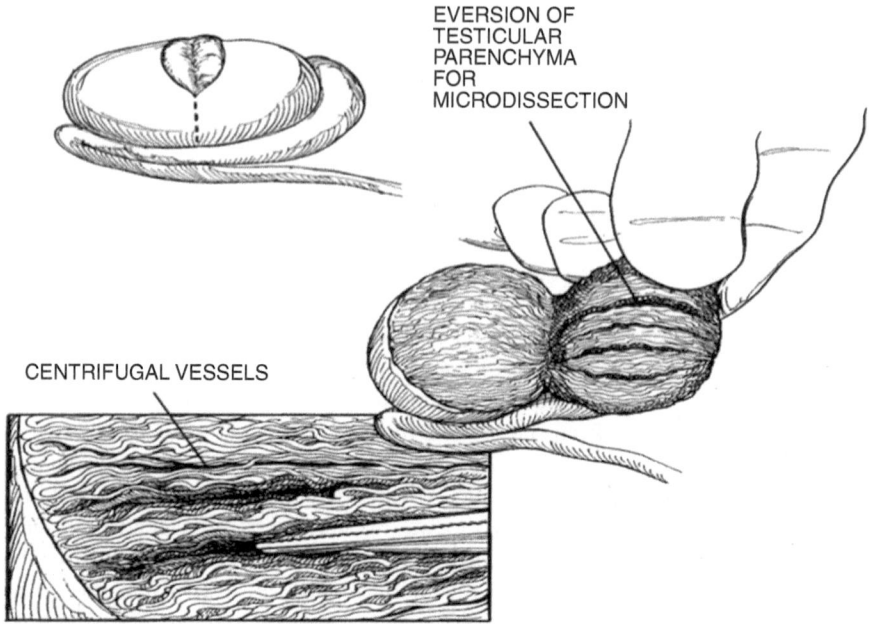

EVERSION OF
TESTICULAR
PARENCHYMA
FOR
MICRODISSECTION

CENTRIFUGAL VESSELS

Fig. 19.1 An area of the tunica albuginea is incised and microdissected (Copyright, Brady Urology Foundation 2005)

One major disadvantage of FNAB is the potential risk of disruption of testicular vascular supply. Given the nature of the procedure, subtunical or intraparenchymal testicular bleeding cannot by directly stopped and must be allowed to progress and resolve with the treatment of ice packs. Another negative consequence of the blind technique is the high chance of failure simply due to sampling error. To address this issue in a systematic manner, Turek et al. introduced the technique of testis mapping. In mapping, the skin over the testis is pulled taut and secured in place by wrapping a sponge or Penrose drain behind the testis. A sterile pen is used to mark four to nine evenly distributed sites, depending on testis size, on the skin surface. A wheal of local anesthesia, and subsequently the aspiration needle, is then directed at each marked site [8].

Microdissection TESE

Microdissection TESE is most sophisticated method for retrieving spermatozoa in men with NOA (Fig. 19.1). With the benefit of optical magnification, an avascular area of the tunica albuginea is incised. Small areas of bleeding are selectively coagulated with a microbipolar forceps, thereby minimizing damage to adjacent testicular tissue. Microscopic foci of healthy-appearing tubules are identified among the much great numbers of Sertoli cell-only or sclerotic tubules typically seen in NOA patients. Normal tubules are usually larger and more opaque than those that do not produce sperm and can be carefully dissected out along their entire length. They are then extracted from the testis without disrupting blood supply or removing an extraneous volume of tissue.

Microdissection TESE requires advanced microsurgical training. An embryologist must be available in the operating room to evaluate processed testis parenchymal samples as they are passed off the operating table. By evaluating testicular samples in real time, the surgeon can stop the procedure as soon as the presence of sperm is confirmed, thereby minimizing operative time and removal of testicular tissue. Patience is essential since thorough microscopic dissection of tubules can require up to 2 h per testis if sperm is not identified during the case.

In an early prospective study from our institution, we reported a sperm retrieval rate of 45% (10/22) for patients undergoing conventional TESE compared with 63% (17/27) of patients undergoing microdissection TESE ($p < 0.05$). We further showed that the average of 64,000 spermatozoa yielded by conventional TESE biopsy samples were obtained in samples averaging 720 mg each, compared with an average of 160,000 spermatozoa in the microdissected samples that averaged only 9.4 mg ($p < 0.05$ for all comparisons) [6].

In another prospective study, Amer et al. performed conventional TESE on one testis and microdissection TESE on the other in 100 patients with NOA. The authors reported a significantly higher sperm retrieval of 47% for the microdissection TESE side than the 30% obtained on conventional TESE side ($p < 0.05$). Follow-up ultrasound testing demonstrated significantly fewer acute and chronic complications on the testes that underwent microdissection TESE, presumably due to improved vascular control as described previously [7].

Genetic Screening for TESE Candidates

Along with the revolutionary fertility potential associated with the development of advanced reproductive techniques, some novel concerns have been raised. In previous eras, the state of azoospermia ensured that some abnormalities (including infertility traits themselves) would not typically be vertically transmitted. With the advent of ICSI in conjunction with sperm retrieval techniques, it has now become possible for these genetic abnormalities to be passed on to offspring.

In an analysis of patients with NOA who were candidates for the TESE procedure at Weill-Cornell Medical College, 17% (33/190) were found to have abnormalities on Y chromosome microdeletion analysis and/or karyotypic testing [9]. Given the high rate of genetic abnormalities and the potential for genetic transmission, we believe that genetic screening should be conducted on all TESE candidates prior to attempts at assisted reproduction. Karyotype evaluation and Y chromosome microdeletion analysis are indicated for men with sperm concentrations lower than 10×10^6/cc.

Men with abnormalities detected on screening should be referred to a genetics counselor for a thorough discussion of the potential implications prior to undergoing attempts at sperm retrieval. Depending on the likelihood of passing infertility traits or other genetic defects to offspring, some couples may elect to use donor spermatozoa. Genetic screening of TESE candidates also facilitates specific genetic testing and subsequent selection of embryos prior to implantation.

Cytogenetic Analysis

Common abnormalities seen in men with NOA includes Klinefelter's syndrome (47, XXY), autosomal translocations, and other sex chromosome anomalies (i.e., 46, XX). Of 190 sequential TESE candidates who underwent genetic evaluation at Weill-Cornell, 33 (17%) were found to have genetic abnormalities. Of the 183 patients who underwent molecular analysis for Y chromosome partial deletion, defects were detected in 17 (9%). Of the 101 patients who underwent karyotype testing, 21 (21%) had cytogenetic abnormalities, including 13 with KS. Five men with sex chromosome anomalies detected on karyotyping also had Y chromosome deletions. Of the 33 men in whom genetic anomalies were discovered, 31 underwent counseling with their partners. Knowledge of the specific genetic defect affected the choice of clinical treatment in 7 of the 33 couples (21%), including donor insemination, adoption, and delaying treatment. The remainder of couples elected to proceed with TESE/ICSI and was counseled to use the preimplantation diagnosis to allow selection of genetically unaffected embryos for transfer [9].

Y Microdeletion Testing

Submicroscopic deletions in the Y chromosome are also prevalent in patients with severely impaired spermatogenesis. Partial Y chromosome deletion analysis is recommended for all men who are TESE candidates, along with karyotype testing, prior to assisted reproductive techniques. Microdeletion testing involves polymerase chain reaction (PCR) of Y-chromosome sequence-tagged sites.

Girardi et al. evaluated 160 men referred for evaluation of male factor infertility who consented to genetic testing. Azoospermic men had a 7% prevalence of Y chromosome microdeletions. Microdeletions were found in 10% of men who were virtually azoospermic ($0-1 \times 10^6$) and 8% of severely oligozoospermic ($1-5 \times 10^6$) men. No microdeletions were detected in men who were moderately oligozoospermic ($5-20 \times 10^6$) or normozoospermic ($>20 \times 10^6$) [10].

Most Y chromosome deletions relating to fertility partially or completely involve the AZFa, AZFb, or AZFc regions. Although sperm can often be found with isolated AZFc deletions, complete AZFa and AZFb deletions are highly associated with failure of sperm retrieval techniques. The likelihood of failing to find sperm in these patients is high enough that we do not recommend that they undergo sperm retrieval procedures. If they do elect to undergo a sperm retrieval procedure despite the dismal odds of sperm retrieval, then the couple should plan to use donor sperm as a backup.

Microdissection TESE Technique

Surgical Approach

After general anesthesia is induced and a first-generation cephalosporin is given the scrotum is shaved. The decision of which testicle to address first is based on several factors. The intent is to maximize the likelihood of adequate sperm retrieval on the first testicle incised and avoid opening the contralateral testis. If the patient has had previous biopsy or TESE that shows better sperm production on a given side then that side is addressed first. Size of the testes is also considered, since larger testis size is usually attributed to fuller seminiferous tubules and thereby better sperm production. Patients who have had previous testis procedures have preoperative ultrasounds to determine scarring. Significantly more scar tissue in one side gives cause for starting with the contralateral side. If all else is equal, the right testis is incised first. It has been our clinical experience that the likelihood of finding sites of spermatogenesis tends to be better on the right than the left side. In some cases, this may be related to left-sided varicoceles, but we have found it to be true even in the absence of a clinical varicocele.

The testis is manipulated to the midline and an incision is made along the median raphe with a 15-blade. The scrotal layers are divided and the testis is delivered. Many patients undergoing microdissection TESE have had one or more prior testicular procedures. In these patients, the tunica vaginalis is often scarred down and adherent to the tunica albuginea. In some cases, a curved scissors can be used to separate the layers. If there are extensive adhesions, then it is advisable to bring in the microscope with 6–8× power magnification. The flat edge of the bovie is used to gently cauterize the lateral aspect of the vaginalis, which is gently spread away from the testis by the assistant. Care is taken to avoid thermal injury to the epididymis. It is necessary to completely free the testis from any adhesions so that it is easily manipulated in the latter parts of the operation.

Under microscopic vision, a 15° ultrasharp ophthalmic knife is used to widely incise the testis horizontally. Subtunical blood vessels can be visualized under the microscope and should be avoided. The testis should be divided as evenly as possible since an eccentric cut makes it harder to subsequently separate the tissue. The knife is lightly applied so that the albuginea is completely incised but the tubules are not disrupted. Using both hands, with the thumbs applying pressure outwards, the testis is bivalved. Bipolar electrocautery is used sparingly to coagulate bleeding at the cut edges of the tunica layer. It is crucial to avoid separating the tubules from the inner surface of the tunica albuginea, since this can result in bleeding that is difficult to control. With extremely small testes that are difficult to manipulate (as is characteristic of azoospermic patients) clamps are placed on either edge of the tunica albuginea inclusive of a portion of the underlying tubules to help prevent such separation.

The testis, which is held in the nondominant hand with the arm in a comfortable position, can be safely twisted up to 180° on its cord as needed during the procedure. The entire superficial surface of exposed seminiferous tubules is scanned to identify large and/or opaque tubules. Magnification is then increased to 20× for tubule dissection. Applying pressure with fingers helps expose tubules of interest while excluding others. The thumb and index finger is used to apply gentle pressure to expose an area of interest between them, while the middle finger of the same hand applies gentle counterpressure in the opposite direction (see diagram). Tension should be applied parallel to the wedges of seminiferous tubules (that is, perpendicular to the incision).

Maintaining proper visualization and exposure of the tubules is a dynamic process that requires constant readjustment so that the entire field, with the tubule of interest in the center, remains in focus. Since the depth of focus is very shallow, and perfect focus is imperative for visualization of the tubules, only one pair of gloves should be used to ensure sufficient tactile feedback. When a promising tubule is found among sclerotic tubules, it is individually teased and dissected out for its entire length before being passed off the field. This is best accomplished by repetitive lateral sweeping motions, whereby a portion of the tubule is mobilized to the side before another area is picked up and then also brought over the side.

In addition to the tubules that are dissected for fertility purposes, a random sample of testis should be separately removed with Iris scissors for histological diagnosis. This sample should be removed without individual dissection of tubules or any other distortion to preserve the histological architecture.

An important adjunct to the treatment of microdissection TESE is the presence of a skilled embryologist in the operating room during the procedure. The role of the embryologist is to review tissue under microscopic vision and immediately give an initial report on the presence, number, and quality of sperm directly to the surgeon. The yield of the tissue is greatly increased by surgeon processing just prior to evaluation by the embryologist. Once a sufficient sperm concentration has been identified (taking into account morphology and motility), there is no need for further dissection. The procedure is terminated with the expectation that more sperm will be found by the laboratory after formal processing. If adequate sperm numbers are not seen by the embryologist, then the surgeon proceeds until the entire testis has been thoroughly sampled. At that point, the contralateral testis will be opened and the procedure will be repeated on that side.

Once extraction is finished on a given testis, the edges of the tunica albuginea are brought together and secured with multiple mosquito clamps under 4× magnification. Special care is taken to avoid manipulation of testicular tissue, since movement of the testicular tissue off of the tunica albuginea can result in substantial bleeding under the surface of the testis resulting in substantial scarring. The incision is closed with nonabsorbable 5-0 polypropylene suture, which is chosen to minimize inflammatory response as well as for immediate identification of the original incision site if repeat microdissection TESE is required. The dartos layer and skin are then closed in the usual fashion. Bacitracin ointment and fluff dressing is applied within a scrotal support.

Sperm Processing

Excised biopsy samples are placed in human tubular fluid with 5% Plasmanate and the testicular region from which it was dissected is noted. Since spermatazoa are normally within seminiferous tubules, mechanical dispersion with fine scissors is required to release sperm that can be identified on wet-prep in the operating room. A few drops of medium (up to 400 μL) should be used to keep the tissue from drying out during the mincing process, but adding too much saline will dilute the sample. Once the tissue has been processed into a suspension, the entire sample drawn up into a syringe and passed several times through a 24-gage angiocatheter to assure adequate dispersion of the tubules. This aggressive dispersion approach can increase sperm yield up to 300-fold [11].

To avoid accidentally losing any volume, the tubule suspension is injected into a 1.5-cc microfuge Eppendorf tube instead of a Petri dish. Since each drop of processed tissue placed on the wet-prep slide contains about 5 μL, the number of sperm in the Eppendorf can be estimated based on number of sperm counted under the microscope. For example, if three spermatozoa are seen on microscopy from a sample containing a total volume of 500 μL, multiplying by 100 gives an estimated number of 300 individual sperm in the Eppendorf.

Each specimen containing the best-appearing seminiferous tubules should be sequentially processed and examined in the operating room until either sperm is found or all areas of the testis have been thoroughly examined. Detecting sperm under the microscope allows the procedure to stop and unnecessary removal of testicular tissue can be avoided. Since there may be a sampling error, the procedure continues until the surgeon feels that adequate sperm have been confirmed to be present to inject all eggs. It is fruitful to continue working in the same area of the testis where sperm were positively identified. However, even a single spermatozoon seen on wet-prep can represent sufficient spermatozoa to end the procedure and proceed with ICSI.

Microdissection TESE Results

Sperm Retrieval Rates

Rates of successful microdissection TESE–ICSI rates have been encouraging in our institutional experience of more than 1,000 attempted treatment cycles for couples in whom the man had NOA. Sperm were retrieved by microdissection TESE in 58% of attempts. For cycles in which sperm was retrieved, clinical pregnancies (as defined by fetal heartbeat on ultrasound) were established at a 45% rate.

The risk of postoperative hematoma following microdissection TESE is approximately 2–3%. One of the advantages of the microdissection TESE technique is the ability of removing minimal tissue with an eye toward future attempts at retrieval, if necessary. Indeed, repeat microdissection TESE following prior successful retrieval has been shown to yields a 96% sperm retrieval rate. If sperm are not found on prior micro-dissection TESE, the success rate of repeat microdissection TESE drops to 33% [12].

Histopathologic Findings

Three testicular histologic architectural patterns can be found in men with NOA: hypospermatogenesis, maturation arrest, and Sertoli cell-only [11]. Hypospermatogenesis represents abnormally decreased sperm production. While germ cells are present within seminiferous tubules, only limited numbers of sper-matids are found. In maturation arrest, both Sertoli cells and immature germ cells are present in seminiferous tubules. In Sertoli cell-only pattern, no germ cells are present and, the name describes, only Sertoli cells are seen.

As previously noted, men with NOA often have heterogeneous patterns of function within their testicular tissue, with microscopic foci of germ cells present among more abundant sclerotic or Sertoli cell-only tubules. The results of microdissection TESE are related to the most advanced pattern of spermatogenesis, rather than the predomi-nant pattern. In 2007, we evaluated the microdissection results for men who have had prior unsuccessful biopsies in men with NOA. There was no statistically significant difference between sperm retrieval rates in men with a diagnosis of either maturation or hypospermatogenesis regardless of the number of previous biopsies. In men with at least one prior biopsy showing Sertoli cell-only as the most advanced pattern, how-ever, sperm retrieval rates were lower than among men with no previous biopsies [13].

Endocrine Evaluation and Treatment

Men with testicular failure typically have abnormally elevated follicle-stimulating hormone (FSH) levels, as a result of decreased germ cells within the testis as a result of poor sperm production, along with normal or near-normal testosterone levels. Randomized controlled trials have not yet demonstrated a fertility benefit from manipulating hormone levels in these patients. Many men with severely impaired spermatogenesis, however, demonstrate a low testosterone (ng/dL) to estradiol (pg/mL) ratio (T/E2 ratio). High intratesticular testosterone is necessary for spermatogene-sis, and estradiol may impair spermatogenesis by decreasing pituitary luteinizing hormone (LH) and FSH [14].

Pavlovich et al. compared T/E2 ratios of fertile men, used for reference, with those with of patients with severe male factor infertility [15]. While normal fertile men had an average T/E2 ratio of 16 ± 3, men with NOA had a ratio of 7. Men with KS had an even lower T/E2 ratio of 4. Patients were treated with the aromatase inhibitor testolactone, resulting in significant increases in testosterone and decreases in estradiol. In 12 oligozoospermic patients, the hormonal changes were associated with significant improvements in sperm concentration and motility compared with initial semen analyses. Of men who were initially azoospermic, however, no sperm was found on semen analysis after testolactone treatment.

At our institution, we now routinely obtain testosterone and estradiol levels in men with NOA or severe oligozoospermia. Men with KS who have low testosterone and low T/E2 ratios are treated with 50–100 mg of testolactone per day. For non-KS patients, T/E2 ratio and estradiol level responses were found to be even better with the use of 1 mg of oral anastrazole per day [16].

Structural Changes to Testis

The testicular artery enters the posterior aspect of the testis beneath the epididymis and continues inferiorly to the lower pole of the testis. From the lower pole, multiple branches course superiorly along the anterior testis in the subtunical space, periodically giving off branches to supply the parenchyma. FNAB and conventional TESE provide no visualization of these microscopic vessels and therefore engender an increased risk of vascular disruption. Testicular bleeding can lead to hematoma, devascularization of parenchymal tissue, and intratesticular scarring. Since the tunica albuginea is a non-flexible enclosure surrounding the testicular parenchyma, even small amounts of bleeding can quickly lead to significant increases in intratesticular pressure with possible subsequent atrophy [17].

In contrast with conventional open TESE or FNAB, microdissection TESE allows avoidance of subtunical and parenchymal blood vessels and provides for microscopic hemostatic control of any bleeding sites that may arise. Several comparative studies have confirmed that the likelihood of acute and chronic complications, including structural changes to the testes, is minimized with microdissection TESE compared with conventional TESE. FNAB has not been directly compared with TESE. Okada et al. retrospectively reviewed 147 TESE consecutive cases for patients with azoospermia [18]. All patients underwent testicular ultrasound 1 month after TESE. Diffuse heterogeneic patterns or hypoechoic areas on ultrasound were considered indicative of hematoma. Among the 47 patients who underwent conventional TESE, 24 (51%) showed evidence of hematoma. Of the 100 patients who underwent microdissection TESE, only 12 (12%) had ultrasound findings consistent with hematoma. On follow-up ultrasound at 6 months, hematoma was identified in 3/40 (7.5%) of conventional TESE patients and 2/80 (2.5%) of microdissection patients.

The relative safety of microdissection TESE was also demonstrated in a retrospective review from our institution. Patients who underwent either conventional (83 attempts) or microdissection TESE (460 attempts) were followed with serial Color Doppler scrotal ultrasounds at 3 and 6 months following surgery. Diffuse heterogeneic patterns or hypoechoic areas were considered acute changes consistent with hematoma or inflammation and calcifications were considered chronic changes. Acute and chronic changes were both significantly lower for the patients who underwent microdissection TESE than conventional TESE. Although no evidence of permanent testicular devascularization was found in any patient after 6 months, the findings suggest that microdissection TESE is relatively safer than conventional TESE, in addition to providing an improved sperm retrieval rate as discussed elsewhere [19].

Predictors of Microdissection TESE Success

Microdissection TESE is typically carried out in conjunction with ICSI cycles. TESE–ICSI cycles are financially and emotionally burdensome for infertile couples. It is, therefore, important to predict, to the extent possible, the likelihood of successful sperm retrieval before committing to treatment. Several factors, including prior biopsy, FSH levels, and genetic screening have been studied to determine their associated probabilities of spermatozoa retrieval.

Effect of Prior Biopsy or Conventional TESE Procedure

Successful sperm retrieval is often possible in men with NOA in the context of multiple prior negative biopsies. Ostad et al. reported that half of these patients required multiple (range 2–14) biopsies to retrieve sperm. The effect of prior negative biopsies or conventional TESE procedures on the rate of sperm retrieval with microdissection TESE in men with NOA was evaluated at Weill-Cornell. Successful sperm retrieval in patients who underwent no prior biopsies (56%) was higher than for those who had underwent 1–2 biopsies per testis (51%) or 3–4 biopsies per testis (23%) ($p = 0.04$) [20]. In addition to causing scarring and parenchymal fibrosis, diagnostic testicular biopsy can cause parenchymal devascularization with subsequent deleterious effects for spermatogenesis. These changes may explain the lower rates of sperm retrieval associated with more frequent prior biopsies.

Testicular Histology on Diagnostic Biopsy

Diagnosis of NOA can only be definitively made with histopathologic evaluation. Testis biopsy can also be useful for ruling out intratubular germ cell neoplasia (carcinoma in situ). Although the diagnosis is unlikely, it is more common (approximately 3%) in patients who present with NOA and biopsy is required by some centers prior to surgical sperm retrieval procedures. In addition to the role of diagnostic biopsy in identifying rare cases of intratubular germ cell neoplasia (carcinoma in situ) and confirming the diagnosis of nonobstructive azoospermia, diagnostic biopsy helps to predict the chance that a TESE procedure will obtain sperm.

Since diagnostic biopsy does not sample all areas of the testis, small foci of more advanced patterns may be missed. However, the likelihood of successful sperm retrieval in patients with NOA who undergo microdissection TESE can be estimated by the most advanced (as opposed to most predominant) histopathological pattern if a previous testicular biopsy has been performed. In men with at least on area of hypospermatogenesis on prior biopsy, 81% had sperm retrieved with microdissection TESE. In patients with maturation arrest at the most advanced pattern on biopsy, 44% had successful sperm retrieval [19].

If Sertoli cell-only is found without any areas of more advanced spermatogenesis, however, the sperm retrieval rate drops to approximately 30%. This has important counseling implications. Some couples may decide that they would be unwilling to undergo the process of a simultaneous IVF cycle, if there is only a 30% chance of sperm retrieval on microdissection TESE. In these cases, then the male partner is encouraged to undergo a diagnostic biopsy. If a uniform pattern of Sertoli-cell only is demonstrated the couple can avoid ovarian hyperstimulation as well as the financial and emotional costs of an IVF cycle.

Microdissection TESE in Setting of Elevated FSH Levels

Elaboration of inhibin by Sertoli cells is decreased in the setting of testicular failure. With less negative feedback mediated by inhibin, production of FSH from the anterior pituitary increases. Elevated serum FSH levels are, therefore, generally associated with impaired spermatogenesis. In a study of predictors of sperm retrieval and probability of fertilization using open testis biopsy methods, receiver operating characteristics showed FSH levels of ≥ 20 IU/L as cutoff for treatment success [21].

FSH levels are less relevant for predicting success of microdissection TESE. Even though serum FSH indirectly reflects the global histology of the testes, microdissection TESE is much more sensitive than open techniques for finding isolated foci of sperm production. This hypothesis was tested in a retrospective study of nearly 800 men with NOA who underwent microdissection TESE. Patients were divided into four groups by serum FSH levels (<15, 15–30, 31–45, and >45 IU/mL). Contrary to previous studies and conventional wisdom, sperm retrieval rates were higher for men with elevated FSH than those in the normal range. Sperm retrieval rates were maintained as FSH levels increased, furthermore, even for several patients with FSH >90 IU/mL [22]. These findings underscore the concept that FSH levels are not predictive of sperm retrieval success with microdissection. Azoospermic patients with normal FSH may represent a distinct infertility population. Indeed, it has been reported that many patients with diffuse maturation arrest have normal FSH levels (and testicular volume) [23].

AZF Deletions

PCR-based analysis of Y chromosome sequence-tagged sites is prognostically important and is routinely performed for microdissection TESE candidates. The Y chromosome microdeletions that relate to infertility are seen in part of all of the AZFa, AZFb, or AZFc regions of the DAZ (deleted in azoospermia) gene and are found in 6–18% of men presenting with NOA or oligozoospermia [24–28].

In men with isolated AZFc deletions, sperm production found in the testis at similar rates as for other patients with NOA. At Weill-Cornell, in a retrospective analysis of 1,591 men with sperm concentrations less than 5 million sperm/mL, a total of 149 microdeletions (9.4%) were found. Of the 718 patients who underwent microdissection TESE, sperm retrieval failed in all men with AZFa, AZFb, AZFb + c, and complete Yq deletions. Presence of an AZFc microdeletion, in contrast, was associated with a 71.4% sperm retrieval rate. Of the 15 patients with AZFc deletions with successful sperm retrieval, ten of them achieved clinical pregnancy. AZFc deletions were reported, for the first time, to be favorably associated with sperm retrieval in comparison to 385 patients with idiopathic azoospermia, for whom microdissection TESE yielded a 48.8% retrieval rate [28].

Given the exceptionally poor prognosis for patients with complete AZFa or AZFb deletions, primary utilization of donor sperm is advised rather than microdissection TESE. Men with AZFc deletions have a favorable likelihood of successful sperm retrieval on microdissection TESE. Genetics counseling for the couple is mandatory, since potential male offspring will carry the same infertility trait as the father and eventually face similar reproductive issues themselves.

Microdissection TESE in Patient Subpopulation

There are several patient populations that may particularly benefit from microdissection TESE, including KS, post-chemo, and NOA associated with cryptorchidism.

Klinefelter's Syndrome

Klinefelter syndrome (KS), or hypergonadotropic hypogonadism, is, at 11%, the most frequently diagnosed karyotype abnormality in infertile men [29]. The genetic abnormality results from a meiotic nondisjunction event that most commonly results in classic 47,XXY genotype, but 3% of men with KS are mosaic 46,XX/47,XXY.

KS patients have traditionally been considered a difficult group to retrieve sperm from because they typically have small testes, high FSH levels, and a predominant expression of tubular sclerosis on testicular histopathology. Several studies, however, have reported successful sperm retrieval rates of 40–48% in KS patients [30, 31]. More recently, even higher retrieval rates have been demonstrated. In 2005, we retrospectively reviewed a series of 42 patients with KS who underwent 54 attempted microdissection TESE procedures. Patients had mean FSH levels of 33.2 IU/L and a successful sperm retrieval rate of 72% per TESE attempt [32].

There are several possible reasons for the higher sperm retrieval rates in these data. Patients at Weill-Cornell are screened for hormonal profiles prior to undergoing sperm retrieval procedures. We have previously shown that while normal fertile men have an average T/E2 ratio of 16 ± 3, patients with KS have an average T/E2 ratio of 4 [15]. We treat patients with low T/E2 ratios with aromatase inhibition and have found dramatic improvements in sperm concentration and motility in patients with severe oligozoospermia. Men with KS respond best to testolactone 50–100 mg per day. Testolactone treatment of these KS patients boosted testosterone levels from 190 to 332 ng/dL during the time period evaluated, with improved T/E2 ratios [16].

Other possible explanations for our better sperm retrieval rates in KS patients include use of the more effective surgical technique of microdissection TESE versus standard TESE procedures, as well as the benefits inherent with a substantial single-surgeon (PNS) experience. It has been our clinical observation that in KS patients, for example, there may often exist short segments of normal-appearing tubule, even while the vast majority of the remainder of the tubule (and adjacent tubules) is sclerotic. In this situation, when such tiny amounts of partial tubule is recovered, we do not process the sample as we usually do in the operating room, to avoid any risk of losing or otherwise disrupting the miniscule sample.

Postchemotherapy Azoospermia

As screening and treatment for various types of cancer continue to improve, a growing population of cancer patients has the opportunity to focus on quality of life issues. Cancer patients are at an elevated risk for infertility even before treatment. Although the importance of the concept of fertility preservation has been increasingly recognized, fewer than half of oncologists in the USA routinely refer patients to a fertility specialist prior to treatment that will further threaten their patients' fertility potential [33]. Systemic chemotherapeutic agents are associated with dose-dependent toxicity to germinal epithelium and posttreatment azoospermia. Alkylating agents are particularly destructive and typically render patients severely oligozoospermic or azoospermic. Vinca alkaloids and high-dose antimetabolites are also known to impair spermatogenesis.

A subset of patients with persistent postchemotherapy azoospermia has been treated at Weill-Cornell. Of 20 attempts of TESE–ICSI performed for 17 patients, 45% (9/20) resulted in successful sperm retrieval. The mean time period between chemotherapy and microdissection TESE was 16.3 years (range, 6–34 years). Clinical pregnancy was established for a third (3/9) of patients with sperm retrieved with two live deliveries. Sertoli cell-only pattern was demonstrated in 76% of patients, with hypospermatogenesis as the most advanced pattern seen in the remainder of patients. Sperm was retrieved in 23% of men with Sertoli cell-only pattern. There was no association between TESE–ICSI outcomes and the underlying conditions treated with chemotherapy or with the specific chemotherapeutic agents used [34].

The use of microdissection TESE–ICSI for patients with persistent postchemotherapy azoospermia has enabled conception and delivery of healthy children. Although certain chemotherapeutic agents are known to be particularly toxic to germinal epithelium, specific regimens have not been shown to clearly predict success of sperm retrieval with microdissection TESE. Although patients should ideally be encouraged to bank ejaculated sperm prior to treatment when possible, patients with long-standing postchemotherapy azoospermia may now be success-fully treated with advanced reproductive techniques.

NOA Associated with Cryptorchidism

Failure of testicular descent is associated with impaired sperm counts, sperm qual-ity, and fertility rates. Cryptorchid testes are also associated with an increased risk of eventual testicular germ cell cancer. There is no evidence that orchiopexy decreases the risk of cancer, although it facilitates testicular examination. In con-trast, subfertility secondary to cryptorchidism appears to be a duration-dependent process. Increased age at orchiopexy, as well as bilateral cryptorchidism, has been associated with worsening fertility parameters [35].

Several mechanisms for increased risk of infertility with cryptorchidism have been proposed. The first step in postnatal spermatogenic development, maturation of gono-cytes to type A spermatagonia, is believed to be deficient in infants with cryptorchi-dism. Gonocytes that fail to mature degenerate and consequently yield a decreased total number of germ cells. Androgen production, which is impaired within a few months of birth, may be either a primary or secondary defect. Poor steroid secretion may be a causative factor in deficient germ cell maturation. Finally, cryptorchid testes are subject to an increased temperature of several degrees compared with the normal scrotal temperatures. Temperature-induced degeneration of germ cells in cryptorchid testes is also believed to contribute to decreased fertility potential [36].

In 2003, we reported on our experience at Weill-Cornell with sperm retrieval in men with NOA associated with cryptorchidism. A total of 38 men (mean age 36.7 ± 6.5 years) underwent a total of 8 conventional and 39 microdissection TESE procedures. Successful retrieval of sperm was achieved in 63% (5/8) of open TESE procedures and 77% (30/39) of microdissection TESE procedures for a combined rate of 74%.

Spermatozoa were retrieved in all patients (9/9) with a history of unilateral crypt-orchidism and 68% (26/38) patients with a history of bilateral cryptorchidism. For cases of successful sperm retrieval, couples achieved clinical pregnancy for 46% (16/35) cycles. Serum FSH was not correlated with successful sperm retrieval, but larger testicular volume ($p < 0.05$) and younger patient age at orchiopexy ($p < 0.001$) were independent predictors for spermatozoa recovery [37].

Expert Commentary

The story of fertility potential for men with NOA represents one of the greatest medical achievements of the past 20 years. In the recent past, men with NOA were considered sterile and child adoption was the only option for those seeking parent-hood. Today many patients with the same diagnosis have successfully fathered chil-dren with the assistance of advanced reproductive techniques.

The advent of ICSI has created the potential for oocyte fertilization even with a single, nonmotile sperm. It has been clinically recognized that sperm retrieved directly from the testis can be used for ICSI. It has also been recognized that many men with NOA, including even those with Sertoli cell-only pattern as the most advanced pattern on diagnostic biopsy, may harbor microscopic testicular foci of spermatogenesis. Finally, microdissection TESE has yielded a superior sperm retrieval rate compared with open TESE by allowing visualization of individual normal-appearing seminiferous tubules. The use of an operating microscope that characterizes microdissection TESE, a procedure we developed at Weill-Cornell, also serves to minimize bleeding, devascularization, and subsequent scarring, thereby increasing likelihood of successful sperm retrieval should a repeat procedure become necessary.

Five-Year View

The use of an operating microscope represents a significant improvement in the mechanical sophistication of sperm retrieval compared with conventional TESE or FNAB. Improving fertility rates in the near future will likely relate to the development of treatment options in gene therapy, stem cell therapies, and possibly in vitro spermatogenesis. Screening TESE candidates for Y chromosome microdeletions associated with infertility has facilitated appropriate counseling and improved prognostic accuracy, but approximately 50% of men with NOA have an idiopathic underlying etiology. At Weill-Cornell, we are currently addressing this issue by seeking to identify novel underexpressed genes and mutations in testicular tissue samples taken from men with idiopathic NOA.

Key Issues

Microdissection TESE is an advanced sperm retrieval procedure that requires microscopic training. Patience in the operating room is necessary as the procedure almost invariably takes more time to perform than conventional TESE or FNAB. An embryologist is required in the operating room for real-time wet-prep analysis of testicular specimens so that the procedure may be terminated as soon as spermatozoa are identified. Increased operating times, use of an operating room, and utilization of an operating room embryologist increase financial costs for the procedure.

However, microdissection TESE has distinct and important advantages over conventional open TESE or FNAB. These include a superior sperm retrieval rate with much less tissue removed. Microscopic vision allows for avoidance of subtunical vessels and improved hemostasis with a resultant decrease in acute and chronic complications. Microdissection TESE is an extremely sensitive technique for locating isolated foci of spermatogenesis in testes that may otherwise be overwhelmingly composed of sclerotic tubules. The most advanced pattern of spermatogenesis, rather than the predominant one, is associated with likelihood of sperm retrieval on microdissection TESE.

Microdissection TESE has been successfully used in subpopulations with NOA, including postchemotherapy patients and those with KS. Correctable factors that may impact spermatogenesis, such as presence of a varicocele or low T/E2 ratio, should be treated prior to attempting microdissection TESE. There are no absolute predictors of successful sperm retrieval on microdissection TESE, but genetic screening of operative candidates and results from prior biopsies provide useful prognostic information.

References

1. Schoysman R, Vanderzwalmen P, Nijs M, Segal L, Segal-Bertin G, Geerts L, van Roosendaal E, Schoysman D. Pregnancy after fertilisation with human testicular spermatozoa. Lancet. 1993; 342(8881):1237.
2. Silber SJ, Nagy Z, Liu J, et al. The use of epididymal and testicular spermatozoa for intracytoplasmic sperm injection: the genetic implications for male infertility. Hum Reprod. 1995;10: 2031–43.
3. Devroey P, Liu J, Nagy Z. Pregnancies after testicular sperm extraction and intracytoplasmic sperm injection in non-obstructive azoospermia. Hum Reprod. 1995;10:1457–60.
4. Levine LA, Dimitri RJ, Fakouri B. Testicular and epididymal percutaneous sperm aspiration in men with either obstructive or nonobstructive azoospermia. Urology. 2003;62:328–32.
5. Lewin A, Reubinoff B, Porat-Katz A, Weiss D, Eisenberg V, Arbel R, et al. Testicular fine needle aspiration: the alternative method for sperm retrieval in nonobstructive azoospermia. Hum Reprod. 1999;14:1785–90.
6. Schlegel PN. Testicular sperm extraction: microdissection improves sperm yield with minimal tissue excision. Hum Reprod. 1999;14:131–5.
7. Amer M, Ateyah A, Hany R, Zohdy W. Prospective comparative study between microsurgical and conventional testicular sperm extraction in nonobstructive azoospermia: follow-up by serial ultrasound examinations. Hum Reprod. 2000;15:653–6.
8. Turek PJ, Cha I, Ljung BM. Systematic fine-needle aspiration of the testis: correlation to biopsy and results of organ "mapping" for mature sperm in azoospermic men. Urology. 1997;49:734–48.
9. Rucker GB, Mielnik A, King P, Goldstein M, Schlegel PN. Preoperative screening for genetic abnormalities in men with non-obstructive azoospermia prior to testicular sperm extraction. J Urol. 1998;160:2068–71.
10. Girardi SK, Mielnik A, Schlegel PN. Submicroscopic deletions in the Y chromosome of infertile men. Hum Reprod. 1997;12:1635.
11. Ostad M, Liotta D, Ye Z, Schlegel PN. Testicular sperm extraction (TESE) for non-obstructive azoospermia: results of a multi-biopsy approach with optimized tissue dispersion. Urology. 1998; 52:692–7.
12. Haimov-Kochman R, Lossos F, Nefesh I, et al. The value of repeat testicular sperm retrieval in azoospermic men. Fertil Steril. 2009;91(4 Suppl):1401–3.
13. Ramasamy R, Schlegel PN. Microdissection testicular sperm extraction: effect of prior biopsy on success of sperm retrieval. J Urol. 2007;177(4):1447–9.
14. Veldhuis JD, Sowers JR, Rogol AD, et al. Pathophysiology of male hypogonadism associated with endogenous hyperestrogenism. Evidence for dual defects in the gonadal axis. N Engl J Med. 1985;312:1371.
15. Pavlovich CP, King P, Goldstein M, Schlegel PN. Evidence for a treatable endocrinopathy in infertile men. J Urol. 2001;165:837–41.

16. Raman JD, Schlegel PN. Aromatase inhibitors for male infertility. J Urol. 2002;167(2 Pt 1):624–9.
17. Silber SJ. Microsurgical TESE the distribution of spermatogenesis in non-obstructive azoospermia. Hum Reprod. 2000;15:2278.
18. Okada H, Dobashi M, Yamazaki T, Hara I, Fujisawa M, Arakawa S, Kamidono S. Conventional versus microdissection testicular sperm extraction for nonobstructive azoospermia. J Urol. 2002;168(3):1063–7.
19. Ramasamy R, Yagan N, Schlegel PN. Structural and functional changes to the testis after conventional versus microdissection testicular sperm extraction. J Urol. 2007;177(4):1447–9.
20. Ostad M, Liotta D, Ye Z, et al. Testicular sperm extraction with optimized tissue dispersion. Urology. 1998;52:692–7.
21. Zitzmann M, Nordhoff V, von Schönfeld V, Nordsiek-Mengede A, Kliesch S, Schüring AN, Luetjens CM, Kamischke A, Cooper T, Simoni M, Nieschlag E. Elevated follicle-stimulating hormone levels and the chances for azoospermic men to become fathers after retrieval of elongated spermatids form cryopreserved testicular tissue. Fertil Steril. 2006;86(2): 339–47.
22. Ramasamy R, Lin K, Gosden LV, Rosenwaks Z, Palermo GD, Schlegel PN. High serum FSH levels in men with nonobstructive azoospermia does not affect success of microdissection testicular sperm extraction. Fertil Steril. 2009;92(2):590–3.
23. Tsujimura A, Matsumiya K, Miyagawa Y, Takao T, Fujita K, Koga M, et al. Prediction of successful outcome of microdissection testicular sperm extraction in men with idiopathic nonobstructive azoospermia. J Urol. 2004;172:1944–7.
24. Vogt PH, Edelmann A, Kirsch S, Henegariu O, Hirschmann P, Kiesewetter F, Kohn FM, Schill WB, Farah S, Ramos C, et al. Human Y chromosome azoospermia factors (AZF) mapped to different subregions in Yq11. Hum Mol Genet. 1996;5:933–43.
25. Reijo R, Alagappan R, Patrizio P, Page DC. Severe oligospermia resulting from deletions of asoospermia factor gene on Y chromosome. Lancet. 1996;347:1290–3.
26. Brandell RA, Mielnik A, Liotta D, Ye Z, Veeck LL, Palermo GD, Schlegel PN. AZFb deletions predict the absence of spermatozoa with testicular sperm extraction: preliminary report of a prognostic genetic test. Hum Reprod. 1998;13:2812–5.
27. Martinez MC, Bernabe MJ, Gomez E, Ballesteros A, Landeras J, Glover G, Gil-Salom M, Remohi J, Pellicer A. Screening for AZF deletion in a large series of severely impaired spermatogenesis patients. J Androl. 2000;21:651–5.
28. Stahl PJ, Masson P, Mielnik A, Marean MB, Schlegel PN, Paduch DA. A decade of experience emphasizes that testing for Y microdeletions is essential in American men with azoospermia and severe oligozoospermia. Fertil Steril. 2010;94:1753–6.
29. Foresta C, Galeazzi C, Bettella A, Marin P, Rossato M, Grolla A, Ferlin A. Analysis of meiosis in intratesticular germ cells from subjects affected by classic Klinefelter's syndrome. J Clin Endocrinol Metab. 1999;84:3807–10.
30. Friedler S, Raziel A, Strassburger D, Schachter M, Bern O, Ron-El R. Outcome of ICSI using fresh and cryopreserved thawed testicular spermatozoa in patients with non-mosaic Klinefelter's syndrome. Hum Reprod. 2001;16:2616–20.
31. Levron J, Aviram-Goldring A, Madgar I, Raviv G, Barkai G, Dor J. Sperm chromosome analysis and outcome of IVF in patients with non-mosaic Klinefelter's syndrome. Fertil Steril. 2000;74:925–9.
32. Schiff JD, Palermo GE, Veeck LL, Goldstein M, Rosenwaks Z, Schlegel PN. Success of testicular sperm extraction and intracytoplasmic sperm injection in men with Klinefelter syndrome. J Clin Endocrinol Metab. 2005;90(11):6263–7.
33. Quinn GP. Physician referral for fertility preservation in oncology patients: a national study of practice behaviors. J Clin Oncol. 2009;27(35):5952.
34. Chan PT, Palermo GD, Veeck LL, Rosenwaks Z, Schlegel PN. Testicular sperm extraction combined with intracytoplasmic sperm injection in the treatment of men with persistent azoospermia postchemotherapy. Cancer. 2001;92(6):1632–7.
35. Trsinar B, Muravec UR. Fertility potential after unilateral and bilateral orchidopexy for cryptorchidism. World J Urol. 2009;27(4):513–9.

36. Hutson JM, Hasthorpe S, Heyns CF. Anatomical and functional aspects of testicular descent and cryptorchidism. Endocr Rev. 1997;18(2):259–80.
37. Raman JD, Schlegel PN. Testicular sperm extraction with intracytoplasmic sperm injection is successful for the treatment of nonobstructive azoospermia associated with cryptorchidism. J Urol. 2003;170:1287–90.

Further Reading

Goldstein M, Tanrikut C. Microsurgical management of male infertility. Nat Clin Pract Urol. 2006;3(7):381–91.
Schlegel PN. Nonobstructive azoospermia: a revolutionary surgical approach and results. Semin Reprod Med. 2009;27:165–70.
Su LM, Palermo GD, Goldstein M, Veeck LL, Rosenwaks Z, Schlegel PN. Testicular sperm extraction with intracytoplasmic sperm injection for nonobstructive azoospermia: testicular histology can predict chance of sperm retrieval. J Urol. 1999;161(1):112–6.
Turunc T, Gul U, Haydardedeoglu B, Bal N, Kuzgunbay B, Peskircioglu L, Ozkardes H. Conventional testicular sperm extraction combined with the microdissection technique in nonobstructive azoospermic patients: a prospective comparative study. Fertil Steril. 2010;94:2157–60.

Chapter 20
Best Practice Guidelines for the Use of Antioxidants in Male Infertility

Francesco Lanzafame, Sandro La Vignera, and Aldo E. Calogero

Oxidative stress (OS), an imbalance between the production of radical oxygen species (ROS) and antioxidant scavenging activities in which the former prevails [1], causes male and female infertility. The role of OS in the pathophysiology of human sperm function has been extensively explored. Indeed, spermatozoa are extremely sensitive to ROS because of their high content of polyunsaturated fatty acids (PUFA) and their limited ability to repair deoxyribonucleic acid (DNA) damage [2, 3]. Therefore, the administration of many antioxidants has been proposed in the attempt to improve sperm quality.

Treatments varied over the years involving the use of many different compounds, such as carnitines, phosphatidylcholine, kallikrein, pentoxifylline, vitamins A, C, and E, etc. [4]. The administration of antioxidants to infertile men represents a great challenge for the andrologist. Indeed, a correct and complete diagnostic workup should not be ignored, because different andrological diseases may respond to antioxidant administration in a different manner [5]. Furthermore, it should be reminded that no standardized markers have been developed which may help to identify those patients who may benefit from a scavenging treatment. Additionally, reliable, prognostic, and not expensive tests to evaluate the effects of ROS exposure or to determine the total antioxidant capacity (TAC) are not yet available for the clinical practice.

The efficacy of antioxidant administration would positively benefit from the use of markers that can reliable measure OS before treatment and/or of markers which evaluate the damage caused by OS on the sperm membrane and DNA. Many studies

F. Lanzafame, M.D. (✉)
Centro Territoriale di Andrologia, Siracusa, Italy

S. La Vignera, M.D. • A.E. Calogero, M.D.
Department of Medical and Pediatrics Sciences,
University of Catania Medical School, Catania, Italy
e-mail: sandrolavignera@unict.it; acaloger@unict.it

S.J. Parekattil, A. Agarwal (eds.), *Male Infertility for the Clinician,*
© Springer Science+Business Media New York 2013

have not taken into account the measurement of OS, a primary endpoint, and its possible improvement after treatment. Moreover, diseases which impair fertility have often a subclinical development with few or no symptoms and/or signs; consequently, the patients consult the andrologist after a long time from their onset. This often causes an irreparable OS-induced damage in spermatozoa. Therefore, the first step before antioxidant treatment is prescribed is to consider the clinical history and laboratory and instrumental data to understand if a given patient is suitable for a scavenging treatment or whether a different therapeutic strategy should be undertaken. A suitable strategy would be to eradicate all causes that increase ROS production and/or reduce seminal plasma scavenging action.

Regardless of the discrepant findings reported [6, 7], antioxidant treatment seems to be helpful both in vitro and in vivo to ameliorate sperm quality. Experimental data in laboratory and farm animals support this statement [8, 9]. Glutathione (GSH) administration plays a fundamental action in improving sperm motility and consequently in enhancing fertilization in asthenozoospermic bulls with varicocele and in rabbits with dispermy due to cryptorchidism [10]. In lead-injected mice, vitamin C, given at a concentration equivalent to the human therapeutic dose (10 mg/kg body weight), significantly decreases the concentration of testicular malondialdehyde (MDA), an important marker of OS, with a concurrent improvement in sperm concentration and a significant decline in the percentage of abnormal spermatozoa. Vitamin E (100 mg/kg body weight) and vitamin C have a comparable scavenging power, but the later has a poorer effectiveness. Given together at the above indicated dosages, they induce the most important fall in the content of MDA in lead-treated mice with a concomitant increase of sperm concentration and amelioration of sperm morphology [11]. An analogous protective effect of vitamin E has been shown in mice with mercury-induced decrease of sperm count and function [12]. The presence of an elevated quantity of α-tocopheryl acetate in the rabbit diet significantly enhances the semen amount of vitamin E and its oxidative firmness subsequent to cryoconservation [13].

Thus, many studies carried out in animal models suggest a possible successful use of antioxidants in humans. Unfortunately, contrasting evidences have been published from several uncontrolled trials, often performed to sustain the efficacy of some type of treatment even if its usefulness is not yet confirmed [14]. Heavy smokers [15] and infertile patients [16] who received an antioxidant supplementation ameliorate sperm quality. In addition, antioxidants improve the fertilizing capability of healthy men with elevated seminal ROS concentration [17] and also increase the fertilization rate of fertile normozoospermic men with low fertilization rates in previous IVF cycles, by significantly decreasing the levels of MDA [18].

Despite many studies describe positive results following administration of antioxidants on sperm parameters, there is no well-defined scavenging approach during OS, and often the experimental design is not double blind and/or placebo controlled. In addition, nonhomogenous cohorts of patients have been enrolled in some studies. Finally, a large number of compounds have been used, but for many of them scanty evidence have been published. All this makes the scientific literature very

Table 20.1 List of antioxidants reviewed in this chapter

Antioxidants
Ascorbic acid (vitamin C)
α-Tocopherol (vitamin E)
Ascorbic acid (vitamin C) plus α-tocopherol (vitamin E)
α-Tocopherol (vitamin E) plus selenium
Glutathione
L-Carnitine plus L-acetyl-carnitine
Coenzyme Q10
Lycopene
Pycnogenol
N-acetyl-cysteine
Vitamin A and vitamin E
Pentoxifylline
Selenium
Shao-Fu-Zhu-Yu-Tang
Astaxanthin
Lepidium meyenii
α-Linolenic acid and lignans
Vitamin C and E, lycopene, selenium, folic acid, garlic oil plus zinc
Morindae officinalis extract

Table 20.2 Evidence classification of the National Clinical Guidelines for Type 2 Diabetes (the Royal College of General practitioners, Effective Clinical Practice Unit, ScHAAR University of Sheffield) used in this chapter

Evidence classification	
Ia	Evidence from meta-analysis of randomized controlled trials
Ib	Evidence from at least one randomized controlled trial
IIa	Evidence from at least one controlled study without randomization
IIb	Evidence from at least one other type of quasi-experimental study
III	Evidence from nonexperimental descriptive studies, such as comparative studies, correlation studies, and case–control studies
IV	Evidence from expert committee reports or opinions and/or clinical experience of respected authorities

Adapted from Agency for Health Care Policy and Research [82]

heterogeneous with a consequent difficulty to get an ultimate conclusion, as also suggested by Patel and Sigman [19].

Because of the difficulty to clearly distinguish which antioxidant can play a better role to reduce OS generation and/or to prevent the OS-mediated sperm damage, we decided to use an evidence-based medicine (EBM) method to better understand the role of the various antioxidants for the treatment of infertile men (Table 20.1). To accomplish this, the National Clinical Guidelines for Type 2 Diabetes, formulated by the Royal College of General practitioners, Effective Clinical Practice Unit, ScHAAR University of Sheffield (http://www.nice.org.uk/nicemedia/live/10911/28998/28998.pdf) were used as they seem more suitable for pharmacological trials. These guidelines classify evidences and recommendations as indicated in Tables 20.2 and 20.3.

Table 20.3 Recommendations of the National Clinical Guidelines for Type 2 Diabetes (the Royal College of General practitioners, Effective Clinical Practice Unit, ScHAAR University of Sheffield) used in this chapter

Recommendation grading
A Directly based on category I evidence
B Directly based on category II evidence, or extrapolated recommendation from category I evidence
C Directly based on category III evidence, or extrapolated recommendation from category I or II evidence
D Directly based on category IV evidence, or extrapolated recommendation from category I, II, or III evidence

From Eccles et al. [83], with permission

Ascorbic Acid

Ascorbic acid (vitamin C) is ten times higher in the seminal plasma than in serum [20]. It is an effective scavenger if peroxyl radicals are in an aqueous phase [21], but does not have the some powerful scavenging action within membrane lipids [22]. The amount of vitamin C in the seminal plasma decreases significantly when the concentration of ROS increases [23]. Also in leucocytospermic samples, the concentrations of seminal ascorbic acid are significantly depleted. When this occurs, a significantly higher sperm DNA fragmentation index (DFI) has been found compared with semen samples with normal or high levels of ascorbic acid [24]. Interestingly, vitamin C plays an antioxidant action at low concentrations, but it can start auto-oxidation processes at higher concentrations [25]. Moreover, in humans, the vitamin C plasma saturation occurs at daily dose of 1 g. Higher amounts could promote the development of kidney stones, because of the enhanced excretion of oxalate [26].

The administration of vitamin C (1 g/day) increases ascorbic acid level by 2.2-fold [27]. In addition, it has been reported that seminal plasma vitamin C concentrations positively correlates with the number of normal spermatozoa, in a controlled clinical trial [28] (IIa). In earlier studies, vitamin C (1 g/day) supplementation has been proposed to ameliorate the sperm quality in infertile men [15] (III), [29] (Ib). Sperm parameters also increases with a higher vitamin C intake, as shown by the higher sperm concentration and total progressive motile sperm count (TPMS) [30] (IIb). In a placebo-controlled study, vitamin C given to heavy smokers at a dose of 200 or 1,000 mg/day for 4 months improved sperm parameters. The group that took the dose of 1,000 mg/day had a higher increase [29] (Ib). In addition, vitamin C safeguards human spermatozoa from endogenous oxidative DNA damage [31] (IIb).

α-Tocopherol

In a single-blinded study, eight patients treated with 100 mg of α-tocopherol (vitamin E) tid for 4 months did not show any sperm parameter improvement [32] (IIa). While the administration of vitamin E, at a dose of 100 mg three times per day, produced a slight increase in seminal plasma vitamin E concentration. In a study performed on 15 subjects, the number of spermatozoa, the percentage of sperm with forward motility, the half-life of the percentage displaying forward motility, and the rate of swollen spermatozoa in hypo-osmotic medium did not show any significant enhancement during vitamin E administration. The authors explained the lack of effects on these parameters with the small increase of vitamin E achieved in the seminal plasma. They hypothesized that higher doses of vitamin E may be more effective [33] (Ib). When in infertile men, vitamin E is administered at doses ranging between 300 and 1,200 mg/day for 3 weeks, seminal plasma vitamin E levels increase weakly [34]. The sperm α-tocopherol concentration is independent from the concentration or the total amount present in the seminal plasma. On the other hand, the percentage of motile spermatozoa relates significantly with sperm α-tocopherol content [35].

Many trials have been conducted to ameliorate sperm parameters of infertile men by vitamin E administration. In a double-blind randomized, placebo-controlled, crossover trial, 30 healthy men with elevated semen ROS concentrations and healthy female partners were given vitamin E (600 mg/day) or placebo for 3 months. Vitamin E increased significantly blood serum α-tocopherol concentrations and sperm function evaluated by the zona-binding assay [17] (Ia). Some other reports utilized lower doses of vitamin E. For example, a single-blinded study took into account eight patients receiving 300 mg/day of vitamin E, divided in three daily doses of 100 mg each, for 4 months. Patients receiving α-tocopherol did not show any improvement [32] (IIa). A placebo-controlled, double-blind study showed that the elevated sperm MDA in asthenozoospermic and oligoasthenozoospermic men decreased significantly after vitamin E administration which also improved sperm motility in asthenozoospermic patients. In addition, 11 of 52 wives (21%) of the treated group got pregnant during the 6-month treatment; 9 of them had a normal term deliveries, while 2 aborted in the first trimester. No pregnancy was reported in the placebo group [36] (IIa). Moreover, elevated MDA concentrations significantly dropped to normal levels, and the fertilization rate per cycle increased significantly following administration of 200 mg/day of vitamin E for 3 months, in a prospective study conducted in 15 fertile normozoospermic men. The elevated MDA concentrations significantly decreased to normal levels and the fertilization rate per cycle increased significantly after 1 month of treatment [18] (IIa). Furthermore, an elevated consumption of daily nutrients with scavenging potential (food and nutraceutical complements such as zinc, folate, vitamins C and E, and β-carotene) proposed to 97 healthy, nonsmoking men, showed that the vitamin E intake correlated with the highest progressive motility and TPMS [30] (IIb).

Ascorbic Acid and α-Tocopherol

Ascorbic acid (vitamin C) and α-tocopherol (vitamin E) may be administered together to decrease the peroxidative injury on spermatozoa, taking advantage of their hydrophilicity and lipophilicity, respectively. In addition, if these compounds act directly on spermatozoa to prevent ROS-induced damage, the improvement could be rapid, given that the two vitamins reach spermatozoa both within the epididymis and following ejaculation.

A double-blind, placebo-controlled, randomized trial has been performed in asthenozoospermic or moderate oligoasthenozoospermic men. Vitamins C (1 g) and E (800 mg) were prescribed simultaneously for 2 months, but no improvement of semen parameters was reported [37] (Ib). These unsatisfactory findings match with the findings of other studies [32, 33], but diverge from other published data [18, 38]. It is also possible that the duration of the treatment was too short to produce an effect, particularly if the action occurs within the testis.

Sixty-four patients with idiopathic infertility and an increased ($\geq$15%) proportion of spermatozoa with DNA fragmentation were randomly divided into two groups: one was given vitamins C (1 g) and E (1 g) daily and the other one, placebo. After a 2 months of treatment, the proportion of DNA-fragmented spermatozoa decreased significantly in the antioxidant-treated group, while no variation was detected in the placebo group [39] (Ib). An additional trial was performed on 38 patients with a raised ($\geq$15%) percentage of DNA-fragmented spermatozoa in the ejaculate. They were prescribed vitamins C (1 g) and E (1 g) daily for 2 months following one ICSI cycle failure. In 29 of them (76%), the scavenging therapy led to a decline in the proportion of DNA-fragmented spermatozoa and a successful ICSI attempt with a higher clinical pregnancy (48.2% vs. 6.9%) and implantation (19.6% vs. 2.2%) rates [40] (IIb).

α-Tocopherol and Selenium

Few studies have been performed using the association between vitamin E and selenium [41, 42]. A trial was conducted in nine oligoasthenoteratozoospermic patients who were prescribed vitamin E (400 mg) plus selenium (100 μg) daily for 1 month. Thereafter, selenium supplementation was increased to 200 μg/day for the next 4 months. This kind of association produced a significant improvement of sperm motility, morphology, and vitality [41] (Ib). The other study, using the same association, was performed in 28 men who were given vitamin E (400 mg) and selenium (225 μg) daily for 3 months. Other 26 patients assumed vitamin B (4.5 g/day) for the same length of time, as control. The administration of vitamin E and selenium resulted in a significant reduction in MDA concentrations and an enhancement of sperm kinetic parameters [42] (Ib).

Glutathione

GSH is one of the most commonly used drugs; thanks to its antitoxic and scavenging action in different diseases. Although it cannot cross cell membranes, its concentration increases in biological fluids following a systemic intake. GSH is able to reach the seminal plasma and to play an action at this level. Here, it safeguards spermatozoa from ROS attack; hence, GSH may play a beneficial function in several andrological diseases, particularly during male genital tract inflammation [16].

GSH (600 mg/day i.m.) has been prescribed to 11 patients with dyspermia associated with different andrological diseases in a 2-month pilot trial. Sperm kinetics improved, particularly in men with male accessory gland infections (MAGI) and in men with varicocele [43] (III), two circumstances wherein ROS or other noxious substance may play a pathogenic role. Following these encouraging findings, the same investigators conducted a placebo-controlled, double-blind, crossover study on infertile men experiencing unilateral varicocele and amicrobial MAGI. The patients were allocated to treatment with GSH, 600 mg i.m. on alternate days, or placebo ampoules. Men who received GSH showed higher sperm number, motility, kinetic parameters, and percentage of normal forms. These effects on sperm motility and morphology lasted for some time after the treatment was discontinued. The authors hypothesized that these findings may relate to a post-spermatocyte action of GSH, since the length of the treatment did not cover the full length of a complete spermatogenesis [16] (Ib). This kind of sperm modification can be partially corrected by GSH administration when cell membrane injury is not too critical [44] (IIa).

The above reported data indicate that, at least to some extent, the beneficial effect of GSH is suitable for the biochemical changes in membrane organization and its following defensive action on the lipid components of the cell membrane. The decline of lipoperoxide levels in seminal plasma let to consider that GSH minimizes the consequence of lipoperoxidation generated by vascular or inflammatory diseases.

Carnitines

Carnitines are involved in many metabolic pathways in several cellular organelles. These compounds play a primary function in sperm maturation within the male genital organs and a relevant role in the metabolism of spermatozoa by furnishing immediately accessible energy to be utilized by spermatozoa. This positively correlates with sperm motility and concentration [45]. An increase of sperm progressive motility occurs simultaneously to L-carnitine augmentation and storage in the epididymal lumen [46].

Several different kinds of studies (controlled, uncontrolled, human, and animal) have been carried out to evaluate the potential application of carnitines as scavenging molecules. In 1992, a study was conducted on the male partners of 20 couples affected by idiopathic oligoasthenozoospermia (concentration $<20 \times 10^6$ spermatozoa/ml, progressive motility <50%) who were given 4 g/day of L-acetyl-carnitine for 2 months. No significant effect on sperm concentration, total motility, and morphology resulted, whereas a significant improvement of progressive motility ($21.7 \pm 3.2\%$ vs. 38.2 ± 4.7) was appreciated [47] (IIb). Afterwards, a multicentre open study was performed on 100 men with idiopathic asthenozoospermia. L-carnitine was administered orally at the dose of 1 g three times per day for 4 months with a significant improvement of several sperm kinetic parameters [48] (IIb). Another study came to similar results, giving an oral solution of L-carnitine (1 g) three times a day for 3 months, to 47 patients with idiopathic asthenozoospermia [49] (IIb). A review article proposed carnitines treatment as an alternative method in the broader medical treatment of patients with infertility due to OS [50].

Some clinical evidence suggests that a selective group of infertile men, those with prostato-vesiculo-epididymitis (PVE), benefit from carnitines administration, since antimicrobial and/or nonsteroidal anti-inflammatory drugs, although effective to eliminate microbial infection, have a poor scavenging action [51] (Ib). Another study conducted on 98 men with PVE and leukocytospermia showed that carnitine scavenging treatment was totally successful once they were pretreated with nonsteroidal anti-inflammatory compounds [52] (Ib).

In a placebo-controlled, double-blind, crossover trial, L-carnitine was capable to enhance sperm parameters, even if it was unsuccessful to reduce LPO concentrations. These findings suggested an incomplete action of L-carnitine to counteract the ROS attack [53] (Ib). The same group proposed a double-blind, randomized, placebo-controlled trial. They gave a combined treatment with L-carnitine (2 g/day) and L-acetyl-carnitine (1 g/day) or placebo to 60 infertile males with oligoasthenoteratozoospermia. All sperm parameters improved, but the most important enhancement was found in both progressive and total sperm motility particularly in men with the highest degree of asthenozoospermia [54] (Ib). Another placebo-controlled study conducted also in patients with oligoasthenoteratozoospermia showed that the same treatment improved sperm concentration, motility, and morphology, particularly when cinnoxicam (1 suppository every 4 days) was added [55] (Ib). Furthermore, 60 patients with asthenozoospermia were enrolled in a double-blind clinical trial with L-carnitine (3 g/day), L-acetyl-carnitine (3 g/day), a combination of L-carnitine (2 g/day) plus L-acetyl-carnitine (1 g/day), or placebo, for 6 months. Total and forward motility, including kinetic parameters analyzed by computer-assisted sperm analysis, improved in men receiving either L-ACETYL-CARNITINE alone or in association with L-carnitine. The total oxyradical scavenging capacity of the semen towards hydroxyl and peroxyl radicals also improved and correlated with the enhancement of sperm kinetics. Patients with lower motility and total oxyradical scavenging capacity of the seminal fluid had more chances of responding to the treatment [56] (Ib). In another trial, L-carnitine (2 g/day) and L-acetyl-carnitine (1 g/day) were given orally tid for 3 months to 90 men with oligoasthenozoospermia. In the treatment group, ten female partners (11.6%) achieved pregnancy, whereas only two pregnancies (3.7%) were recorded in the control group. Moreover, their percentage of forward and total motile spermatozoa increased significantly [57] (Ib). In the trial lead by De Rosa and colleagues, 66 patients with <50% motility receiving L-carnitine (1 g/day) and L-acetyl-carnitine (500 mg tid), for 6 months, had a significant increase in sperm total motility, viability, membrane integrity, and linearity of sperm movement, both after 3 and 6 months of treatment, and in the ability to penetrate the cervical mucus increased after 6 months [58] (IIb). Twenty-one patients with infertility and with sperm motility ranging from 10 to 50% were given carnitines (2 g of L-carnitine and 1 g of L-acetyl-carnitine per day) orally for 6 months, but differently from the other studies, no significant effects on sperm motility resulted [59] (Ib). In a further trial, L-carnitine (2 g/day) and L-acetyl-carnitine (1 g/day) were administered for 3 months in men with PVE and increased ROS production. Carnitines showed to be a successful treatment once seminal leukocytes were within the normal range [60] (IIb).

On the light of the many studies exploring the effects of carnitines on sperm parameters, a systematic review has been recently published. The meta-analysis compared L-carnitine and/or L-acetyl-carnitine treatment to placebo reported significant improvement in total and forward sperm motility, atypical sperm cells, and pregnancy rate. No significant difference has been found in sperm concentration [61] (Ia).

Coenzyme Q10

Coenzyme Q10 (CoQ10) is a lipid-soluble constituent of the respiratory chain. Ubiquinol is the reduced form and the active one. It behaves as a powerful scavenger in some biological components, for instance lipoproteins and membranes. The concentrations of reduced and oxidized forms of CoQ10 (ubiquinol/ubiquinone) and of hydroperoxide have been measured in the seminal plasma and seminal fluid of 32 infertile men. A positive correlation between ubiquinol concentration and sperm count has been observed, whereas a negative correlation was reported between sperm count and ubiquinol concentration or hydroperoxide levels. An important correlation between sperm concentration, motility, and seminal fluid ubiquinol-10 content has been found, whereas, in total fluid, an inverse correlation between ubiquinol/ubiquinone ratio and the severity of teratozoospermia has been reported. These findings indicate that ubiquinol-10 impedes hydroperoxide occurrence in seminal fluid and in seminal plasma [62].

CoQ10 has been given orally at the dose of 60 mg/day to 17 men with low fertilization rate after ICSI for male infertility for an average of 103 days previously the subsequent ICSI procedure. The results showed a significant enhancement of the fertilization rate [63] (IIb).

In the human seminal fluid, CoQ10 has been found at relevant concentrations and it shows a direct association with sperm concentrations and kinetics. Differently, in men with varicocele, despite a higher proportion of CoQ10 in the seminal plasma, the correlation with sperm motility was not observed [64]. Elevated CoQ10 levels have been found in spermatozoa of oligozoospermic and asthenozoospermic patients without varicocele. This correlation was not detected in men with varicocele, who additionally showed slightly lower intracellular absolute concentrations of CoQ10. Higher intracellular levels could be linked to a spermatozoa protective system. In men with varicocele, this kind of system could be inadequate, leading to an excessive susceptivity to OS [64].

Very recently a double-blind, randomized trial has been carried out in 60 infertile patients with idiopathic asthenozoospermia. Patients underwent a double-blind therapy with CoQ10 (200 mg/day) or placebo for 6 months. After treatment, CoQ10 and ubiquinol raised appreciably in seminal plasma as well as in spermatozoa. Interestingly, spermatozoa improved their motility. Men with a poorer sperm motility and lower concentrations of CoQ10 had a statistically significant more elevated chance to better respond to its administration [65] (Ib).

Lycopene

Lycopene is an element of human redox defensive system against oxidative stress. Oral lycopene administration appears to have a function in the treatment of patients with idiopathic infertility. Following the administration of 2 g of lycopene, twice a day, for 3 months, a significant increase occurs in the sperm number and motility, but the sperm concentration increase is present only in men with a sperm concentration >5 million/ml [66] (IIb).

Pycnogenol

Pycnogenol is a substance obtained from the bark of the "Pinus maritima." Pycnogenol's constituents inhibit cyclooxygenases that release inflammatory prostaglandins [67]. A study has been conducted in subfertile men who were administered pycnogenol (200 mg/day), for 3 months. The results showed a mean sperm morphology improvement by 38% of the pretreatment values and the mannose receptor binding assay score augmented by 19% [68] (IIb).

Other Compounds

N-Acetyl-Cysteine or Vitamin A Plus Vitamin E and Essential Fatty Acids

An open, prospective study, conducted in 27 infertile men who were given a combined oral antioxidants treatment with N-acetyl-cysteine (NAC) or vitamin A plus vitamin E and essential fatty acids, showed an increase of sperm concentration in oligozoospermic patients. Moreover, this treatment significantly reduced ROS and 8-OH-dG production, and in the mean time, it increased the percentage of acrosome-reacted spermatozoa, the quantity of PUFA in phospholipids, and sperm membrane [69] (IIb). Very recently, 120 idiopathic infertile men were randomly given NAC alone (600 mg/day orally) or placebo for 3 months. NAC increased semen volume and sperm motility as well as semen viscosity [70] (Ib).

Pentoxifylline

Spermatozoa from 15 patients with asthenozoospermia and high ROS levels were treated in vitro with pentoxifylline to evaluate the effects of this compound on ROS generation and sperm movement. Pentoxifylline was able to reduce the production of ROS by spermatozoa, and it slowed down the in vitro decline of the curvilinear velocity and the beat cross frequency for 6 h. These same 15 patients and 18 asthenozoospermic patients, whose spermatozoa did not generate ROS at steady state, were then prescribed pentoxifylline at two distinct doses (300 and 1,200 mg daily) to validate its in vivo outcome on ROS generation, sperm kinetics, and sperm fertilizing competence. Pentoxifylline administration had no effects on spermatozoon-induced ROS formation, and it did not show any effect on sperm motility and fertilizing capacity. Nevertheless, it increased motility and beat cross frequency at the dose of 1,200 mg daily [71].

Selenium

Selenium supplementation has been given alone to 33 subfertile men for 3 months, but it did not produced any improvement of sperm count, motility, and morphology [72] (IIa). Subsequently, a trial was performed on 69 asthenozoospermic patients who received either placebo, selenium alone, or selenium plus vitamins A, C, and E daily for 3 months. Treatment did not show any improvement of sperm concentration, while sperm motility increased in both selenium-treated groups. This study showed that oral selenium administration is effective especially in patients with a low selenium [73] (Ib). Recently, a clinical trial investigated the usefulness of selenium (200 µg) and/or NAC (600 mg) in 468 infertile men with idiopathic oligoasthenoteratozoospermia for 6 months. This treatment showed to be effective on all sperm parameters measured and a clear correlation between seminal plasma selenium concentrations, NAC, and semen characteristics [74] (Ib).

Shao-Fu-Zhu-Yu-Tang

Shao-Fu-Zhu-Yu-Tang has been proposed to have antiaging and sperm scavenging properties. Its administration, for 60 days to 36 patients with chronic prostatitis, revealed a significant increase in sperm motility as evaluated by computer-assisted semen analysis [75] (IIb).

Zinc, Folic Acid, Astaxanthin, and Acetyl-Carnitine

Sperm parameters ameliorated following the intake of a mixture of zinc and folic acid, or the antioxidant astaxanthin, or a so-called energy-providing combination including (acetyl)-carnitine (Proxeed®). Furthermore, a double-blind study showed that the latter two compounds increase spontaneous or intrauterine insemination-assisted conception rates [76] (Ib). Astaxanthin appears to act significantly to decrease ROS and inhibin B concentrations and to increase sperm linear velocity and pregnancy rate [76].

Lepidium meyenii

The extracts of the Peruvian plant *Lepidium meyenii* appeared to be useful to increase the sperm number and the percentage of normal forms in an uncontrolled trial [77] (IIb).

α-Linolenic Acid and Lignans

Linseed oil includes α-linolenic acid and lignans. α-linolenic acid adjusts the poor intake of omega-3 essential fatty acids that is connected with reduced sperm motility among patients with fertility problems [78] (IV).

Vitamin C and Vitamin E, Lycopene, Selenium, Folic Acid, Garlic Oil, and Zinc

Menevit®, an antioxidant preparation combining vitamins C and E, lycopene, selenium, folic acid, garlic oil, and zinc, has been prescribed to 60 couples with severe male infertility for 3 months, in a prospective randomized, double-blind, placebo-controlled trial, before undergoing an IVF cycle. Men who assumed Menevit® had a significant improvement of the pregnancy rate (38.5%) compared to the men who assumed placebo (16% pregnancy) [79] (Ib).

Morindae Officinalis Extract

Morindae officinalis extract, taken at the concentrations of 0.25 or 0.5 g/ml, showed to be more effective than vitamin C in enhancing SOD vitality of sperm suspension and in decreasing MDA concentration. It has been shown to take part in a defensive action in the ROS-mediated damage of sperm membrane. Moreover, at higher dosage (0.5 mg/ml), Morindae officinalis particularly safeguards sperm membrane function [80].

Zinc

Zinc therapy has been shown valuable in decreasing OS, sperm apoptosis, and DFI in asthenozoospermic men. Zinc associated with vitamin E or with vitamin E plus vitamin C did not result in any further significant effect [81].

Expert Commentary

Many studies have been performed using different antioxidant compounds with the aim to improve semen parameters. Unfortunately the endpoints taken into account by these studies are often different and this does not help in understanding the efficacy of a given antioxidant. Moreover, it should be kept in mind that any andrological disease, independently of the OS, may be reversible or not according to the degree of the damage that has developed at the time of the therapeutical intervention. A prolonged exposure to OS can also cause an extensive damage that, over the time, can compromise the efficiency of the male accessory glands on sperm function. This represents an additional bias for many trials that have not considered the duration of the disease. All these reasons make the scavenging therapy a great challenge for the andrologist.

Bearing this in mind, we attempted a primary distinction dividing the antioxidants into compounds which play positive effects and compounds which play negative effects, as reported in Table 20.4. Using an EBM method, we proposed that some compounds may be considered as first-line treatment, because of the extensive investigation and the higher EBM evidences. These include vitamins C and E and carnitines. The efficacy of other antioxidants is not yet supported by a sufficient number of studies. These include pycnogenol, lycopene, etc., which need additional controlled trials. Other scavenging molecules, such as CoQ10 and GSH, can be proposed as second-line treatment because of the well-done, though few, studies performed on them. Nevertheless, also for these compounds studies that can clarify the dark points previously analyzed are welcome.

Five-Year View and Key Issues

Two major issues need, in the next future, to be further implemented to allow a clear evaluation of the true effectiveness of the antioxidant treatment in the infertile men. First of all, studies should be carried out in homogeneous cohorts of patients. This requires a careful andrological screening aimed at exactly diagnosing the disease which increases the oxidative stress. The second issue relates to the development of

Table 20.4 Summary of the evidences and grading of the recommendations of the effects of each antioxidant used alone or combination on sperm quality and function, according to the National Clinical Guidelines for Type 2 Diabetes (the Royal College of General practitioners, Effective Clinical Practice Unit, ScHAAR University of Sheffield)

Compound	Classification of evidences		Grading of recommendations
	Positive effects	Any or negative effects	
Vitamin C			
Dawson et al. [15]	III		B
Fraga et al. [31]	IIb		C
Dawson et al. [29]	Ib		A
Thiele et al. [28]	IIa		B
Eskenazi et al. [30]	IIb		B
Vitamin E			
Giovenco et al. [32]		IIa	B
Moilanen et al. [33]		Ib	A
Kessopoulou et al. [17]	Ia		A
Suleiman et al. [36]	IIa		B
Geva et al. [18]	IIa		B
Eskenazi et al. [30]	IIb		B
Vitamin C plus vitamin E			
Rolf et al. [37]		Ib	A
Greco et al. [39]	Ib		A
Greco et al. [40]	IIb		B
Vitamin E plus selenium			
Vezina et al. [41]	Ib		A
Keskes-Ammar et al. [42]	Ib		A
N-acetyl-cysteine plus vitamin E			
Comhaire et al. [69]	IIb		
Selenium plus N-acetyl-cysteine			
Safarinejad and Safarinejad [74]	Ib		
N-acetyl-cysteine			
Ciftci et al. [70]	Ib		
Glutathione			
Lenzi et al. [43]	III		C
Lenzi et al. [16]	Ib		A
Carnitines			
Moncada et al. [47]	IIb		B
Costa et al. [48]	IIb		B
Vitali et al. [49]	IIb		B
Vicari et al. [51]	Ib		A
Vicari and Calogero [60]	IIb		A
Vicari et al. [52]	Ib		A
Lenzi et al. [53]	Ib		A
Lenzi et al. [54]	Ib		A
Cavallini et al. [55]	Ib		A
Balercia et al. [56]	Ib		A
Li et al. [57]	Ib		B

Table 20.4 (continued)

Compound	Classification of evidences		Grading of recommendations
	Positive effects	Any or negative effects	
De Rosa et al. [58]	IIb		A
Sigman et al. [59]		Ib	A
Zhou et al. [61]	Ia		B
Coenzyme Q10			
Lewin and Lavon [63]	IIb		B
Balercia et al. [65]	Ib		A
Lycopene			
Gupta and Kumar [66]	IIb		B
Pycnogenol			
Roseff [68]	IIb		B
Selenium			
Iwanier and Zachara [72]		IIa	B
Scott et al. [73]	Ib		A
Shao-Fu-Zhu-Yu-Tang			
Yang et al. [75]	IIb		B
Astacarox®			
Comhaire et al. [76]	Ib		A
Proxeed®			
Comhaire et al. [76]	Ib		A
Lepidium meyenii			
Gonzales et al. [77]	IIb		B
Linseed oil			
Comhaire and Mahmoud [78]	IV		None
Menevit®			
Tremellen et al. [79]	Ib		A

more precise and hopefully inexpensive and non-cumbersome methods to estimate the oxidative stress in the semen samples. Finally, keeping these issues in mind, there is an absolute need of additional double-blind, placebo-controlled, randomized, crossover, multicenter clinical trials to gain more information about the effectiveness of an antioxidant (or a combination of them) over another one in men with infertility due to an increased oxidative stress.

References

1. Sikka SC. Relative impact of oxidative stress on male reproductive function. Curr Med Chem. 2001;8:851–62.
2. Griveau JF, Le Lannou D. Reactive oxygen species and human spermatozoa: physiology and pathology. Int J Androl. 1997;20:61–9.
3. Shen H, Ong C. Detection of oxidative DNA damage in human sperm and its association with sperm function and male infertility. Free Radic Biol Med. 2000;28:529–36.

4. Lanzafame F, Chapman MG, Guglielmino A, et al. Pharmacological stimulation of sperm motility. Hum Reprod. 1994;9:192–9.
5. Vicari E. Effectiveness and limits of antimicrobial treatment on seminal leukocyte concentration and related reactive oxygen species production in patients with male accessory gland infection. Hum Reprod. 2000;15:2536–44.
6. Ten J, Vendrell FJ, Cano A, et al. Dietary antioxidant supplementation did not affect declining sperm function with age in the mouse but did increase head abnormalities and reduced sperm production. Reprod Nutr Dev. 1997;37:481–92.
7. Ménézo YJ, Hazout A, Panteix G, et al. Antioxidants to reduce sperm DNA fragmentation: an unexpected adverse effect. Reprod Biomed Online. 2007;14:418–21.
8. Chew BP. Effects of supplemental β-carotene and vitamin A on reproduction in swine. J Anim Sci. 1993;71:247–52.
9. Luck MR, Jeyaseelan I, Scholes RA. Ascorbic acid and fertility. Biol Reprod. 1995;52:262–6.
10. Tripodi L, Tripodi A, Mammi C, et al. Pharmacological action and therapeutic effects of glutathione on hypokinetic spermatozoa for enzymatic-dependent pathologies and correlated genetic aspects. Clin Exp Obstet Gynecol. 2003;30:130–6.
11. Mishra M, Acharya UR. Protective action of vitamins on the spermatogenesis in lead-treated Swiss mice. J Trace Elem Med Biol. 2004;18:173–8.
12. Rao MV, Sharma PS. Protective effect of vitamin E against mercuric chloride reproductive toxicity in male mice. Reprod Toxicol. 2001;15:705–12.
13. Castellini C, Lattaioli P, Bernardini M, et al. Effect of dietary alpha-tocopheryl acetate and ascorbic acid on rabbit semen stored at 5 degrees C. Theriogenology. 2000;54:523–33.
14. Agarwal A, Said TM. Carnitines and male infertility. Reprod Biomed Online. 2004;8:376–84.
15. Dawson EB, Harris WA, Rankin WE, et al. Effect of ascorbic acid on male fertility. Ann N Y Acad Sci. 1987;498:312–23.
16. Lenzi A, Culasso F, Gandini L, et al. Placebo-controlled, double blind, cross-over trial of glutathione therapy in male infertility. Hum Reprod. 1993;8:1657–62.
17. Kessopoulou E, Powers HJ, Sharma KK, et al. A double-blind randomized placebo cross-over controlled trial using the antioxidant vitamin E to treat reactive species associated male infertility. Fertil Steril. 1995;64:825–31.
18. Geva E, Bartoov B, Zabludovsky N, et al. The effect of antioxidant treatment on human spermatozoa and fertilization rate in an in vitro fertilization program. Fertil Steril. 1996;66:430–4.
19. Patel SR, Sigman M. Antioxidant therapy in male infertility. Urol Clin North Am. 2008;35: 319–30.
20. Jacob RA, Pianalto FS, Agee RE. Cellular ascorbate depletion in healthy men. J Nutr. 1992;122: 1111–8.
21. Frei B, England L, Ames BN. Ascorbate is an outstanding antioxidant in human blood plasma. Proc Natl Acad Sci USA. 1989;86:6377–81.
22. Doba T, Burton GW, Ingold KU. Antioxidant and co-antioxidant activity of vitamin C. The effect of vitamin C, either alone or in the presence of vitamin E or a water-soluble vitamin E analogue, upon the peroxidation of aqueous multilamellar phospholipid liposomes. Biochim Biophys Acta. 1985;835:298–303.
23. Lewis SE, Sterling ES, Young IS, et al. Comparison of individuals antioxidants of sperm and seminal plasma in fertile and infertile men. Fertil Steril. 1997;67:142–7.
24. Song GJ, Norkus EP, Lewis V. Relationship between seminal ascorbic acid and sperm DNA integrity in infertile men. Int J Androl. 2006;29:569–75.
25. Wayner DD, Burton GW, Ingold KU. The antioxidant efficiency of vitamin C is concentration-dependent. Biochim Biophys Acta. 1986;884:119–23.
26. Levine M, Conry-Cantilena C, Wang Y, et al. Vitamin C pharmacokinetics in healthy volunteers: evidence for a recommended dietary allowance. Proc Natl Acad Sci USA. 1996;93:3704–9.
27. Wen Y, Cooke T, Feely J. The effect of pharmacological supplementation with vitamin C on low-density lipoprotein oxidation. Br J Clin Pharmacol. 1997;44:94–7.
28. Thiele JJ, Friesleben HJ, Fuchs J, et al. Scorbic acid and urate in human seminal plasma: determination and interrelationships with chemiluminescence in washed semen. Hum Reprod. 1995;10:110–5.

29. Dawson EB, Harris WA, Teter MC, et al. Effect of ascorbic acid supplementation on the sperm quality of smokers. Fertil Steril. 1992;58:1034–9.
30. Eskenazi B, Kidd SA, Marks AR, et al. Antioxidant intake is associated with semen quality in healthy men. Hum Reprod. 2005;20:1006–12.
31. Fraga CG, Motchnik PA, Shigenaga MK, et al. Ascorbic acid protects against endogenous oxidative DNA damage in human sperm. Proc Natl Acad Sci USA. 1991;88:11003–6.
32. Giovenco P, Amodei M, Barbieri C, et al. Effects of kallikrein on the male reproductive system and its use in the treatment of idiopathic oligozoospermia with impaired motility. Andrologia. 1987;19 Spec No:238–41.
33. Moilanen J, Hovatta O, Lindroth L. Vitamin E levels in seminal plasma can be elevated by oral administration of vitamin E in infertile men. Int J Androl. 1993;16:165–6.
34. Moilanen J, Hovatta O. Excretion of alpha-tocopherol into human seminal plasma after oral administration. Andrologia. 1995;27:133–6.
35. Therond P, Auger J, Legrand A, et al. Alpha-tocopherol in human spermatozoa and seminal plasma: relationships with motility, antioxidant enzymes and leukocytes. Mol Hum Reprod. 1996;2:739–44.
36. Suleiman SA, Ali ME, Zaki ZM, et al. Lipid peroxidation and human sperm motility: protective role of vitamin E. J Androl. 1996;17:530–7.
37. Rolf C, Cooper TG, Yeung CH, et al. Antioxidant treatment of patients with asthenozoospermia or moderate oligoasthenozoospermia with high-dose vitamin C and vitamin E: a randomized, placebo-controlled, double-blind study. Hum Reprod. 1999;14:1028–33.
38. De Lamirande E, Gagnon C. Reactive oxygen species and human spermatozoa. I. Effects on the motility of intact spermatozoa and on sperm axonemes. J Androl. 1992;13:368–78.
39. Greco E, Iacobelli M, Rienzi L, et al. Reduction of the incidence of sperm DNA fragmentation by oral antioxidant treatment. J Androl. 2005;26:349–53.
40. Greco E, Romano S, Iacobelli M, et al. ICSI in cases of sperm DNA damage: beneficial effect of oral antioxidant treatment. Hum Reprod. 2005;20:2590–4.
41. Vézina D, Mauffette F, Roberts KD, et al. Selenium-vitamin E supplementation in infertile men. Effects on semen parameters and micronutrient levels and distribution. Biol Trace Elem Res. 1996;53:65–83.
42. Keskes-Ammar L, Feki-Chakroun N, Rebai T, et al. Sperm oxidative stress and the effect of an oral vitamin E and selenium supplement on semen quality in infertile men. Arch Androl. 2003;49:83–94.
43. Lenzi A, Lombardo F, Gandini L, et al. Glutathione therapy for male infertility. Arch Androl. 1992;29:65–8.
44. Lenzi A, Picardo M, Gandini L, et al. Glutathione treatment of dyspermia: effect on the lipoperoxidation process. Hum Reprod. 1994;9:2044–50.
45. Tang LF, Jiang H, Shang XJ, et al. Seminal plasma levocarnitine significantly correlated with semen quality. Zhonghua Nan Ke Xue. 2008;14:704–8.
46. Jeulin C, Soufir JC, Marson J, et al. Acetylcarnitine and spermatozoa: relationship with epididymal maturation and motility in the boar and man. Reprod Nutr Dev. 1988;28:1317–27.
47. Moncada ML, Vicari E, Cimino C, et al. Effect of acetyl carnitine treatment in oligoasthenospermic patients. Acta Eur Fertil. 1992;23:221–4.
48. Costa M, Canale D, Filicori M, et al. L-carnitine in idiopathic asthenozoospermia: a multicenter study. Andrologia. 1994;26:155–9.
49. Vitali G, Parente R, Melotti C. Carnitine supplementation in human idiopathic asthenospermia: clinical results. Drugs Exp Clin Res. 1995;21:157–9.
50. Dokmeci D. Oxidative stress, male infertility and the role of carnitines. Folia Med (Plovdiv). 2005;47:26–30.
51. Vicari E, Rubino C, De Palma A, et al. Antioxidant therapeutic efficiency after the use of carnitine in infertile patients with bacterial or non bacterial prostato-vesiculo-epididymitis. Arch Ital Urol Androl. 2001;73:15–25.
52. Vicari E, La Vignera S, Calogero AE. Antioxidant treatment with carnitines is effective in infertile patients with prostatovesiculoepididymitis and elevated seminal leukocyte

concentrations after treatment with nonsteroidal anti-inflammatory compounds. Fertil Steril. 2002;78:1203–8.

53. Lenzi A, Lombardo F, Sgrò P, et al. Use of carnitine therapy in selected cases of male factor infertility: a double-blind crossover trial. Fertil Steril. 2003;79:292–300.

54. Lenzi A, Sgrò P, Salacone P, et al. A placebo-controlled double-blind randomized trial of the use of combined L-carnitine and L-acetyl-carnitine treatment in men with asthenozoospermia. Fertil Steril. 2004;81:1578–84.

55. Cavallini G, Ferraretti AP, Gianaroli L, et al. Cinnoxicam and L-carnitine/acetyl-L-carnitine treatment for idiopathic and varicocele associated oligoasthenospermia. J Androl. 2004;25:761–70.

56. Balercia G, Regoli F, Armeni T, et al. Placebo-controlled double-blind randomized trial on the use of L-carnitine, L-acetylcarnitine, or combined L-carnitine and L-acetylcarnitine in men with idiopathic asthenozoospermia. Fertil Steril. 2005;84:662–71.

57. Li Z, Chen GW, Shang XJ, et al. A controlled randomized trial of the use of combined L-carnitine and acetyl-L-carnitine treatment in men with oligoasthenozoospermia. Zhonghua Nan Ke Xue. 2005;11:761–4.

58. De Rosa M, Boggia B, Amalfi B. Correlation between seminal carnitine and functional spermatozoal characteristics in men with semen dysfunction of various origins. Drugs R&D. 2005;6:1–9.

59. Sigman M, Glass S, Campagnone J, et al. Carnitine for the treatment of idiopathic asthenospermia: a randomized, double-blind, placebo-controlled trial. Fertil Steril. 2006;85:1409–14.

60. Vicari E, Calogero AE. Effects of treatment with carnitines in infertile patients with prostato-vesiculo-epididymitis. Hum Reprod. 2001;16:2338–42.

61. Zhou X, Liu F, Zhai S. Effect of L-carnitine and/or L-acetyl-carnitine in nutrition treatment for male infertility: a systematic review. Asia Pac J Clin Nutr. 2007;16 Suppl 1:383–90.

62. Alleva R, Scararmucci A, Mantero F, et al. Protective role of ubiquinol content against formation of lipid hydroperoxide in human seminal fluid. Mol Aspects Med. 1997;18:S221–8.

63. Lewin A, Lavon H. The effect of coenzyme Q10 on sperm motility and function. Mol Aspects Med. 1997;18:S213–9.

64. Mancini A, Conte G, Milardi D, et al. Relationship between sperm cell ubiquinone and seminal parameters in subjects with and without varicocele. Andrologia. 1998;30:1–4.

65. Balercia G, Buldreghini E, Vignini A, et al. Coenzyme Q10 treatment in infertile men with idiopathic asthenozoospermia: a placebo-controlled, double-blind randomized trial. Fertil Steril. 2009;91:1785–92.

66. Gupta NP, Kumar R. Lycopene therapy in idiopathic male infertility: a preliminary report. Int Urol Nephrol. 2002;34:369–72.

67. Baumann J, Wurm G, von Bruchhausen F. Prostaglandin synthetase inhibition by flavonoids and phenolic compounds in relation to their O_2—scavenging properties. Arch Pharm (Weinheim). 1980;313:330–7.

68. Roseff SJ. Improvement in sperm quality and function with French maritime pine tree bark extract. J Reprod Med. 2002;47:821–4.

69. Comhaire FH, Christophe AB, Zalata AA, et al. The effects of combined conventional treatment, oral antioxidants and essential fatty acids on sperm biology in subfertile men. Prostaglandins Leukot Essent Fatty Acids. 2000;63:159–65.

70. Ciftci H, Verit A, Savas M, et al. Effects of N-acetylcysteine on semen parameters and oxidative/antioxidant status. Urology. 2009;74:73–6.

71. Okada H, Tatsumi N, Kanzaki M, et al. Formation of reactive oxygen species by spermatozoa from asthenospermic patients: response to treatment with pentoxifylline. J Urol. 1997;157:2140–6.

72. Iwanier K, Zachara BA. Selenium supplementation enhances the element concentration in blood and seminal fluid but does not change the spermatozoal quality characteristics in subfertile men. J Androl. 1995;16:441–7.

73. Scott R, MacPherson A, Yates RW, et al. The effect of oral selenium supplementation on human sperm motility. Br J Urol. 1998;82:76–80.

74. Safarinejad MR, Safarinejad S. Efficacy of selenium and/or N-acetyl-cysteine for improving semen parameters in infertile men: a double-blind, placebo controlled, randomized study. J Urol. 2009;181:741–51.

75. Yang CC, Chen JC, Chen GW, et al. Effects of Shao-Fu-Zhu-Yu-Tang on motility of human sperm. Am J Chin Med. 2003;31:573–9.
76. Comhaire FH, El Garem Y, Mahmoud A, et al. Combined conventional/antioxidant "Astaxanthin" treatment for male infertility: a double blind, randomized trial. Asian J Androl. 2005;7:257–62.
77. Gonzales GF, Cordova A, Gonzales C, et al. *Lepidium meyenii* (Maca) improved semen parameters in adult men. Asian J Androl. 2001;3:301–3.
78. Comhaire FH, Mahmoud A. The role of food supplements in the treatment of the infertile man. Reprod Biomed Online. 2003;7:385–91.
79. Tremellen K, Miari G, Froiland D, et al. A randomised control trial examining the effect of an antioxidant (Menevit) on pregnancy outcome during IVF-ICSI treatment. Aust N Z J Obstet Gynaecol. 2007;47:216–21.
80. Yang X, Zhang YH, Ding CF, et al. Extract from Morindae officinalis against oxidative injury of function to human sperm membrane. Zhongguo Zhong Yao Za Zhi. 2006;31:1614–7.
81. Omu AE, Al-Azemi MK, Kehinde EO, et al. Indications of the mechanisms involved in improved sperm parameters by zinc therapy. Med Princ Pract. 2008;17:108–16.
82. Agency for Health Care Policy and Research. Acute pain management: operative or medical procedures and trauma. Rockville: Agency for Health Care Policy and Research/US Department of Health and Human Services, Public Health Service; 1992.
83. Eccles M, et al. North of England evidence based guideline development project: guideline for angiotensin converting enzyme inhibitors in primary care management of adults with symptomatic heart failure. BMJ. 1998;316:1369.

Chapter 21
Harmful Effects of Antioxidants

Adam F. Stewart and Edward D. Kim

Oxidative stress has an integral role in the pathophysiology of most human diseases. With a rapidly aging population, increased attention and study have been directed toward the use of antioxidant therapy. The appeal is that these agents are considered "natural" substances and are associated with a healthy diet. The hypothesis has been that decreasing oxidative stress may prevent disease processes such as cancer or coronary heart disease [1, 2]. Because much of the general population use is in relatively healthy patients, it is critically important that these supplements are free of toxicity and side effects.

While initial studies of antioxidant supplementation suggested a beneficial role in disease prevention, more recent clinical trials and a meta-analysis have questioned the benefit of these therapies. Several studies have suggested that excess supplementation may in fact be harmful [3–6]. Recent attention has also focused on the use of antioxidants for the treatment of male infertility. The focus of this chapter is the potentially harmful effects of antioxidant therapy.

Risks of Dietary Antioxidants

Certain vegetables have high contents of oxalic acid, phytic acid, and tannins. These relatively strong reducing acids may have antinutrient effects by binding to dietary minerals in the gastrointestinal tract and diminishing their absorption [7, 8]. Calcium and iron deficiencies are not uncommon in developing countries where less meat is

A.F. Stewart, MD (✉) • E.D. Kim, MD
Division of Urology, Department of Surgery,
University of Tennessee Medical Center, 1928 Alcoa Highway,
Suite 222, Knoxville, TN 37920, USA
e-mail: afstewart@utmck.edu; ekim@utmck.edu

S.J. Parekattil, A. Agarwal (eds.), *Male Infertility for the Clinician*,
© Springer Science+Business Media New York 2013

Table 21.1 Dietary antioxidants	Foods	Reducing acid present
	Cocoa bean and chocolate, spinach, turnip, and rhubarb	Oxalic acid
	Whole grains, maize, legumes	Phytic acid
	Tea, beans, cabbage	Tannins

eaten, and there is high consumption of phytic acid from beans and unleavened whole grain bread [9]. In modern, industrialized nations where balanced diets are more common, the adverse effects of excessive dietary antioxidant intake are minimal. Table 21.1 lists foods containing oxalic acid, phytic acid, and tannins.

Oxalic Acid

Oxalic acid impairs calcium absorption by forming an insoluble salt of calcium oxalate. Cases of calcium deficiency have been associated with a high content of oxalates in foods [10]. A high level of oxalate intake constitutes a health risk for infants and metabolically disposed adults. Spinach is among the vegetables richest in oxalate. Sweet potatoes and peanut greens are also high in oxalic acid [11].

Phytic Acid

Phytic acid is a strong inhibitor of iron absorption in both infants and adults [12]. Iron and zinc deficiencies are widespread in infants and young children in developing countries where vegetable protein sources are often mixed with cereals. This iron deficiency in infants can lead to reduced psychomotor and mental development. Complementary foods increase the protein content and improve the protein quality of cereal-based foods. Cereals and common legumes, such as soybean, mung bean, black bean, lentils, and chick peas, are high in phytic acid. Decreasing phytic acid by 90% (approximately 100 mg/100 g dried product) would be expected to increase iron absorption about twofold. Complete enzymatic degradation of phytic acid with cooking methods such as blanching has been recommended for at-risk populations [7, 11].

Tannins

Tannins, which include condensed tannins (proanthocyanidins) and derived tannins, belong to the flavonoid family [13]. Tannins are found in a wide variety of foods, that is, apples, berries, chocolate, red wines, and nuts. Derived tannins are formed during food handling and processing and are found primarily in black and oolong teas, red wine, and coffee. Flavonoids and tannins are quite sensitive to oxidative enzymes and cooking conditions.

Condensed tannins inhibit herbivore digestion by binding to consumed plant proteins and making them more difficult for animals to digest and by interfering with protein absorption and digestive enzymes. Tannins have traditionally been considered antinutritional, but it is now known that their beneficial or antinutritinal properties depend upon their chemical structure and dosage. If ingested in excessive quantities, tannins inhibit the absorption of minerals such as iron, which may, if prolonged, lead to anemia [14]. In sensitive individuals, a large intake of tannins may cause bowel irritation, kidney irritation, liver damage, irritation of the stomach, and gastrointestinal pain.

Others

Nonpolar antioxidants such as eugenol, a major component of oil of cloves, have toxicity limits that can be exceeded with the misuse of undiluted essential oils. Toxicity associated with high doses of water-soluble antioxidants such as ascorbic acid is less of a concern as these compounds can be excreted rapidly in urine.

Risk of Antioxidant Supplements

It is well established that certain amounts of antioxidants, vitamins, and minerals are required in the diet. However, the benefit, dosing requirements, and risk profile of most antioxidant supplements are largely unknown. When used for disease prevention, the doses are severalfold greater than the recommended daily allowance (RDA). The hypothesis that antioxidant supplements can prevent diseases has been proven false by researchers. In spite of this information, many companies manufacture and sell dietary supplements with antioxidants in a variety of different formulations. Common ones include the "ACES" (Vitamins A, C, E, and selenium), resveratrol (found in grape seeds and knotweed roots), and herbs like green tea and jiaogulan.

The potential for harmful effects of antioxidant therapy has been suggested, such as in the β-Carotene and Retinol Efficacy Trial (CARET) which was a randomized, double-blinded, placebo-controlled chemoprevention trial in 18,314 men and women at high risk of developing lung cancer [15]. The study was initiated due to the observation of other studies that found people who have high serum β-carotene concentrations had lower rates of lung cancer [15]. The hypothesis of the CARET study was that these antioxidants would decrease the risk of lung cancer in an already high-risk population. Subjects were treated for up to 6 years. This study demonstrated that smokers who ingested a combination of 30 mg β-carotene and 25,000 IU retinyl palmitate (vitamin A) taken daily had 28% more lung cancer and 17% more deaths than placebo subjects. The CARET intervention was stopped 21 months early because of clear evidence of no benefit and substantial evidence of possible harm.

Other studies have found similar findings of adverse events. Table 21.2 lists observed side effects of supplemental antioxidants. The α-Tocopherol (Vitamin E) β-Carotene Cancer Prevention Study Group (ATBC) reported on a randomized,

Table 21.2 Observed side effects with supplemental antioxidants

Antioxidant metabolite	Recommended daily allowance (RDA)	Reported side effects
Glutathione	250 mg/day or 600 mg IM QOD for male infertility	Acute: gastrointestinal disturbances
Carotenes	15–30 mg/day	Acute: skin color changes
		Chronic: possible increased risk of death and certain cancers
α-Tocopherol (vitamin E)	22.4 IU/day	Acute: headache, fatigue, muscle weakness, creatinuria
		Chronic: impaired bone mineralization, increased bleeding, cardiovascular disease; increased overall mortality
Ascorbic acid (vitamin C)	75–90 mg/day	Acute: diarrhea
		Chronic: hyperoxaluria, urinary stone formation, iron overload
Ubiquinol (coenzyme Q)	60–90 mg/day	Acute: gastrointestinal disturbances, heartburn, abdominal discomfort
		Chronic: hemorrhagic toxicity
Selenium	55 mcg/day	Acute: fatigue, gastrointestinal disturbances, skin rashes, irritability
		Chronic: concern for diabetes, loss of hair and nails, neuropathy
Melatonin	10 mg/day (bedtime)	Acute: diarrhea, rash, dizziness, headache, heartburn, nausea
		Chronic: sleep disturbance
Zinc	8–11 mg/day	Acute: gastrointestinal disturbance, anosmia (intranasal)
		Chronic: concern for increased risk prostate cancer, copper deficiency, suppression of immune system, anemia

double-blind, placebo-controlled primary prevention trial [16]. The objective was to determine whether daily supplementation with vitamin E, β-carotene, or both would reduce the incidence of lung cancer and other cancers. A total of 29,133 male smokers 50–69 years of age from southwestern Finland were randomly assigned to one of four regimens: α-tocopherol (50 mg/day) alone, β-carotene (20 mg/day) alone, both α-tocopherol and β-carotene, or placebo. These patients were followed for 5–8 years. There was no reduction in the incidence of lung cancer among male smokers after 5–8 years of dietary supplementation with vitamin E. Those men given β-carotene had an 18% increase in the incidence of lung cancer compared to placebo. There was also an increased number of deaths due to ischemic heart disease and lung cancer in the β-carotene group compared to placebo. The vitamin E group had an increased incidence of death due to hemorrhagic stroke and an increased incidence of other cancers compared to placebo. While these data suggest that there may be harmful effects of these supplements, the authors state that further studies would need to be performed in order to validate these results [16].

Observation of these adverse effects was not limited to smokers. Bjelakovic's meta-analysis from 2007 included 68 randomized trials with 232,606 participants. This publication showed that treatment with β-carotene, vitamin A, and vitamin E may increase all-cause mortality and the potential roles of vitamin C and selenium on mortality may need further study [3].

These results were later confirmed by the same authors with an additional publication using the Cochrane Colla-boration methodology [3]. In this systematic review, several key findings were noted: (1) β-carotene, vitamin A, and vitamin E given singly or combined with other antioxidant supplements appeared to significantly increase mortality, (2) there was no evidence that vitamin C increases longevity, (3) selenium tended to reduce mortality, and (4) trials with inadequate bias control overestimated intervention effects [17–20]. It should be noted that only all-cause, not the cause of the increased mortality, was assessed. It is likely that increased cancer and cardiovascular mortality are the main reasons for the increased all-cause mortality [21, 22].

Several other publications have disagreed with the Bjelakovic meta-analysis [17, 21, 23, 24] and reported no effect on all-cause mortality. The Supplementation en Vitamines et Mineraux Antioxydants (SU.VI.MAX) study by Hercberg et al. was a randomized, double-blind, placebo-controlled primary prevention trial. A total of 13,017 participants took a single daily capsule of a combination of 120 mg of ascorbic acid, 30 mg of vitamin E, 6 mg of β-carotene, 100 mcg of selenium, and 20 mg of zinc or a placebo. After a mean of 7.5 years, there were no major differences found between the groups in total cancer incidence, ischemic cardiovascular disease incidence, or all-cause mortality [23].

Miller et al. performed a meta-analysis on the dose–response relationship between vitamin E supplementation and total mortality by evaluating randomized, controlled trials. Vitamin E doses ranged from 16.5 to 2,000 IU/day, and there were 135,967 who took vitamin E alone or in combination with other vitamins and minerals. While the results showed that there very well may be an increased risk of all-cause mortality with high doses of vitamin E (greater than or equal to 400 IU/day), lower doses did not reveal this same concern [24].

Although Bjelakovic et al. found no compelling evidence that antioxidant supplements have a significant beneficial effect on primary or secondary prevention of colorectal adenoma formation, in their meta-analysis of eight randomized clinical trials comparing antioxidant supplements with placebo or no intervention, they found no statistically significant effects of supplementation with β-carotene, vitamins A, C, E, and selenium alone or in combination. Antioxidant supplements seemed to increase the development of colorectal adenoma in three low-bias risk trials (1.2, 0.99–1.4) and significantly decrease its development in five high-bias risk trials (0.59, 0.47–0.74). There was also no significant difference between the intervention groups regarding adverse events including mortality (0.82, 0.47–1.4) [17].

The mechanism of the possible negative impact of antioxidant supplements is speculative. First, it is known that oxidative stresses are a part of the pathogenesis of different chronic diseases; however, could the oxidative stress be the cause of the chronic disease or the chronic disease causing the oxidative stress [25]? Second, some essential defense mechanisms, such as phagocytosis, detoxification, and apoptosis, depend on free radicals. If impaired, a negative impact on homeostasis may ensue [26–28]. Third, unlike prescription drugs, antioxidant supplements are not put through the same thorough toxicity studies in order to be sold to consumers [29]. A better understanding of the mechanisms and actions of antioxidants toward specific disease processes is needed [30].

Finally, if antioxidants reduce the redox stress in cancer cells, then they may decrease the effectiveness of chemotherapy and radiation therapy. However, other researchers argue that the antioxidants would reduce the unintentional side effects of the cancer treatment and increase survival times [31, 32].

β-*Carotene*

α-Carotene, β-carotene, and β-cryptoxanthin are provitamin A carotenoids. In the human body, these carotenoids can be converted to retinol (vitamin A). The essential function of carotenoids is that of provitamin A carotenoids (α-carotene, β-carotene, and β-cryptoxanthin) to serve as a source of vitamin A. Because of its vitamin A activity, β-carotene may be used to provide all or part of the vitamin A in multivitamin supplements. The vitamin A activity of β-carotene from supplements is much higher than that of β-carotene from foods [33].

As previously mentioned, the use of β-carotene was tested for its ability to prevent lung cancer in two large trials, the ATBC trial and the CARET trial. Surprisingly, an increased incidence of lung cancer was observed in the study groups. In CARET, it was not feasible to distinguish whether β-carotene or vitamin A was to blame for the negative results. In ATBC, there was a clear distinction that β-carotene was responsible for the increased incidence of lung cancers and increased overall mortality. Of note, there was no benefit of preventing other cancers, including gastric, pancreatic, breast, bladder, colorectal, and prostate cancer as well as leukemia, mesothelioma, and lymphoma [15, 16].

A large randomized, double-blind, placebo-controlled trial of β-carotene (50 mg on alternate days) involved 22,071 United States male physicians. The results after 12 years showed practically no early or late differences in the overall incidence of malignant neoplasms, cardiovascular disease, or in overall mortality. At initial glance, it seemed there was an increased incidence of thyroid cancer (16 vs. 2) and bladder cancer (62 vs. 41) in the β-carotene versus placebo group; however, after adjustment for multiple comparisons, neither of these differences was statistically significant. Overall, the only adverse side effects reported in the β-carotene group were yellowing of the skin and upset stomach [34].

Two other trials [35, 36] studied the ability of β-carotene to prevent nonmelanoma skin cancer. Neither found a beneficial effect on subsequent skin cancer incidence or reported any adverse effects of β-carotene supplementation.

The Women's Health Study was a large study of 39,876 healthy American women over 45 years old which found no effect of β-carotene on cancer incidence, but there was a suggestion of increased stroke risk during the study duration of 4.1

years (2.1 years treatment plus another 2.0 years follow-up). While it did not show statistical significance, the number of women who suffered a stroke was 61 (0.31%) for the β-carotene group versus 43 (0.22%) for the placebo group [37].

Minor side effects associated with the use of β-carotene include yellowing of the skin, also known as hypercarotenemia, when doses of greater than 30 mg/day are used for more than several weeks. This side effect is reversible upon cessation and has been observed in patients with photosensitivity disorders using these doses. Infrequently, mild gastrointestinal distress with gas and bloating may be seen.

Carotenemia is the ingestion of excessive amounts of vitamin A precursors in food, mainly carrots. It is manifested by a yellow–orange coloring of the skin. This differs from jaundice because the sclerae are still white in carotenemia. Other than the cosmetic effect, carotenemia has no adverse consequences because the conversion of carotenes to retinol is not sufficient to cause toxicity [38].

Tocopherols and Tocotrienols

Vitamin E, also known as α-tocopherol, refers to a set of eight related tocopherols and tocotrienols which are fat-soluble vitamins with antioxidant properties. Adequate amounts of this vitamin are typically present in Western diets. Multivitamins often contain about 30 international units (IU) of vitamin E, but supplements often contain 200, 400, or 1,000 IU. While research suggests that taking vitamin E supplements may boost immune systems and prevent heart disease and some types of cancer [39], large amounts of vitamin E may increase the risk for bleeding problems and death.

Miller et al. published a meta-analysis in 2005 that included 135,967 adults who had participated in 19 placebo-controlled studies of over a 1-year duration [24]. Approximately 60% of subjects had heart disease or risk factors for heart disease. Vitamin E in amounts of 400 IU or more daily for longer than 1 year increased the risk for death compared with placebo or no treatment. Limitations of the study were that trials which tested high amounts of vitamin E often involved older adults with chronic diseases. Therefore, findings from these trials may not apply to younger adults. Also, multivitamin combinations rather than vitamin E alone were often studied. This meta-analysis also did not find the exact lowest amount of vitamin E that was associated with increased risk for death.

In the HOPE and HOPE-TOO trials, the daily administration of 400 IU of natural source vitamin E for a median of 7 years had no clear impact on fatal and nonfatal cancers, major cardiovascular events, or deaths [39]. Unexpectedly, a consistent increase in the risk of heart failure was observed. A regression analysis identified vitamin E as an independent predictor of heart failure and supportive mechanistic evidence from an echocardiographic substudy of the HOPE trial found that vitamin E decreased left ventricular ejection fraction. Based on these findings, the authors recommended that vitamin E supplements should not be used in patients with vascular disease or diabetes mellitus.

A double-blind, placebo-controlled trial by Hemila et al. evaluated 652 Dutch subjects aged greater than or equal to 60 years [40]. These authors identified a greater severity of respiratory infections among participants supplemented with 200 mg vitamin E daily than among those not given vitamin E. These findings suggest that some population groups may be harmed by vitamin E supplementation. In contrast, Hathcock et al. supported the safety of vitamin E supplementation. They concluded that "at present, the evidence is not convincing that vitamin E supplementation up to the UL (i.e., the tolerable upper intake level, or 1,000 mg/day) increases the risk of death due to cardiovascular disease or other causes" [41].

Adults should consider avoiding taking vitamin E preparations in amounts of 400 IU or more. In November 2004, the American Heart Association stated that high amounts of vitamin E can be harmful. Taking 400 IU/day, or higher, may increase the risk of death. Taking smaller amounts, such as those found in a typical multivitamin, was not harmful.

Ascorbic Acid

Ascorbic acid, also known as vitamin C, is a monosaccharide antioxidant that is found in plants and animals. It functions specifically as a substrate for the antioxidant enzyme ascorbate peroxidase. Reactive oxygen species can be neutralized by ascorbic acid because it is a reducing agent [42, 43]. In humans, vitamin C is required for the synthesis of collagen. It is also a component of blood vessels, tendons, ligaments, and bone. Vitamin C also plays an important role in the synthesis of the neurotransmitter norepinephrine. Also, vitamin C is required for the synthesis of carnitine, a small molecule that is essential for the transport of fat into cellular organelles called mitochondria where the fat is converted to energy [44].

In a 15-year study of postmenopausal women, Lee et al. found that diabetic women who reported taking at least 300 mg/day of vitamin C from supplements were at significantly higher risk of death from coronary heart disease and stroke than those who did not take vitamin C supplements. Overall, vitamin C supplement use was not associated with a significant increase in cardiovascular disease mortality in the cohort as a whole [45]. Although a number of observational studies have found that higher dietary intakes of vitamin C are associated with lower cardiovascular disease risk, randomized controlled trials have not found antioxidant supplementation that included vitamin C to reduce the risk of cardiovascular disease in diabetic or other high-risk individuals [46].

Some studies have attempted to reveal if vitamin C supplementation would benefit athletes. While there does not seem to be an increased demand for vitamin C in athletes, there is the idea that if vitamin C is taken, it can allow the athlete a longer more strenuous exercise with less muscle damage. In fact, some research has found that amounts of vitamin C as high as 1,000 mg inhibits recovery theoretically by causing a decrease in mitochondria production and hampering endurance capacity [47].

Excessive doses of vitamin C not absorbed by the gastrointestinal tract can lead to mild diarrhea and indigestion. Large doses of ascorbic acid over prolonged periods can lead to urinary oxalate stone formation, although this effect is minimal and inconsistent [48, 49].

Glutathione

Glutathione is a cysteine-containing peptide made in human cells from specific amino acids. Glutathione is an endogenous intracellular antioxidant. Glutathione has a thiol group in its molecular structure which gives it antioxidant properties that allows it to be reversibly oxidized and reduced [50, 51]. Glutathione is touted by some to be the most important cellular antioxidant due to its high concentration and its main role in keeping the cell's redox state. Thorough literature review has failed to find any reported adverse effects of taking glutathione [52].

Melatonin

Melatonin is a unique antioxidant in that it can easily cross cell membranes including the blood–brain barrier. Another reason it is unique is because it does not undergo redox cycling which allows the antioxidant to undergo repeated reduction and oxidation. This repeated reduction and oxidation functions as a prooxidant and may allow the formation of free radicals [53, 54].

The recommended dose for melatonin is 10 mg by mouth at bedtime. Melatonin has been reported to cause sleep disruption, daytime fatigue, irritability, mood changes, depression, paranoia, hyperglycemia, headaches, dizziness, abdominal cramps, chest pain, and even tachycardia or seizures at higher doses [55, 56]. Several drug interaction precautions should be noted. First, there is caution with the use of systemic steroids and melatonin due to the interference with immunosuppressive activity of the steroid. Second, there is a caution with the use of ginkgo biloba due to the increased risk of seizures. Third, there is a caution with the use of melatonin and other CYP1A2 substrates. Lastly, a caution should be given with concomitant use of any CNS depressing drugs, sedatives, or hypnotics [56].

Antioxidant Nutrients: Selenium and Zinc

Selenium and zinc, commonly referred to as antioxidant nutrients, have no antioxidant action themselves and are instead required for the activity of some antioxidant enzymes. Selenium protects against oxidative damage by means of selenium-dependent proteins called selenoproteins including glutathione peroxidase. At serum levels of 70–90 ng/mL, a maximum level of activity is reached for the selenoproteins with the possible exception of one named selenoprotein P. The dietary intake of selenium in the USA is enough so that 99% of Americans have a serum selenium level greater than 90 ng/mL [57].

The Selenium and Vitamin E Cancer Prevention Trial (SELECT) was a large randomized, placebo-controlled trial set up to evaluate the potential benefit of selenium and vitamin E for the prevention of prostate cancer. Over 35,000 men enrolled and were divided into four groups (selenium, vitamin E, selenium + vitamin E, or placebo). After a mean follow-up of 5.46 years, there was no significant effect on the prevention of prostate cancer or any other prespecified cancer end points. However, in the selenium alone group, there was a statistically insignificant increased risk of type 2 diabetes mellitus. Further prospective, randomized studies would be needed to delineate the effect of supplemental and dietary selenium on the risk for developing diabetes. Because of the lack of benefit on prostate cancer and the potential risk of therapy, this trial was terminated [58].

While long-term use of zinc supplements at the upper limit of tolerability (40 mg/day) in adults is not considered unsafe, there are some common adverse effects of excessive zinc intake. These include metallic taste, nausea, vomiting, abdominal cramping, urinary tract infection, and diarrhea. Extended intake of amounts above the tolerable upper intake level may suppress immunity, decrease high-density lipoprotein cholesterol levels, and cause hypochromic microcytic anemia and copper deficiency [59, 60]. Interestingly, Leitzmann et al. evaluated zinc intake and the risk of prostate cancer in the Health Professionals Follow-up Study [61]. Results showed that in the 46,974 adult men studied, there was a 2.3 increased relative risk of advanced prostate cancer in men using elemental zinc in amounts of 100 mg/day or more. There was not an associated risk of prostate cancer in men who consumed less than 100 mg/day. While the authors could not rule out residual confounding by supplemental calcium intake or some unmeasured correlate of zinc supplement use, the evidence that chronic zinc ingestion above 100 mg/day may play a role in prostate carcinogenesis justifies further investigation.

Zinc may alter the way the body processes some drugs and other vitamins and minerals. For example, it may inhibit the absorption of tetracyclines, penicillamine, and quinolones. On the other hand, the absorption of zinc can be impaired by iron supplements and phytates, which are found in grains and legumes. Therefore, zinc supplements should be taken at least 2 h from iron and phytate ingestion [60].

Expert Commentary

Antioxidant supplements are widely used with the belief their use may improve health and have beneficial effects on disease prevention. These supplements are used in addition to the adequate amounts obtained in the typical Western diet. Recent meta-analyses and large-scale placebo-controlled trials suggest that long-term antioxidant supplements such as β-carotene, vitamin A, and vitamin E may increase overall all-cause mortality. The significance of these adverse effects is controversial as other meta-analyses, using many of the same studies, have provided mixed results depending on the criteria used for study inclusion. Although speculative, it is likely that increased cancer risk and cardiovascular disease risks are the main reasons for the increased mortality. Long-term indiscriminate use of antioxidant supplements should be avoided as the true benefit cannot be determined without further study.

Five-Year View

Although antioxidant supplements have been extensively studied, further large-scale randomized clinical trials with sufficient safety analyses will be necessary to determine their true long-term safety profile. Short-term use appears to be without significant adverse events. While supplements are not subject to the rigorous study required for FDA labeling of pharmaceutical agents, numerous clinical trials of their efficacy in specific disease states are ongoing as indicated by a search of http://www.clinicaltrials.gov. Some insight into harmful effects can be obtained from these studies, although clinical safety is usually a secondary end point of such investigations.

Key Issues

- Antioxidant supplements are increasingly used in the general population. Very high doses of some antioxidants, both dietary and as supplements, may have harmful long-term effects.
- β-Carotene, vitamin A, and vitamin E given singly or combined with other antioxidant supplements may increase all-cause mortality. Meta-analyses on this topic have yielded mixed results.
- Although speculative, it is likely that increased cancer and cardiovascular mortality are the main reasons for the increased all-cause mortality seen with β-carotene, vitamin A, and vitamin E.

Acknowledgment We acknowledge Joy Nicely and Kathy Gribble for manuscript preparation.

References

1. Halliwell B. Antioxidant defense mechanisms: from the beginning to the end (of the beginning). Free Radic Res. 1999;31:261–72.
2. Willcox JK, Ash SL, Catignani GL. Antioxidants and prevention of chronic disease. Crit Rev Food Sci Nutr. 2004;44:275–95.
3. Bjelakovic G, Nikolova D, Gluud LL, Simonetti RG, Gluud C. Mortality in randomized trials of antioxidant supplements for primary and secondary prevention: systematic review and meta-analysis. JAMA. 2007;297(8):842–57.
4. Bjelakovic G, Nikolova D, Simonetti RG, Gluud C. Antioxidant supplements for preventing gastrointestinal cancers. Cochrane Database Syst Rev. 2004;1(4):CD004183.

5. Bjelakovic G, Nikolova D, Simonetti RG, Gluud C. Antioxidant supplements for prevention of gastrointestinal cancers: a systematic review and meta-analysis. Lancet. 2004;364: 1219–28.
6. Stanner SA, Hughes J, Kelly CN, Buttriss J. A review of the epidemiological evidence for the "antioxidant hypothesis". Public Health Nutr. 2004;7:407–22.
7. Hurrell R. Influence of vegetable protein sources on trace element and mineral bioavailability. J Nutr. 2003;133(9):2973S–7S.
8. Hunt J. Bioavailability of iron, zinc, and other trace minerals from vegetarian diets. Am J Clin Nutr. 2003;78(3 Suppl):633S–9S.
9. Gibson R, Perlas L, Hotz C. Improving the bioavailability of nutrients in plant foods at the household level. Proc Nutr Soc. 2006;65(2):160–8.
10. Kelsay JL. Effect of oxalic acid on bioavailability of calcium. In: Kies C, editor. Nutritional bioavailability of calcium. Washington, DC: American Chemical Society; 1985.
11. Mosha TC, Gaga HE, Pace RD, Laswai HS, Mtebe K. Effect of blanching on the content of antinutritional factors in selected vegetables. Plant Foods Hum Nutr. 1995;47:361–7.
12. Hallberg L, Brune M, Rossander L. Iron absorption in man: ascorbic acid and dose-dependent inhibition by phytate. Am J Clin Nutr. 1989;49:140–4.
13. Beecher G. Overview of dietary flavonoids: nomenclature, occurrence and intake. J Nutr. 2003;133(10):3248S–54S.
14. Brune M, Rossander L, Hallberg L. Iron absorption and phenolic compounds: importance of different phenolic structures. Eur J Clin Nutr. 1989;43(8):547–57.
15. Omenn GS, Goodman GE, Thornquist MD, et al. Risk factors for lung cancer and for intervention effects in CARET, the Beta-Carotene and Retinol Efficacy Trial. J Natl Cancer Inst. 1996;88(21):1550–9.
16. Heinonen OP, Huttuten JK, Albanes D, et al. The effect of vitamin E and beta carotene on the incidence of lung cancer and other cancers in male smokers. The Alpha-Tocopherol, Beta Carotene Cancer Prevention Study Group. N Engl J Med. 1994;330(15):1029–35.
17. Bjelakovic G, Nagorni A, Nikolova D, Simonetti RG, Bjelakovic M, Gluud C. Meta-analysis: antioxidant supplements for primary and secondary prevention of colorectal adenoma. Aliment Pharmacol Ther. 2006;24:281–91.
18. Moher D, Pham B, Jones A, et al. Does quality of reports of randomized trials affect estimates of intervention efficacy reported in meta-analysis. Lancet. 1998;352:609–13.
19. Schulz KF, Chalmers I, Hayes RJ, Altman DG. Empirical evidence of bias: dimensions of methodological quality associated with estimates of treatment effects in controlled trials. JAMA. 1995;273: 408–12.
20. Kjaergard LL, Villumsen J, Gluud C. Reported methodologic quality and discrepancies between large and small randomized trials in meta-analyses. Ann Intern Med. 2001;135: 982–9.
21. Caraballoso M, Sacristan M, Serra C, Bonfill X. Drugs for preventing lung cancer in healthy people. Cochrane Database Syst Rev. 2003;2:CD002141.
22. Vivekananthan DP, Penn MS, Sapp SK, Hsu A, Topol EJ. Use of antioxidant vitamins for the prevention of cardiovascular disease: meta-analysis of randomized trials. Lancet. 2003;361: 2017–23.
23. Hercberg S, Galan P, Preziosi P, et al. The SU.VI.MAX Study: a randomized, placebo-controlled trial of the health effects of antioxidant vitamins and minerals. Arch Intern Med. 2004;164(21):2335–42.
24. Miller E, Pastor-Barriuso R, Dalal D, Riemersma R, Appel L, Guallar E. Meta-analysis: high-dosage vitamin E supplementation may increase all-cause mortality. Ann Intern Med. 2005;142(1):37–46.
25. Halliwell B. Free radicals, antioxidants, and human disease: curiosity, cause, or consequence? Lancet. 2000;344:721–4.
26. Salganik RI. The benefits and hazards of antioxidants: controlling apoptosis and other protective mechanisms in cancer patients and the human population. J Am Coll Nutr. 2001;20 (5 Suppl):464S–72S.

27. Simon HU, Haj-Yehia A, Levi-Schaffer F. Role of reactive oxygen species (ROS) in apoptosis induction. Apoptosis. 2000;5:415–8.

28. Kimura H, Sawada T, Oshima S, Kozawa K, Ishioka T, Kato M. Toxicity and roles of reactive oxygen species. Curr Drug Targets Inflamm Allergy. 2005;4:489–95.

29. Bast A, Haenen GR. The toxicity of antioxidants and their metabolites. Environ Toxicol Pharmacol. 2002;11:251–8.

30. Ratnam DV, Ankola DD, Bhardwaj V, Sahana DK, Kumar MN. Role of antioxidants in prophylaxis and therapy: a pharmaceutical perspective. J Control Release. 2006;113:189–207.

31. Seifried H, McDonald S, Anderson D, Greenwald P, Milner J. The antioxidant conundrum in cancer. Cancer Res. 2003;63(15): 4295–8.

32. Lawenda BD, Kelly KM, Ladas EJ, Sagar SM, Vickers A, Blumberg JB. Should supplemental antioxidant administration be avoided during chemotherapy and radiation therapy? J Natl Cancer Inst. 2008;100(11):773–83.

33. Institute of Medicine, Food and Nutrition Board. Beta-carotene, other carotenoids. Dietary reference intakes for vitamin C, vitamin E, selenium, and carotenoids. Washington, DC: National Academy; 2000. p. 325–400.

34. Hennekens CH, Buring JE, Manson JE, et al. Lack of effect of long-term supplementation with beta carotene on the incidence of malignant neoplasms and cardiovascular disease. N Engl J Med. 1996;334:1145–9.

35. Green A, Williams G, Neale R, et al. Daily sunscreen application and betacarotene supplementation in prevention of basal-cell and squamous-cell carcinomas of the skin: a randomized controlled trial. Lancet. 1999;354:723–9.

36. Greenberg ER, Baron JA, Karagas MR, et al. Mortality associated with low plasma concentration of beta carotene and the effect of oral supplementation. JAMA. 1996;275:699–703.

37. Lee IM, Cook NR, Manson JE, Buring JE, Hennekens CH. Beta-carotene supplementation and incidence of cancer and cardiovascular disease: the Women's Health Study. J Natl Cancer Inst. 1999;91:2102–6.

38. Penniston KL, Tanumihardjo S. The acute and chronic toxic effects of vitamin A. Am J Clin Nutr. 2006;83:191–201.

39. Lonn E, Bosch J, Yusuf S, et al. Effects of long-term vitamin E supplementation on cardiovascular events and cancer: a randomized controlled trial. JAMA. 2005;293:1338–47.

40. Hemila H. Potential harm of vitamin E supplementation [letter]. Am J Clin Nutr. 2005;82(5): 1141–2.

41. Hathcock JN, Azzi A, Blumberg J, et al. Vitamins E and C are safe across a broad range of intakes. Am J Clin Nutr. 2005;81:736–45.

42. Padayatty S, Katz A, Wang Y, et al. Vitamin C as an antioxidant: evaluation of its role in disease prevention. J Am Coll Nutr. 2003;22(1):18–35.

43. Linster CL, Van Schaftingen E. Vitamin C biosynthesis, recycling and degradation in mammals. FEBS J. 2007;274(1):1–22.

44. Carr AC, Frei B. Toward a new recommended dietary allowance for vitamin C based on antioxidant and health effects in humans. Am J Clin Nutr. 1999;69(6):1086–107.

45. Lee DH, Folsom AR, Harnack L, Halliwell B, Jacobs Jr DR. Does supplemental vitamin C increase cardiovascular disease risk in women with diabetes? Am J Clin Nutr. 2004;80(5):1194–200.

46. Waters DD, Alderman EL, Hsia J, et al. Effects of hormone replacement therapy and antioxidant vitamin supplements on coronary atherosclerosis in postmenopausal women: a randomized controlled trial. JAMA. 2002;288(19):2432–40.

47. Mastaloudis A, Traber M, Carstensen K, Widrick J. Antioxidants did not prevent muscle damage in response to an ultramarathon run. Med Sci Sports Exerc. 2006;38(1):72–80.

48. Peake J. Vitamin C: effects of exercise and requirements with training. Int J Sport Nutr Exerc Metab. 2003;13(2):125–51.

49. Massey LK, Liebman M, Kynast-Gales SA. Ascorbate increases human oxaluria and kidney stone risk. J Nutr. 2005;135(7): 1673–7.

50. Meister A. Glutathione metabolism and its selective modification. J Biol Chem. 1988;263(33): 17205–8.

51. Meister A. Glutathione-ascorbic acid antioxidant system in animals. J Biol Chem. 1994;269(13): 9397–400.
52. Meister A, Anderson M. Glutathione. Annu Rev Biochem. 1983;52:711–60.
53. Reiter RJ, Carneiro RC, Oh CS. Melatonin in relation to cellular antioxidative defense mechanisms. Horm Metab Res. 1997;29(8): 363–72.
54. Tan DX, Manchester LC, Reiter RJ, Qi WB, Karbownik M, Calvo JR. Significance of melatonin in antioxidative defense system: reactions and products. Biol Signals Recept. 2000;9(3–4): 137–59.
55. Taylor SR, Weiss JS. Review of insomnia pharmacotherapy options for the elderly: implications for managed care. Popul Health Manag. 2009;12(6):317–23.
56. Buscemi N, Vandermeer B, Hooton N, et al. Efficacy and safety of exogenous melatonin for secondary sleep disorders and sleep disorders accompanying sleep restriction: meta-analysis. BMJ. 2006;332(7538):385–93.
57. Bleys J, Navas-Acien A, Guallar E. Selenium and diabetes: more bad news for supplements. Ann Intern Med. 2007;147(4):271–2.
58. Lippman SM, Klein EA, Goodman PJ, et al. Effect of selenium and vitamin E on risk of prostate cancer and other cancers: the Selenium and Vitamin E Cancer Prevention Trial (SELECT). JAMA. 2009;301(1):39–51.
59. Fosmire GJ. Zinc toxicity. Am J Clin Nutr. 1990;51(2):225–7.
60. Saper RB, Rash R. Zinc: an essential micronutrient. Am Fam Physician. 2009;79(9):768–72.
61. Leitzmann MF, Stampfer MJ, Wu K, Colditz GA, Willet WC, Giovannucci EL. Zinc supplement use and risk of prostate cancer. J Natl Cancer Inst. 2003;95(13):1004–7.

Index

S.J. Parekattil, A. Agarwal (eds.), *Male Infertility for the Clinician,*
© Springer Science+Business Media New York 2013